MCQs in General Med

Volume 1

693

CW01010962

MCQs in General Medicine

Volume 1

Edited by

J. R. Lawrence FRACP FACP

J. D. Hunter FRACP FRCP

from

The Board of Continuing Education of
The Royal Australasian College of Physicians

Churchill Livingstone

MELBOURNE EDINBURGH LONDON AND NEW YORK 1986

CHURCHILL LIVINGSTONE
Medical Division of Longman Group UK Limited

Distributed in Australia by Longman Cheshire Pty Limited, Longman House, Kings Gardens, 95 Coventry Street, South Melbourne 3205, and by associated companies, branches and representatives throughout the world.

© Longman Group UK Limited 1986

All rights reserved. No part of this publication may be reproduced, stored in a retrieval system, or transmitted in any form or by any means, electronic, mechanical, photocopying, recording or otherwise, without the prior permission of the publishers (Churchill Livingstone, Robert Stevenson House, 1–3 Baxter's Place, Leith Walk, Edinburgh EH1 3AF).

First published 1986

ISBN 0-443-03425-7

British Library Cataloguing in Publication Data

MCQs in general medicine. — (MCQ)
Vol. 1
1. Medicine — Problems, exercises, etc.
I. Lawrence, J. R. II. Hunter, J. D.
III. Series
610'.76 R834.5

Produced by Longman Singapore Publishers (Pte) Ltd.
Printed in Singapore

Preface

This book contains 200 multiple choice questions in general medicine. The answers are explained by brief critiques and selected references for further reading. In the selection of topics emphasis has been placed on clinical relevance. The questions have been chosen and edited from the first four Australian Self Assessment Programmes for Physicians which have been prepared since 1980 by subcommittees of the Board of Continuing Education of The Royal Australasian College of Physicians. The primary objective of the programme is to facilitate continuing self-education, and the main aims are to encourage physicians:

- to obtain a clearer insight into their personal standard of professional knowledge;
- to compare their personal standard with peer group performances;
- to identify areas of deficiency on which they might profile some of their continued learning;
- to be aware of recent advances and of recently published outstanding reviews on important topics.

While it is widely acknowledged that continuing medical self-education is a major personal responsibility for all physicians, there are many difficulties. The exponential growth of knowledge has been accompanied by an uncontrolled proliferation of opportunities for various forms of educational activities of variable quality. The conscientious individual is confronted by a choice which is bewildering in its complexity and magnitude. Despite the increasing range of educational activities including meetings, computerised programmes, video and audio cassettes, etc., most studies have shown that reading remains the most popular form of 'keeping up' for medical professionals. Adult learning also tends to be most effective if stimulated by perceived need.

By combining the challenge of the familiar multiple choice question format with critiques and selected references, this volume will assist physicians and trainees to direct their reading and learning most effectively. Because the aim is educational, some controversial answers have been included.

This book should be useful to all students preparing for examinations in internal medicine and also to physicians interested in sustaining awareness of recent advances in the whole broad field of general medicine.

The Board of Continuing Education of
The Royal Australasian College of Physicians

J. R. L.
J. D. H.

Acknowledgements

The advisory committees who have prepared and selected questions and critiques, many of which were submitted for consideration by Fellows of the College, spent many hours discussing relevance, accuracy and editing. They are listed below, represent most specialties in internal medicine, and include many practising physicians. Invaluable professional assistance was given by Ms Robin Wines BSc MEd. Mrs Loloma Wren and Miss Tracey Kelly have also made invaluable contributions.

Advisory Committee Members:

E. G. Wilmshurst FRACP (Chairman 1984–85)
J. R. Lawrence FRACP FACP (Chairman 1981–83)
W. J. Benson FRACP FRCPA
R. Bradbury FRACP FRCPA
P. R. Davis FRACP
D. J. de Carle FRACP
J. P. Edmonds FRACP
J. Fowler FRACP
R. Garrick FRACP
P. Gianoutsos FRACP FCCP
K. J. Goulston FRACP
M. R. Joseph FRACP FRCP FCCP
P. S. Morey FRACP MPH FRACMA
G. M. Shenfield FRCP FRACP
C. I. Smith FRACP
G. M. Stathers FRACP
C. E. Storey FRACP
J. Yiannikas FRACP
I. H. Young PhD FRACP

Contents

PART I: QUESTIONS

1. **Which of the following tests is/are useful as a screening procedure to identify persons with a heavy alcohol intake?**
   A Serum alkaline phosphatase level
   B Mean corpuscular volume
   C Serum gamma glutamyl transpeptidase level (GGTP)
   D Serum aspartate amino transferase level (AST)
   E Serum uric acid level.

2. **Which of the following drugs cause physical dependence, leading to abstinence symptoms (indistinguishable from the alcohol withdrawal syndrome) on withdrawal of the drug?**
   A Pentobarbitone
   B Oxazepam
   C Diazepam
   D Cocaine
   E Marihuana.

3. **In the management of chronic severe pain due to advanced malignancy**
   A the standard 'Brompton mixture' contains morphine, cocaine and alcohol.
   B pain relief from the 'Brompton mixture' can be expected to last for 8 hours.
   C regular administration of analgesics is preferable to p.r.n. medication.
   D phenothiazines or anti-depressants should usually be given simultaneously with a narcotic analgesic.
   E tolerance to narcotic analgesics develops rapidly, necessitating an escalation in dosage.

4. When a patient presents in an emergency situation with paracetamol overdosage, which of the following statements is/are correct?

- **A** It is safe to discharge the patient who has taken a 15 g overdose of paracetamol after 24 hours if there are no apparent clinical effects.
- **B** If hepatic damage occurs it will be clinically apparent within 36 hours.
- **C** An accurate method for the prediction of possible hepatic damage is by the rapid estimation of blood levels of paracetamol.
- **D** Severe overdoses of paracetamol exhaust hepatic glutathione levels.
- **E** Intravenous N-acetylcysteine can be recommended as an adjunct in the treatment of paracetamol overdose.

5. Concerning hypothermia in man, which of the following statements is/are correct?

- **A** It may be associated with ethanol excess, anorexia nervosa and diffuse erythroderma as well as with hypothyroidism.
- **B** Profound blood volume depletion is commonly present.
- **C** A characteristic ECG abnormality has been described but is not always present.
- **D** The patient may survive relatively long periods of cardiac arrest.
- **E** External reheating is more effective treatment than rewarming with peritoneal dialysis.

6. A girl aged 10 years is stung by a bee. Within minutes she has severe swelling at the site of the sting and begins to complain of difficulty getting her breath. Her mother notices swelling of the lips and tongue.
Which of the following statements is/are correct?

- **A** Her response is due to an IgE-mediated reaction to bee venom.
- **B** Treatment with subcutaneous adrenaline should be given as an emergency.
- **C** Corticosteroids should be administered promptly.
- **D** She, and those close to her, such as family and school teachers, should be instructed in the use of adrenaline kits (such as the 'Anakit').
- **E** Long-term management should consist of confirmation of the allergy by prick testing and hyposensitisation with pure bee venom extract.

7. **Porphyria cutanea tarda**
   A is characterised by bullous skin lesions which may be indistinguishable from those seen in variegate porphyria.
   B is associated with an increased urinary uroporphyrin excretion with a lesser rise in coproporphyrins.
   C occurs in men approximately 4 times as often as in women.
   D is associated with histological abnormalities in the liver in more than 70% of patients.
   E is a common complication of haemochromatosis.

8. **Concerning Marfan's syndrome, which of the following statements is/are correct?**
   A It is inherited as an autosomal dominant trait.
   B Subluxation of the lenses occurs in less than 30% of cases.
   C Body proportions show a decreased upper to lower segment ratio for age.
   D Whether or not there is evidence of a valvular lesion, antibiotic prophylaxis should be given to cover dental extractions.
   E Dilatation of the aortic root is the most common cardiovascular abnormality.

9. **Concerning gallium 67-citrate scanning, which of the following statements is/are correct?**
   A A normal scan excludes the presence of Hodgkin's disease.
   B Its efficacy in abscess detection is decreased by having to delay imaging for 48 hours post-injection.
   C It is a first-line investigation in the detection of causes of pyrexia of unknown origin.
   D It is recommended in abdominal abscess detection when there is no other clue to the site of the abscess.
   E Focal uptake of gallium in the liver indicates the presence of hepatoma.

10. **A young man has a positive result in a screening test used to detect a disease with a prevalence of 1:1000 in the target population. The test is known to have a false positive rate of 5%.**
    Assuming that you know nothing about his clinical status, which of the following percentages is closest to the probability that he actually has the disease?
    A 95%
    B 50%
    C 20%
    D 5%
    E 2%.

11. A clinically healthy woman undergoes a battery of 20 biochemical screening tests. The assumed normal range for each test is mean ±2 standard deviations.
The probability that she will register within the normal range on all 20 tests is closest to which of the following percentages?

A 90%
B 80%
C 60%
D 40%
E 20%.

12. Complaints of insomnia are common in the elderly.
Which of the following statements concerning sleep and ageing is/are correct?

A Elderly people need less total sleep time than the young.
B Ageing is accompanied by an increasing number of EEG-proven arousals during normal sleep.
C Ageing is accompanied by a decrease in those sleep segments which are characterised by a high arousal threshold (stage 4).
D Young and elderly subjects show a basically similar course of the non-REM–REM cycle throughout the night.
E Clinical and experimental studies show all available hypnotic drugs to be effective in idiopathic insomnia for a period of several weeks only.

13. A woman aged 78 years has blood pressure readings of 180/100 mmHg lying down and 130/80 standing.
Concerning this observation, which of the following statements is/are correct?

A It is a normal finding for women of her age.
B It may be caused by diabetes mellitus.
C It may be associated with Parkinson's disease.
D In the aged this fall in blood pressure can result from the use of diuretics.
E Plasma expansion with 9 α-fluorohydrocortisone is an effective form of treatment.

14. A man aged 84 years presents with agitation, forgetfulness, difficulty in concentration, decline in intellectual ability and decreased emotional responsiveness to others.
Which of the following statements is/are correct?

A The condition requires no treatment.
B He should be treated with phenothiazines in the first instance.
C The use of antidepressant drugs should be considered.
D The highest suicide rate in the population is found in depressed elderly males.
E All severely depressed patients complain of depressed mood.

15. A woman aged 84 years, with a previous history of hypertension and two strokes from which she has recovered well, now presents with frequency, nocturia and incontinence.
Which of the following statements is/are correct?

A She has stress incontinence.
B She has an uninhibited neurogenic bladder.
C Cystometrography can establish the diagnosis.
D Urinary infection must be excluded.
E Catheterisation is the only effective management.

16. A woman aged 68 years presents with generalised wasting and weakness. She appears to be depressed and apathetic. She has cold dry skin. There are signs of congestive cardiac failure and atrial fibrillation.
Which of the following statements is/are correct?

A The most likely diagnosis is myxoedema.
B All the findings can be attributed to depression.
C She probably has thyrotoxicosis.
D Her TSH (thyroid-stimulating hormone) level will be greatly elevated.
E Surgical treatment is indicated because of her age.

17. In Paget's disease of bone

A the primary disorder is probably in the osteoclasts.
B the serum alkaline phosphatase level is raised.
C the serum acid phosphatase level may be raised.
D when pain occurs in an area adjoining a joint it should be treated first with a non-steroidal anti-inflammatory drug.
E a drop in urinary hydroxyproline levels and serum alkaline phosphatase during treatment with calcitonin indicates that bone pain probably will be relieved.

18. With regard to therapy with digoxin, which of the following statements is/are correct?

A The intramuscular route for digoxin administration produces a plasma concentration-time profile which is more predictable than that produced following the oral route.
B The plasma digoxin concentration during the 'distribution' phase is thought to correlate well with the concentration of digoxin in cardiac muscle.
C The elimination half-life of digoxin is 6–8 hours.
D The serum creatinine level is an excellent guide to the patient's dose requirement.
E The interpretation of plasma digoxin concentration requires knowledge about the relation between the times of blood collection and last dose, together with details of recent dosage alteration.

19. A woman aged 60 years has been on 0.25 mg digoxin daily because of cardiac failure. Quinidine therapy (1 g daily) is introduced for the control of recurrent atrial arrhythmias. With regard to this patient, which of the following statements is/are correct?

- **A** It is likely that her serum digoxin level will rise.
- **B** If she had been taking digoxin (Lanoxin PG) 62.5 μg daily, a rise in serum digoxin would not have occurred.
- **C** Any rise in serum digoxin level is related to the dose and duration of quinidine therapy.
- **D** If a rise in the serum digoxin level occurs, it will reach a plateau about 5 days after commencement of quinidine.
- **E** If the serum digoxin level rises, it is due partly to a fall in renal digoxin clearance.

20. Prazosin is an antihypertensive agent with vasodilator properties. Which of the following statements about this drug is/are correct?

- **A** It blocks presynaptic alpha 2 receptors.
- **B** It should be used in high initial doses.
- **C** It does not usually cause reflex tachycardia.
- **D** Its use is contraindicated in patients with renal disease.
- **E** It may be beneficial in the treatment of severe congestive heart failure.

21. With regard to therapy with phenytoin (diphenylhydantoin), which of the following statements is/are correct?

- **A** The bioavailability of phenytoin is close to 100%, irrespective of the route of administration.
- **B** If phenytoin is administered orally once daily over a long period there is little fluctuation in the interdosing interval plasma concentration.
- **C** The dosage requirements for children per kg of body weight exceed the adult requirements.
- **D** The clearance of phenytoin remains constant in the same individual regardless of the drug dosage, provided renal function remains constant.
- **E** The interpretation of the total plasma phenytoin concentration is changed in pregnancy.

22. With regard to lithium carbonate therapy, which of the following statements is/are correct?

A The therapeutic range for serum levels is between 0.6 and 1.4 mmol/ℓ .
B The sensitivity of individual patients to the neurotoxicity of lithium is closely related to dose and serum level.
C Lithium therapy must be stopped if a goitre or thyroid nodule develops.
D Diuretics potentiate the action of lithium, with an increased risk of inducing intoxication.
E Persistent tremor is a frequent side-effect which usually does not respond to drugs used for Parkinsonism.

23. Concerning the administration of aspirin, which of the following statements is/are correct?

A Enteric-coated preparations reduce the frequency of gastric blood loss and dyspepsia.
B High-dose aspirin (greater than 3.6 g/day) is associated with urate retention by the kidney.
C Aspirin reduces platelet adhesiveness by irreversibly acetylating the platelet membrane.
D Aspirin reduces plasma levels of other non-steroidal anti-inflammatory drugs when taken concurrently.
E At low and moderate doses, aspirin exhibits linear pharmacokinetics.

24. Drug interactions involving oral contraceptive preparations are now widely recognised. With reference to the use of the combined oestrogen and progesterone pill (OCP), which of the following statements is/are correct?

A Breakthrough bleeding may indicate a reduction of contraceptive effect in subjects with previously regular cycles.
B Reduction of contraceptive effect may be produced by drugs such as phenytoin and barbiturates.
C Antibiotics such as tetracycline reduce OCP efficacy by inducing hepatic microsomal enzymes.
D Commencement of OCP administration may cause increased frequency of fits in an epileptic previously well-controlled on phenytoin.
E Antituberculous drugs do not impair OCP efficacy.

25. Concerning pharmacokinetics in the elderly, which of the following statements is/are correct?

A Gastrointestinal absorption of drugs is not altered to any clinically significant degree in the elderly.
B When given in a dose based on total body weight, drugs which are distributed mainly in body water or in lean body mass are likely to produce lower blood levels in the elderly.
C The elimination half-times of oxazepam and the newer benzodiazepines are less influenced by age than those of diazepam.
D Hepatic clearance of propranolol declines with age.
E Renal tubular secretion, in contrast to glomerular filtration rate, shows little alteration with age.

26. Which of the following drugs may cause mental confusion in the elderly?

A Amantadine
B Indomethacin
C Propranolol
D Digitalis preparations
E Cimetidine.

27. Concerning the side-effects of cimetidine, which of the following statements is/are correct?

A Drowsiness and confusion in a patient aged 70 years with liver disease, being treated with 1 g cimetidine a day for a duodenal ulcer, may be attributable to cimetidine toxicity.
B Cimetidine potentiates the effect of warfarin by decreasing its metabolism in the liver.
C Cimetidine produces drug interactions with all the benzodiazepines.
D Although cardiac arrhythmias have been reported, they are unlikely to be clinically important.
E Ranitidine (a more recently introduced long-acting H2 histamine receptor antagonist) has a similar effect to cimetidine on the metabolism of drugs by the liver.

28. With regard to the effect of ethanol on the gastrointestinal tract, liver and pancreas, which of the following statements is/are correct?

A Most ingested ethanol is metabolised in the liver, where alcohol dehydrogenase oxidises it to acetaldehyde.
B Ethanol ingestion can cause cirrhosis in man even though he also consumes a nutritionally adequate diet.
C For a given daily dose of ethanol, men are more likely to develop cirrhosis than women.
D Ethanol causes a toxic alcoholic gastritis by stimulating gastric acid output and hence gastric secretion.
E Ethanol causes malabsorption of water, electrolytes, folate, thiamine, amino acids and glucose in the small bowel.

29. Ipratropium bromide aerosol (Atrovent) may be useful in the treatment of asthma, because it

A reduces tracheobronchial mucus flow.
B is a phosphodiesterase inhibitor.
C antagonises the effects of acetylcholine on bronchial smooth muscle.
D is used to replace beta agonists (e.g. salbutamol) when they cause muscle tremor.
E blocks the release of histamine within the lung.

30. A man aged 27 years with diabetes presents with a 3-day history of increased thirst, polyuria and vomiting. He is drowsy and dehydrated and is breathing rapidly. Serum electrolytes are measured, with the following results: Na^+ 134 mmol/ℓ (N: 135–145); K^+ 6.0 mmol/ℓ (N: 3.5–5.0); HCO_3^- 3 mmol/ℓ (N: 24–30); urea 18 mmol/ℓ (N: 2–7); creatinine 0.16 mmol/ℓ (N: 0.07–0.12 males) and pH 6.95.
Which of the following statements is/are correct?

A The high K^+ indicates acute tubular necrosis.
B Following treatment with insulin, his serum phosphate will drop to subnormal levels.
C The amount of bicarbonate given should equal the calculated deficit.
D He is unlikely to require K^+ during the first 12 hours of treatment.
E If HCO^-_3 is given, it will correct the cerebrospinal fluid (CSF) acidosis before it corrects the plasma acidosis.

31. A man aged 27 years with diabetes since 15 years of age complains of blurred vision in his left eye. Fundal examination shows recent microaneurysms, blot and flame-shaped haemorrhages, together with soft exudates in both fundi, as well as an area of vitreous opacity in his left fundus. There are new vessels arising from the optic disc in both fundi. In this situation

A the changes are most likely to be caused by complicating hypertension.
B clofibrate has been found to be useful in reversing these changes.
C he should have an urgent hypophysectomy.
D he should be referred urgently to an ophthalmologist, with a view to photocoagulation.
E he needs an urgent vitrectomy.

32. A woman aged 43 years has been referred for assessment of diabetes of recent onset. On initial examination she was noted to have round face, truncal obesity with numerous wide striae, thin extremities, mild hirsutism and a blood pressure of 170/100 mmHg. Her liver was enlarged by 6 cm and was slightly tender. She was taking no medications, smoked 20 cigarettes a day and had a daily alcohol intake of 60–70 g.

After dexamethasone 2 mg at midnight, her plasma cortisol level the following morning was 760 nmol/ℓ (N: below 140) and the 24-hour urinary free cortisol level was 890 nmol/24 h (N: below 300). Gamma glutamyl transpeptidase was 100 U/ℓ (N: below 60).

She has been admitted to hospital for investigation and stabilisation of her diabetes. Her urinary cortisol level on the 6th hospital day is 270 nmoℓ/24 h and the plasma cortisol shows a normal diurnal variation.

Which of the following statements is/are likely to be correct?

A The diagnosis is Cushing's disease with episodic steroid secretion.
B The clinical features have resulted from cortisol hypersecretion induced by alcohol.
C Alcohol interference with the assay for cortisol has resulted in spurious laboratory values.
D The patient was taking dexamethasone surreptitiously.
E Hepatic malfunction has resulted in impaired cortisol metabolism.

33. Hyperosmolar, non-ketotic diabetic coma

A occurs particularly in elderly patients with associated medical or surgical disease.
B commonly presents with fluctuating focal neurological symptoms and signs.
C is often complicated by thromboembolic problems.
D indicates the need for long-term insulin treatment after recovery.
E requires higher insulin doses than ketoacidotic coma.

34. Which of the following features is/are characteristic of diabetic polyradiculopathy (amyotrophy)?

A This condition is usually associated with long-standing insulin-dependent diabetes mellitus.
B Hyperactive tendon reflexes and extensor plantar responses are frequently found.
C Signs of sensory involvement are usually minimal.
D CSF protein concentration may be moderately elevated.
E Resolution occurs spontaneously over a period of several months.

35. A man aged 54 years gives a three month history of progressive proximal muscle weakness, increased skin pigmentation and peripheral oedema. Laboratory investigation shows a serum K^+ concentration of 2.7 mmol/ℓ (N: 3.5–5.0) and serum HCO_3^- concentration of 33 mmol/ℓ (N: 24–30). Chest X-ray shows a hilar mass. It is highly probable that he has

A Addison's disease due to adrenal metastases from a carcinoma of the lung.
B a very high plasma ACTH concentration.
C gross facial and general body habitus changes of Cushing's syndrome.
D a squamous cell carcinoma of the lung.
E an aldosterone secreting carcinoma of the lung.

36. In Cushing's disease due to bilateral adrenal hyperplasia,

A hypertension is unusual.
B plasma adrenocorticotrophic hormone (ACTH) levels measured at midnight equal or exceed early morning values.
C urinary hydroxycorticosteroids are not suppressed following administration of dexamethasone 8 mg daily for 2 days.
D a pituitary adenoma is commonly found.
E pituitary irradiation is the treatment of choice in children.

37. A woman aged 60 years, previously asymptomatic, has a skull X-ray following a minor head injury. This shows no fracture but reveals uniform enlargement of the pituitary fossa.
Which of the following statements is/are correct?

A The probability that she has the 'empty sella syndrome' is about 25%.
B The finding of a visual field disturbance would strongly suggest the presence of a pituitary tumour.
C If an 'empty sella' is present, there is a 50% probability that her serum prolactin level will be elevated.
D A serum prolactin level of 800 μg/ℓ (N: 2–15) would be virtually diagnosic of a prolactin-secreting pituitary tumour.
E Her radiological abnormality could be explained solely on the basis of primary hypothyroidism.

38. In patients with acromegaly

A enlargement of the sella turcica is detectable by standard X-rays of the pituitary fossa in less than 50% of patients.
B clinical features of the disease may be present even though fasting growth hormone levels are normal.
C the most reliable diagnostic test consists of measuring serum growth hormone levels following oral glucose administration.
D serum somatomedin levels are of diagnostic value.
E medical treatment with bromocriptine has a role, even if optic nerve compression with bitemporal visual field defects is demonstrable.

39. A woman aged 27 years presents with a history of secondary amenorrhoea. Physical examination reveals that milk can be expressed from her breasts, but otherwise there is no abnormality. Her serum prolactin level is 84 μg/ℓ (N: 4–16) but she has normal serum levels of luteinising hormone (LH) and follicle stimulating hormone (FSH).
Which of the following statements is/are correct?

A The clinical picture could be due to treatment with chlorpromazine.
B She may have a chromophobe tumour of the pituitary.
C All the features would be explained by premature menopause.
D If no specific cause is demonstrated, the prognosis for her fertility is poor.
E The elevation of the prolactin level could be due to hypothyroidism.

40. A young woman aged 18 years presents with a 6-month history of amenorrhoea and weight loss. She is extremely thin (weight 35 kg, height 162 cm), with quite well preserved breast tissue, but otherwise no abnormalities. Her LH and FSH values are just below the normal range, and thyroid function tests show T_4 100 nmol/ℓ (N: 55–150), T_3 0.7 nmol/ℓ (N: 1.2–2.8) and T_3 resin uptake 102% (N: 80–110%).

In this situation, which of the following statements is/are correct?

A She probably has hypopituitarism due to a chromophobe adenoma.

B The thyroid function tests reflect a protein binding abnormality.

C Similar thyroid function tests may be found in severe lobar pneumonia.

D The picture is not that of 'compensated hypothyroidism'.

E After treatment to reach 90% of ideal body weight, failure of her periods to return within two months would indicate a primary ovarian disorder.

41. A girl aged 19 years presents with facial, truncal and limb hirsutism. Her menstrual periods have been irregular but she is otherwise well.

Which of the following statements is/are correct?

A A moderately raised plasma testosterone level would be very suggestive of an arrhenoblastoma of the ovary.

B Use of the oral contraceptive pill would be expected to make the hirsutism worse.

C A raised plasma LH level would support a diagnosis of the polycystic ovary syndrome.

D Measuring plasma cortisol at 9 a.m. following a midnight dose of 1 mg of dexamethasone is an effective and convenient way of excluding Cushing's syndrome.

E Electrolysis is a rapid, cheap and effective method for improving the cosmetic appearance.

42. A man aged 54 years presents with a three month history of bilateral gynaecomastia. At the age of 29 years, he had severe testicular pain associated with an attack of mumps and was treated in bed for two weeks.

Physical examination revealed bilateral gynaecomastia measuring 6 cm in diameter on the right side and 8 cm in diameter on the left side. Both testes were soft, each with volume approximately 8 ml (3.6 × 2.2 cm). His serum testosterone level was 6.4 nmol/ (N: 13.5–40.0).

Which of the following statements is/are correct?

A His serum prolactin level is likely to be elevated.
B Drug ingestion is the most common cause of gynaecomastia at this age.
C Breast biopsy should be performed to exclude carcinoma.
D Testosterone treatment will probably induce at least partial regression of his gynaecomastia.
E Orchitis develops in about one-third of men who contract mumps and about half of these sustain bilateral testicular atrophy irrespective of whether there was unilateral or bilateral orchitis clinically.

43. A man aged 25 years presents for investigation of infertility. He gives a history of attacks of respiratory illness as a child which were diagnosed as bronchiectasis and treated by numerous courses of antibiotics. Investigations reveal a normal sperm count but less than 5% of sperm are motile.

Regarding diagnosis and prognosis, which of the following statements is/are correct?

A The defect in sperm motility is the result of drug therapy for bronchiectasis.
B Muco-ciliary clearance is delayed and cilial structure is likely to be defective in this man.
C The defect is sperm motility is unimportant as an explanation of his infertility.
D A proportion of men with this combination of disorders have dextrocardia.
E There is likely to be an identical defect in the structure of the cilia in his respiratory tract and in the tail of his spermatozoa.

44. With regard to thyrotoxicosis occurring during pregnancy, which of the following statements is/are correct?

A Maternal thyroid hormones cross the placenta freely.
B Maternal iodide ingestion may result in a large goitre in the fetus.
C Propylthiouracil treatment does not affect the fetal thyroid.
D Thyroid stimulating immunoglobulins from the mother may induce neonatal thyrotoxicosis.
E If carbimazole is given, it will be excreted in breast milk.

45. In subacute (de Quervain's) thyroiditis

- **A** there is usually a prodromal phase with malaise, fever or an upper respiratory tract infection.
- **B** patients characteristically complain of a painful neck and the thyroid is tender.
- **C** enhanced iodine uptake by the thyroid gland occurs.
- **D** symptoms respond to corticosteroids.
- **E** permanent hypothyroidism occurs in most cases.

46. A young woman, delivered of a normal infant 10 days ago, presents with weight loss, tachycardia, tremor and a painless thyroid enlargement. The serum T_3 and T_4 concentrations are elevated and the radioactive iodine uptake is low.
Which of the following statements is/are correct?

- **A** The most likely diagnosis is Graves' disease.
- **B** The clinical course of the illness is likely to be of less than 6 months duration.
- **C** Therapy with beta adrenergic blockade alone is unlikely to be successful.
- **D** A relapse should be anticipated in subsequent pregnancies.
- **E** Thyroid autoantibody titres will be elevated in 90% of such patients.

47. A man aged 35 years presents with a single firm nodule 3 cm in diameter in the thyroid gland. He is clinically euthyroid.
Regarding investigation and management of this patient, which of the following statements is/are correct?

- **A** A technetium scan, showing uptake in the nodule to be equal to the remainder of the gland, justifies a prolonged trial of suppressive therapy with thyroxine.
- **B** The presence of antithyroglobulin antibodies in the serum at a high titre, suggesting Hashimoto's thyroiditis, makes thyroid malignancy extremely unlikely.
- **C** Ultrasound demonstration that the nodule is a thick-walled cyst makes thyroid cancer most unlikely.
- **D** Fine needle aspiration biopsy of the nodule is the most accurate single test in the diagnosis of thyroid cancer prior to surgical removal.
- **E** An elevated serum thyroglobulin concentration will confirm the diagnosis of thyroid cancer.

48. In patients with hypercalcaemia, which of the following statements is/are correct?

- **A** If the patient has primary hyperparathyroidism, oral ingestion of prednisolone 10 mg t.d.s. for 10 days will cause suppression of the plasma calcium to normal.
- **B** Chlorothiazide treatment is likely to increase the serum level of calcium.
- **C** A strong family history of hypercalcaemia and a subnormal urinary calcium supports the diagnosis of primary hyperparathyroidism.
- **D** A normal parathyroid hormone value does not exclude primary hyperparathyroidism.
- **E** The hypercalcaemia may be caused by a squamous cell carcinoma of the lung, even in the absence of bone metastases.

49. A widow aged 74 years presents with a history of pain in her limbs and back. Which of the following features would support the possibility that her symptoms are due to osteomalacia?

- **A** The presence of a proximal myopathy
- **B** A raised serum phosphorus with a normal creatinine level
- **C** A history of drinking no milk and eating table margarine instead of butter
- **D** A raised serum alkaline phosphatase level
- **E** A past history of a partial gastrectomy for peptic ulcer.

50. Concerning herpes zoster infection, which of the following statements is/are correct?

- **A** Shingles occurs exclusively in persons who have had previous infection with varicella-zoster virus.
- **B** The eruption occurs most frequently in the thoracic region.
- **C** Motor neuropathy occurs in up to 30% of patients, corresponds to the dermatome involved and has a good prognosis.
- **D** Dissemination beyond one dermatome is more common in patients with compromised immunological systems.
- **E** If administered during the first 5 days of infection, acyclovir reduces pain and accelerates healing.

51. A man aged 21 years has returned from a skiing holiday in Austria suffering from moderately severe diarrhoea together with anorexia, nausea and epigastric discomfort. He has lost 3 kg in weight in the 4 weeks since symptoms began. Sigmoidoscopy is normal.

In this situation

A the history indicates traveller's diarrhoea and he should be treated with ampicillin.
B normal sigmoidoscopy and absence of blood in the faeces makes a diagnosis of amoebiasis unlikely.
C the most likely cause is *Giardia lamblia* infestation.
D duodenoscopy and duodenal biopsy should be undertaken.
E a therapeutic trial of metronidazole is reasonable.

52. The drug metronidazole ('Flagyl')

A is an effective treatment for giardiasis.
B is an effective treatment for salmonella gastroenteritis.
C produces an 'Antabuse-like' effect.
D causes a metallic taste when taken orally.
E causes mutagenesis in laboratory animals.

53. *Campylobacter jejuni* has been recognised as a cause of intestinal disease in man. In campylobacter enterocolitis, which of the following statements is/are correct?

A The onset of the illness is often sudden with diarrhoea, fever and cramping abdominal pains.
B Gross or occult blood loss in the stool occurs in more than 50% of patients.
C Sigmoidoscopy may show an acute proctitis with features resembling ulcerative colitis.
D The illness runs a prolonged course over several weeks in 50% or more of affected patients.
E In patients with severe or protracted illness, erythromycin may be effective antibiotic therapy.

54. A man aged 64 years receiving 'MOPP' chemotherapy for Hodgkin's disease develops fever, rigors, abdominal pain, diarrhoea and vomiting.
The possibility of disseminated strongyloidiasis is considered, since the patient had been a prisoner of war in South-East Asia during World War II. However, blood cultures are positive for *E. coli* and his peripheral blood eosinophil count is normal.
Which of the following statements is/are correct?

A Strongyloidiasis is unlikely to have persisted in this patient since World War II.
B The peripheral blood eosinophil count is usually elevated in disseminated strongyloidiasis.
C Disseminated strongyloidiasis will be excluded if ova are not found in the faeces.
D Gram-negative bacteraemia commonly occurs in conjunction with disseminated strongyloidiasis.
E Thiabendazole is the treatment of choice for strongyloidiasis.

55. With regard to non-A non-B hepatitis, which of the following statements is/are correct?

A At present it is the most common form of post-transfusion hepatitis.
B Most cases are caused by a hepatitis C virus.
C Carriers can be detected by an immunological screening technique.
D It is seldom complicated by chronic liver disease.
E It is responsible for 40–50% of all cases of fulminant hepatitis with liver failure.

56. A dentist aged 30 years presents with jaundice for three days following malaise, anorexia and fever for 2 weeks.
At this stage of his illness, which of the following statements is/are correct?

A If he has hepatitis A, his faeces are unlikely to contain infectious virus particles.
B Acute hepatitis B infection is confirmed by the presence of antibodies to hepatitis B surface antigen in serum (anti-HBs).
C Lymphadenopathy, together with hepatomegaly and atypical lymphocytes in peripheral blood, makes hepatitis virus infection unlikely.
D It is necessary for all the dental patients he has attended in the last six weeks to receive gammaglobulin injections (pooled human gammaglobulin).
E A mixed aerobic-anaerobic bacterial liver abscess may be present.

57. A chronic asthmatic aged 39 years who has been on steroid therapy for 10 years presents with headaches and vomiting of one month's duration. There are no abnormal physical signs.
Which of the following is the most likely cause of this condition?

A Subacute bacterial endocarditis
B Chronic migraine
C Subarachnoid haemorrhage
D Cryptococcal meningitis
E Tension headaches.

58. Concerning the use of the VDRL (Venereal Disease Research Laboratory) flocculation test and its modification, the rapid plasma-reagin test (RPR), which of the following statements is/are correct?

A A negative serum VDRL or RPR virtually excludes secondary syphilis.
B A negative CSF VDRL is found in more than 30% of patients with neurosyphilis.
C A false-positive serum VDRL or RPR may occur in pregnancy and in narcotic addiction.
D A false-positive CSF VDRL rarely occurs unless positive serum has contaminated the CSF during lumbar puncture.
E After adequate treatment of seropositive primary syphilis, the VDRL remains positive for 12 months or more in over 40% of patients.

59. Concerning the organism *Chlamydia trachomatis*, which of the following statements is/are correct?

A It is associated with the pyuria-dysuria (urethral) syndrome in females, conjunctivitis in neonates and pneumonia in adults.
B It can be grown from the cervix of 25% of female contacts of males with non-specific urethritis.
C Infection may be diagnosed by demonstration of inclusions in polymorphs in pus taken from the affected site.
D The incubation period for infection is approximately 28 days.
E When it causes cystitis in women, the condition may respond to sulphonamide therapy.

60. With regard to dental caries, which of the following statements is/are correct?

- **A** The major bacterium involved in producing caries in man is *Streptococcus mutans.*
- **B** Formation of adhesive extracellular polysaccharides of streptococci is of prime importance in producing dental plaque.
- **C** Frequency of sucrose ingestion is less important in cariogenesis than the total quantity of sucrose ingested daily.
- **D** There is no evidence for any reduction in caries by immunization against *Streptococcus mutans* in primates.
- **E** There is no evidence for any reduction in plaque by use of antiseptic mouthwashes.

61. Acute haemorrhagic conjunctivitis (AHC) has spread recently through much of the South Pacific, as well as the Indian subcontinent and South America. Enterovirus 70 has been implicated as the aetiological agent.
With regard to this disease, which of the following statements is/are correct?

- **A** The incubation period for AHC is only 24 hours.
- **B** The virus is spread from person to person via fingers or fomites.
- **C** Enterovirus 70 can be readily isolated from both the eyes and the faeces of patients with AHC.
- **D** About 2 weeks after the onset of AHC, paralysis of the lower limbs may occur.
- **E** Isolated cranial nerve palsies may be associated with AHC.

62. A man returns from a holiday in South-East Asia with acute urethritis which is shown to be due to *Neisseria gonorrhoeae.*
Which of the following statements is/are correct?

- **A** Intramuscular injection of 2.4 million units of benzathine penicillin with oral probenecid would be acceptable.
- **B** Penicillin G can still be used to treat penicillinase-producing *Neisseria gonorrhoeae* as long as the dosages used are high enough.
- **C** Genital infection preceding disseminated gonococcal disease is usually asymptomatic.
- **D** If his wife is pregnant and allergic to penicillin, she should be treated with erythromycin.
- **E** An initial and a repeat swab for culture and sensitivity should always be taken in gonococcal infections.

63. A man aged 65 years, weighing about 70 kg, presents with a temperature of 38.5°C, a leucocytosis, anaemia and an aortic incompetent murmur. He has splinter haemorrhages in the nail beds of his hands and feet.

Microscopic examination of his urine reveals red blood cells. Five bottles out of six in six sets of blood cultures grow *Streptococcus faecalis*.

Optimal antibiotic treatment would be provided by which of the following?

- **A** intravenous penicillin G (benzyl penicillin) 3 million units four hourly plus intramuscular streptomycin 0.5 g bd.
- **B** intravenous penicillin G 3 million units four hourly plus intravenous gentamicin 80 mg tds.
- **C** intravenous ampicillin 1 g six hourly.
- **D** if he is allergic to penicillin, intravenous vancomycin 500 mg six hourly.
- **E** intravenous cefoxitin 2 g six hourly.

64. A woman aged 71 years, living in a nursing home, has chronic obstructive airways disease and a history of recurrent acute episodes of pneumonia. Two other patients in the nursing home have acute viral respiratory infections at a time when influenza A is known to be occurring frequently in the community.

The antiviral agent, amantadine, is being considered for prophylaxis against influenza A in this woman. With regard to such use, which of the following statements is/are correct?

- **A** Its clinical activity is restricted to influenza A infections.
- **B** Prophylactic administration must continue throughout the period of risk.
- **C** The drug can be started in conjunction with influenza immunisation without interfering with the antibody response.
- **D** The drug accumulates in patients with impaired renal function, increasing the likelihood of toxic effects.
- **E** Side-effects principally involve the central nervous system.

65. A man aged 30 years seeks advice regarding malarial prophylaxis for a trip through South East Asia and Africa.

Which of the following statements is/are correct?

- **A** Chloroquine-resistant *falciparum* malaria is less common in Africa.
- **B** Because most of South-East Asia has chloroquine-resistant strains of *falciparum* malaria, he should take some antimalarial drug in addition to chloroquine.
- **C** Prophylaxis need not begin before departure but should continue for about three months afterwards.
- **D** If he takes his prophylactic drugs, any febrile episode which occurs more than two months after return is most unlikely to be due to malaria.
- **E** If he decides to take his pregnant wife, chloroquine would be the best form of prophylaxis for her.

66. A woman aged 25 years presents with polyarthritis, swelling of fingers, myalgia and muscle weakness, Raynaud's phenomenon and features of scleroderma. Antinuclear antibody is present in a titre of 1/1000 with a speckled pattern, and serum complement levels are normal.

Which of the following statements is/are correct?

A Antibody to double stranded DNA is likely to be present in a high titre.

B Antinuclear antibody specificity is most likely to be directed against the ribonucleoprotein component of extractable nuclear antigen.

C Serious renal and neurological involvement is likely to develop.

D Normal serum complement levels exclude renal damage caused by immune complexes.

E It is probable that she will respond readily to steroids.

67. A variety of drugs, particularly procainamide and hydralazine have been associated with the development of an illness very similar to systemic lupus erythematosus (SLE).

Which of the following statements is/are correct?

A Antinuclear antibodies are always present in a drug-induced lupus.

B Renal and central nervous system disease are rare (less than 10%) in drug-induced lupus.

C Drug-induced lupus occurs only in individuals who have the slow acetylator phenotype.

D Drug-induced lupus, particularly that induced by hydralazine, occurs more frequently in individuals of HLA-DR phenotypes 2 or 3.

E Serum complement levels are usually normal in drug induced lupus.

68. A woman aged 24 years with a five year history of SLE is referred when her family doctor finds that she is 12 weeks pregnant. Previous manifestations of SLE have included arthritis, skin rash, fevers, serositis and thrombocytopenia. However, during the preceding 12 months her disease has been well-controlled on prednisone 5 mg daily and azathioprine 100 mg daily.

At assessment, she is found to have only mild synovitis in her hands, normal renal function, normal complement levels and an elevated DNA binding capacity of 50% (N: up to 30%).

Which of the following statements is/are correct?

A Her pregnancy should be terminated to prevent the onset of renal involvement.

B Azathioprine should be stopped immediately and steroids increased to suppress any resulting exacerbation of disease activity.

C In the absence of renal failure, the prevalence of fetal wastage is around 20–25%.

D During labour and the post-partum period, an increased dose of steroid is indicated to reduce the risk of a post-partum exacerbation.

E If the pregnancy is carried to term, the infant has a greater than normal risk of congenital heart block.

69. Vasculitis may occur as a primary disorder or as a manifestation of systemic disease. Which of the following statements is/are correct?

A Most cases of necrotizing vasculitis are caused by or related to immunological disorders with deposition of immune complexes in the vessel wall.

B In polyarteritis nodosa, an allergic history is uncommon and hepatitis B antigenaemia is commonly found.

C In hypersensitivity vasculitis, the post capillary venules are classically involved and examination of the skin usually reveals palpable purpura.

D In Henoch-Schoenlein disease, immune complexes including IgA are found in vessels in skin, gut and glomerulus.

E In Wegener's granulomatosis, the therapeutic response to cyclophosphamide is usually excellent.

70. A woman aged 47 years has suffered from Raynaud's phenomenon for two years. For 12 months she has complained of dysphagia for solid food and a dry cough with shortness of breath on climbing stairs. She presents to the emergency department of a hospital after a well-documented generalised tonic-clonic seizure.

Examination reveals her to be drowsy and confused, with tight facial skin and multiple telangiectases, dry basal lung crepitations and a blood pressure of 200/160 mmHg. Urinalysis shows ++ blood and +++ protein.

Which of the following statements is/are correct?

A Intravenous pyelogram is likely to show small shrunken kidneys with clubbing of the calyces.
B Renal biopsy will show mesangial glomerulonephritis.
C High-dose steroid therapy is likely to improve mental status and hypertension.
D Renal function may be preserved if blood pressure is effectively controlled.
E Bilateral nephrectomy is indicated.

71. In patients with rheumatoid arthritis, which of the following statements is/are correct?

A In about 20% of them the sacroiliac joints show erosions and periarticular sclerosis.
B Flexor tenosynovitis is a common cause of impaired hand grip.
C Up to 5% of patients with active disease may have a normal ESR.
D If synovial biopsies are undertaken, the histological features are diagnostic of the condition.
E Lymphocytes are the predominant cell in rheumatoid synovial fluid.

72. **A woman aged 54 years with nodular rheumatoid arthritis presents with a pruritic skin rash on the hands, arms and trunk. She is on treatment with enteric-coated aspirin (3 g daily), naproxen (250 mg twice daily) and sodium aurothiomalate (50 mg i.m.i. weekly). Her total dose of gold is 750 mg and she has shown a good clinical response.**

Which of the following statements is/are correct?

A The rash is most likely to be due to aspirin sensitivity, so aspirin treatment should be stopped.
B The rash is unlikely to be due to gold since cutaneous toxicity rarely occurs when the total dose given is less than 1 g.
C If the rash is due to gold it will resolve within one month of stopping treatment.
D Gold should be stopped but since her rheumatoid condition has shown a good response it may be cautiously re-introduced in low doses (e.g. 5 mg, then 10 mg) once the rash has cleared.
E If the rash is due to gold, this side-effect could have been prevented by carefully monitoring serum gold levels.

73. **A woman aged 45 years has had rheumatoid arthritis for 10 years, associated with significant joint damage, nodules and occasional digital vasculitis. She is being treated with sodium aurothiomalate ('Myocrisin') 50 mg monthly, enteric-coated aspirin 1300 mg 8-hourly and indomethacin suppositories at night. Menstruation has stopped and there is no overt gastrointestinal bleeding.**

Her blood count shows haemoglobin 98 g/ℓ, MCV 82 fl (N: 82–92), MCHC 30 g/dℓ (N: 32–36), white cell count 6.9 × 10^9 /ℓ, ESR 68 mm/h, serum iron 4.7 μmol/ℓ (N: 13–32), TIBC 38.7 μmol/ℓ (N: 45–70), serum ferritin 40 μg/ℓ (N: 25–250), serum B_{12} 370 ng/ℓ (N: 150–900). serum folate 4.4 μg/ℓ (N: 3–18), red cell folate 220 μg/ℓ (N: 150–640). The bone marrow biopsy shows normal cellularity.

Which of the following statements is/are correct?

A The anaemia is most likely due to iron deficiency.
B Significant gastric erosion and blood loss may occur in the absence of symptoms of indigestion.
C Her anaemia will respond to oral iron therapy.
D Bone marrow iron stores are likely to be normal or increased.
E The normal serum ferritin level excludes the possibility of iron deficiency.

74. **Which of the following drugs is/are appropriate for use in the management of active polyarticular psoriatic arthritis?**

A Salicylates
B Sodium aurothiomalate
C Indomethacin
D Chloroquine
E Allopurinol.

75. A moderately obese man aged 60 years presents with a four-month history of pain and mild swelling in the left knee. He has a past history of transient cerebral ischaemic attacks for which he takes 0.3 g aspirin daily. On biochemical screening he is found to have a serum uric acid of 0.50 mmol/ℓ (N: 0.18–0.45).

Which of the following statements is/are correct?

- **A** If he had a past history of podagra, the current episode of arthritis in the knee is probably due to gout.
- **B** His symptoms in the left knee are most likely due to osteoarthritis.
- **C** His 24-hour urinary uric acid excretion is probably within the normal range.
- **D** Reduction in aspirin dosage will lead to a fall in the serum uric acid.
- **E** Allopurinol or a uricosuric agent should be used to reduce his serum uric acid to within the normal range.

76. A man aged 22 years presents with a two-month history of inflammatory arthritis involving his left knee, right second and third metatarsophalangeal joints and the interphalangeal joint of his right big toe. Examination reveals marked tenderness over the plantar surface of the left heel and thickening of the left Achilles tendon. The patient recalls having had transient mild dysuria and a slight urethral discharge two weeks prior to the onset of his arthritis.

Synovial fluid aspirated from the involved knee shows a white cell count of 50 000/cmm, 80% of which are neutrophils. Urethral swab culture reveals no significant pathogens. His haemoglobin level and white cell count are normal but his ESR is elevated to 88 mm/h.

Which of the following statements is/are correct?

- **A** If the patient is HLA-B27 negative, the most likely diagnosis is gonococcal arthritis.
- **B** Radiological periostitis along the shafts of the right second and third metatarsals would suggest that he has a low-grade septic polyarthritis.
- **C** The appearance of dystrophic nail changes with subungual hyperkeratosis might be expected, even in the absence of psoriatic skin lesions.
- **D** An episode of dysentery caused by *Shigella flexneri* could have precipitated his present illness.
- **E** He has at least a 30% chance of developing a residual disability.

77. Sjögren's syndrome may occur alone (primary) or in association with other autoimmune diseases such as rheumatoid arthritis or systemic lupus erythematosus (secondary).
Which of the following statements is/are correct?

- **A** The histological changes in the salivary glands are identical in all forms of Sjögren's syndrome.
- **B** Dyspareunia due to vaginitis sicca occurs only in Sjögren's syndrome complicating rheumatoid arthritis.
- **C** Raynaud's phenomenon, purpura and lymphadenopathy occur more commonly in primary Sjögren's syndrome than in Sjögren's syndrome with rheumatoid arthritis.
- **D** The risk of developing lymphoma is increased 40–50 times in both primary and secondary Sjögren's syndrome.
- **E** The HLA antigens B8 and DRw3 occur with equal frequency in primary and secondary Sjögren's syndrome.

78. Concerning calcium pyrophosphate dihydrate deposition disease (CPPD), which of the following statements is/are correct?

- **A** In most patients an underlying metabolic disease can be detected.
- **B** Colchicine may be effective in inducing remissions of acute pseudo-gout.
- **C** About 5% of patients have multiple joint involvement mimicking rheumatoid arthritis.
- **D** Allopurinol is indicated only for patients having multiple attacks of pseudogout.
- **E** Up to 50% of patients show progressive polyarticular osteoarthritis.

79. With respect to the use of D-penicillamine in patients with rheumatoid arthritis, which of the following statements is/are correct?

- **A** D-penicillamine can be used safely despite a past history of penicillin allergy.
- **B** Patients with previous gold-induced proteinuria should not be treated with D-penicillamine.
- **C** Treatment with D-penicillamine is associated with the development or reactivation of peptic ulceration.
- **D** Treatment with low doses of D-penicillamine (to a maximum of 750 mg daily) is usually as effective as with high doses (up to 1.5 g daily).
- **E** Isolated reversible thrombocytopenia is the most common haematological side-effect.

80. In a patient with polymyalgia rheumatica, which of the following is/are likely to be found?

A Jaw and tongue claudication
B A normal EMG
C An elevated serum alkaline phosphatase
D An abnormal bone scan with increased technetium -99 uptake in the shoulders and knees
E A positive antinuclear antibody titre of 1:1000 with a speckled pattern.

81. A woman aged 27 years with systemic lupus erythematosus complains of right groin pain of eight weeks duration. Pain occurs particularly on weight-bearing and on standing up after sitting.

Her disease began when she was 22 years of age, with thrombocytopenia; subsequently she developed arthritis, alopecia, skin rashes and episodes of serositis, some of which required treatment with prednisolone 60–80 mg daily. During the past six months her disease has been relatively quiescent and she has been maintained on prednisolone 7.5 mg daily.

Which of the following statements is/are correct?

A The dose of prednisolone should be increased to 15 mg daily to control right hip synovitis.
B Immediate aspiration of the right hip joint should be undertaken to exclude septic arthritis.
C X-ray of the right hip is most likely to show symmetrical loss of joint space.
D Bone scan may be diagnostically helpful even if an X-ray of the right hip is normal.
E If X-ray shows a translucent subcortical band in the femoral head, steroid withdrawal will not prevent progressive changes in the affected hip.

82. A woman aged 43 years presents with a two-year history of generalised aches, pains and stiffness which become worse with anxiety and in cold or humid weather.

Examination reveals no evidence of joint disease; she is markedly tender along the upper borders of the trapezius muscles, over the humeral epicondyles and the medial aspects of both knees. A full blood count and ESR are normal; rheumatoid factor and antinuclear antibodies are negative.

Which of the following statements is/are correct?

A Even if additional complaints include constant tiredness and poor sleep, primary fibromyalgia is likely to be the diagnosis.
B A history of periodic alterations in bowel habits, with lower abdominal pain or distention relieved by defaecation, would suggest that a colonic neoplasm is responsible for her symptoms.
C The most likely diagnosis is psychogenic rheumatism.
D Rheumatoid arthritis is unlikely in the absence of objective joint changes.
E Thyroid function tests should be included in the screening investigations of this patient.

83. A girl aged 19 years presents with a four-day history of fever and arthritis of the right wrist. There is no history of photosensitivity, Raynaud's phenomenon, morning stiffness, diarrhoea, urethritis or sexual activity for the last 4 weeks.

Examination reveals a warm erythematous and very tender right wrist with associated tenosynovitis and occasional vesiculopustular lesions on the extremities. There is no lymphadenopathy. X-rays of the hand and wrist show only soft tissue swelling with bony changes.

Which of the following statements is/are correct?

A The clinical picture is typical of reactive arthritis following enteric infection (e.g. *Shigella*).
B The presence of rash, fever and arthritis makes systemic lupus erythematosus the most likely diagnosis.
C Synovial fluid should be aspirated from the wrist or tendon sheath for bacterial culture.
D Swabs for culture should be taken from the vesicular skin lesions.
E After appropriate cultures, treatment with parenteral penicillin should be commenced for presumed gonococcal arthritis.

84. A man aged 23 years presents with a history of repeated sinopulmonary infections since childhood, having recently developed polyarthritis. Serum protein estimation shows a greatly reduced globulin and electrophoresis shows a reduced gammaglobulin fraction. Quantitative immunoglobulin determinations show profound reduction in all gammaglobulin classes.

Which of the following statements is/are correct?

- **A** Hypogammaglobulinaemia presenting at this age is always secondary to underlying disease.
- **B** Numbers of circulating B lymphocytes are frequently normal in this condition.
- **C** Because his cell-mediated function is intact, he may receive live attenuated vaccines with safety.
- **D** The risk of malignancy is increased.
- **E** Prophylaxis with gammaglobulin injections 25 mg/kg/week will prevent infection and will reverse the arthritis.

85. Concerning the recognition of autoantibodies directed against specific nuclear components in the delineation of various connective tissue disease syndromes, which of the following statements is/are correct?

- **A** Mixed connective tissue disease is the most likely diagnosis when antibodies to nuclear ribonucleoprotein (nRNP) are present alone in significant titre.
- **B** Anti-centromere antibody is strongly associated with the 'CREST' syndrome (calcinosis, Raynaud's phenomenon, oesophageal involvement, sclerodactyly and telangiectasia).
- **C** In patients with systemic lupus erythematosus, high levels of antibodies to native DNA may be present throughout long periods of inactive disease.
- **D** A speckled pattern of antinuclear antibody is associated typically with antibodies to native DNA.
- **E** Antibodies to single-stranded DNA have the same diagnostic value as antibodies to native DNA.

86. Concerning amyloidosis, which of the following statements is/are correct?

- **A** Amyloid fibrils are beta-pleated proteins, often derived by proteolysis of Bence-Jones protein.
- **B** Patients with acquired systemic (primary) amyloidosis often have Bence-Jones protein in the serum or the urine.
- **C** In reactive systemic (secondary) amyloidosis, amyloid-fibril protein is monoclonal and similar to that found in primary amyloidosis.
- **D** Orthostatic hypotension, a purpuric rash and a polyarthropathy are all recognised features of acquired systemic (primary) amyloidosis.
- **E** In amyloidosis associated with familial Mediterranean fever, colchicine is the treatment of choice.

87. Concerning chronic recurrent urticaria or 'hives', which of the following statements is/are correct?

A Skin-prick tests with a wide variety of potential allergens are generally of little diagnostic value.
B A deficiency of the C1 esterase inhibitor is the basic defect in over 20% of cases.
C It may be associated with episodes of arthralgia and abdominal pain.
D The total haemolytic complement activity assay may be a useful diagnostic measurement.
E Over 70% of cases are caused by substances in the diet which can be confirmed by exclusion and provocation.

88. Concerning mixed cryoglobulinaemia, which of the following statements is/are correct?

A Cryoprecipitates in the serum are usually immune complexes of IgM rheumatoid factor and IgG.
B Cryoglobulinaemia may antedate the detection of lymphoma, macroglobulinaemia or chronic lymphatic leukaemia.
C There is an increased likelihood of HBsAg in the serum.
D Glomerulonephritis and necrotising arteritis of small and medium-sized renal arteries develop in about 50% of patients.
E Detection of cryoglobulinemia is always an indication for treatment.

89. With respect to angioimmunoblastic lymphadenopathy, which of the following statements is/are correct?

A An autoimmune haemolytic anaemia with a positive Coombs' test occurs in some patients.
B Hyperglobulinaemia may be due to polyclonal or monoclonal production of immunoglobulins.
C Vasculitis of small and medium arteries is a common manifestation.
D It is frequently associated with drug allergy.
E Corticosteroid therapy induces a remission in the majority of patients.

90. A man aged 58 years presents with a tender submandibular swelling and enlarged cervical nodes. Biopsy reveals an infected submandibular salivary gland. The lymph node histology was consistent with reactive hyperplasia but another histopathologist raised the possibility of malignant lymphoma (large cell diffuse).

Which of the following findings would be consistent with the diagnosis of lymphoma? (Normal $\kappa:\lambda$ ratio of surface immunoglobulins is 2:1.)

A An increase in bone marrow lymphocytes in which surface immunoglobulin light chains are present in a $k:\lambda$ ratio of 20:1
B Lymph node lymphocytes characterised by both IgM and IgD surface immunoglobulin with a $\kappa:\lambda$ ratio of 2:1
C Lymph node lymphocytes characterised by both IgM and IgD surface immunoglobulin with a $\kappa:\lambda$ ratio of 20:1
D A serum paraprotein of IgM-K type
E Increased serum immunoglobulins of both IgG and IgM type.

91. With reference to the problems associated with high blood pressure, which of the following statements is/are correct?

A Labile systolic blood pressure has no prognostic significance.
B The complications of hypertension (cerebrovascular accidents, cardiac failure, etc.) are related much more closely to diastolic than to systolic elevation of blood pressure.
C Thiazide diuretics are effective in lowering blood pressure because they reduce blood levels of renin and angiotensin.
D High blood pressure levels in chronic renal failure are most closely related to circulating blood volume.
E Elevated renin-angiotensin-aldosterone levels are found in more than 70% of patients with essential hypertension.

92. A man aged 37 years presents with blurred vision, asthma and breathlessness, which have developing over the past four weeks. Previously he has been well with normal blood pressure.

On examination, he has congestive cardiac failure and wheezing expiratory rhonchi in his chest. His blood pressure is 190/135 mmHg, he has retinal haemorrhages and blurred disc margins.

Which of the following statements is/are correct?

A Excessive treatment for asthma with salbutamol could have caused the clinical features.
B Hypertension alone is not likely to be the cause of the cardiac failure.
C An elevated plasma renin activity would be diagnostic of renal artery stenosis.
D Phaeochromocytoma is reliably excluded by normal 24-hour urinary metanephrine levels.
E The presence of circulating hepatitis B antigen is consistent with a primary cause for the presenting problem.

93. Concerning bacterial endocarditis, which of the following statements is/are correct?

- **A** Surgical valve replacement has no place in the management of acute bacterial endocarditis.
- **B** The demonstration of normal valves by echocardiography excludes endocarditis.
- **C** Acute bacterial endocarditis may involve previously normal valves.
- **D** Penicillin prophylaxis is given long-term following rheumatic fever, primarily to prevent bacterial endocarditis.
- **E** When acute aortic incompetence is present, its severity is likely to be underestimated by the usual physical and radiological signs of aortic incompetence.

94. When infective endocarditis occurs in narcotic addicts

- **A** The mitral valve is most commonly affected.
- **B** the tricuspid valve is most commonly affected.
- **C** the most common infecting organism is *Candida albicans.*
- **D** the most common infecting organism is *Staphylococcus aureus.*
- **E** the mortality rate is generally greater than 75%, even with early treatment.

95. An apparently healthy man aged 20 years is found to have multiple tendon xanthomata together with a highly elevated serum cholesterol level of 14 mmol/ℓ (N: 4–7) and a normal triglyceride level. Further lipid estimations confirm a high level of low density lipoprotein (LDL) and a normal level of very low density lipoprotein (VLDL).

Which of the following statements is/are correct?

- **A** He probably has diabetes mellitus.
- **B** A family history of premature coronary heart disease can be expected.
- **C** His fasting serum is probably turbid in appearance.
- **D** This patient will have a defective catabolism of LDL consequent upon an inherited lack of LDL receptors.
- **E** His serum cholesterol level can be expected to fall to within normal limits on a rigid low fat diet without resort to the use of lipid-lowering agents such as cholestyramine.

96. Attacks of coronary artery spasm

- **A** are associated only with attacks of variant angina pectoris (Prinzmetal's angina) when ST segment elevation occurs.
- **B** can be demonstrated by coronary angiography to occur in normal and abnormal coronary vessels.
- **C** can be precipitated by the administration of ergonovine.
- **D** are best treated with large doses of beta blockers.
- **E** are accompanied by acute pain that is often relieved promptly by nitroglycerine.

97. Concerning coronary artery bypass grafting (CABG) performed by competent surgeons, which of the following statements is/are correct?

A CABG is technically more difficult to perform in patients with varicose veins in the legs.
B CABG can be expected to improve left ventricular function when previous left heart failure has been present.
C The effects of CABG on long-term survival are difficult to assess because mortality rates from ischaemic heart disease in the non-operated population continue to decline.
D 85% or more of patients can expect their angina to improve following CABG.
E CABG has a high perioperative mortality rate of 10%, even in those patients with normal preoperative ventricular function.

98. A patient aged 48 years, recovering in the ward from an acute myocardial infarction, suffers a cardiac arrest.
In this situation

A external cardiac massage with a compression to relaxation ratio of 40:60 should be commenced.
B 'blind' defibrillation should be attempted before an ECG diagnosis is obtained.
C cardiac asystole is best treated with sympathomimetic drugs.
D 150 mmol of sodium bicarbonate should be administered routinely.
E methoxamine may be useful if ventricular fibrillation is resistant to other treatment.

99. A loud systolic murmur, maximal at the left sternal edge and accompanied by a thrill, is found in a patient three days after an acute myocardial infarction.
In this situation

A the patient probably has a perforated interventricular septum.
B the infarct is more likely to be anterior than inferior in location.
C the prognosis is poor, despite recent therapeutic advances.
D if cardiogenic shock is also present, the patient should be considered for intra-aortic balloon counter-pulsation.
E the patient should be managed medically until the infarction had healed.

100. A man aged 48 years has moderate angina. A coronary angiogram is performed.
Which of the following statements is/are correct?

A Coronary angiography is associated with a 2% mortality rate.
B If his left main coronary artery is significantly affected, his expected 5 year survival rate after bypass surgery is better than after medical therapy.
C If his angiogram shows a single lesion with 70% obstruction in the proximal anterior descending artery, immediate bypass surgery is indicated.

If he has significant three-vessel disease, but with the left main coronary artery free from disease and evidence of good left ventricular function

D treated medically, the 5-year survival rate is about 80%.
E treatment by coronary artery bypass surgery should improve the 5-year survival rate.

101. In comparison with patients with anterior and inferior transmural myocardial infarction, patients with acute non-transmural myocardial infarction have

A a significantly lower mortality rate during the hospital stay.
B a comparable mortality rate approximately four years later.
C a decreased frequency of atrioventricular and bundle branch block.
D a similar late frequency of angina pectoris — approximately 50%.
E very similar early post-myocardial infarction angiographic findings.

102. With regard to acute myocardial infarction, which of the following statements is/are correct?

A Selective beta blockade beginning a week after the episode increases the mortality.
B There is no difference in overall long-term survival rate between men and women.
C Hypokalaemia reinforces the anti-arrhythmic effect of lignocaine.
D Intravenous atropine should be given urgently to a patient who has a sleeping pulse rate of 40 beats/minute and a blood pressure of 110/60 mmHg.
E Long-term follow-up treatment with beta blockade reduces the incidence of re-infarction.

103. In patients with severe chronic left ventricular failure treated with digoxin and diuretics, which of the following statements is/are correct?

- **A** Systemic vascular resistance is elevated.
- **B** Circulating noradrenaline levels are usually elevated.
- **C** Treatment with arterial vasodilator drugs such as hydralazine may improve cardiac output without significant reduction in blood pressure.
- **D** The venodilator effect of drugs such as prazosin usually results in a marked fall in blood pressure.
- **E** Sinus tachycardia is usually the limiting factor in treatment with vasodilators.

104. In patients with heart block, which of the following statements is/are correct?

- **A** Bifascicular block in symptomatic patients is accompanied by an increased risk of sudden death.
- **B** Left bundle branch block with right axis deviation indicates left anterior hemi-block.
- **C** Permanent cardiac pacing is advisable in symptomatic atrioventricular block.
- **D** Permanent cardiac pacing is advisable in asymptomatic bifascicular block.
- **E** Digoxin toxicity is the most common cause of bifascicular block.

105. In an adult female patient who has undergone mitral valve replacement with a mechanical prosthesis, which of the following statements is/are correct?

- **A** Long-term therapy with oral anticoagulants is indicated to reduce the risk of systemic embolism.
- **B** If the patient is pregnant, coumadin drugs will cross the placenta and increase the risk of fetal haemorrhage.
- **C** Because of the risks to the fetus, oral anticoagulants should be discontinued throughout any pregnancy.
- **D** If a patient such as this develops late prosthetic valve endocarditis, medical therapy can be expected to be curative in only 10% of cases.
- **E** Continued daily suppressant antibiotic therapy is necessary to prevent late endocarditis.

106. Concerning orthostatic hypotension, which of the following statements is/are correct?

- **A** Systolic blood pressure falls by 20 mmHg or more in about 20% of normal elderly persons on standing.
- **B** It may be caused by beta-adrenergic blockers.
- **C** When due to central nervous system disease, plasma noradrenaline levels are normal.
- **D** When drug therapy is indicated, fludrocortisone acetate is often effective.
- **E** If the fall in systolic pressure exceeds 15 mmHg on standing, drug therapy should be instituted, even in the absence of symptoms.

107. Severe aortic stenosis is always accompanied by

- **A** symptoms of angina of effort or syncope.
- **B** a loud aortic systolic murmur (grade 3:4 or 4:4).
- **C** ECG evidence of left ventricular hypertrophy or 'strain'.
- **D** a peak systolic aortic valve gradient of 50 mmHg or more.
- **E** reduced left ventricular function.

108. Concerning the treatment of anginal pain, nitroglycerine

- **A** dilates vascular smooth muscle throughout the body.
- **B** has a dominant venodilatory action.
- **C** is generally ineffective when the angina is associated with coronary artery spasm.
- **D** may be effective when administered in ointment form.
- **E** should not be prescribed if calcium antagonists are also being used.

109. An otherwise healthy patient aged 40 years is found to have ventricular bigeminal rhythm at a routine medical examination. Which of the following statements is/are correct?

- **A** The clinical significance of such ectopics is largely determined by the type and severity of any underlying cardiac disease.
- **B** If the ectopics disappear with exercise, they should be considered as benign.
- **C** This rhythm may be associated with mitral valve prolapse.
- **D** Ectopics presenting in this way should be treated vigorously with anti-arrhythmic drugs.
- **E** Taking regular exercise, stopping smoking, and avoiding coffee and wine will usually result in the abolition of these ectopics.

110. A man aged 38 years is brought to a hospital emergency department. About 45 minutes previously, while eating out, he felt a piece of steak 'lodge in his chest' and 'it would not go down'. He remembers two similar episodes in the preceding two years, but had been asymptomatic between the episodes. Physical examination is normal. In this situation,

A the most likely diagnosis is an oesophageal stricture and he should be admitted for a barium swallow X-ray.
B a coincident history of Raynaud's phenomenon would be expected.
C the most likely diagnosis is a lower oesophageal (Schatzki) ring.
D he should be taken immediately to the operating theatre for oesophagoscopic removal of the foreign body.
E he should be kept in the emergency department for about 4 hours, following the administration of intravenous diazepam (Valium) and hyoscine-N-butylbromide (Buscopan).

111. Concerning gastro-oesophageal reflux and reflux oesophagitis, which of the following statements is/are correct?

A Oesophageal clearance efficiency is an important factor in the pathogenesis of reflux oesophagitis.
B Patients with symptomatic gastro-oesophageal reflux all have an abnormally low pressure in the lower oesophageal sphincter.
C Reflux demonstrated during a barium meal is significant.
D Oesophageal pH measurement and radio-isotope scintillation counting during the swallowing of labelled food are the two most valuable techniques for the measurement of oesophageal reflux.
E Some patients with reflux oesophagitis have no demonstrable hiatus hernia.

112. Flat villous architecture in a small bowel biopsy specimen

A is seen only in coeliac disease.
B may occur in the absence of steatorrhoea.
C occurs in relatives of patients with coeliac disease.
D will often revert to normal villous architecture within two days of institution of a gluten-free diet in a patient with coeliac disease.
E is an essential criterion for a diagnosis of coeliac disease.

113. A jockey aged 28 years is referred because of intermittent tetany and hypocalcaemia which have failed to respond adequately to calcium supplements. Except for vague intermittent diarrhoea during the past few years, his medical history is unremarkable and physical examination is normal. Which of the following statements is/are correct?

A The serum magnesium level should be measured.
B As medullary carcinoma of the thyroid gland is a likely diagnosis, his serum calcitonin level should be measured.
C In the absence of a history of splenectomy, the finding of Howell-Jolly bodies in the blood film is a diagnostic significance.
D In the absence of blood and mucus in the faeces, a sigmoidoscopy is unlikely to contribute to the diagnosis.
E The presence of anaemia in this patient is likely to be associated with folate deficiency.

114. In colonic diverticular disease

A serious complications occur mostly in patients who do not have previous symptoms.
B ingestion of bran increases faecal fat loss, as well as increasing faecal loss of magnesium, phosphorus, calcium and zinc.
C analgesic treatment with morphine is contraindicated.
D complications due to diverticulitis should be treated with non-absorbable antibiotics.
E Angiodysplasia causes 'occult' bleeding as well as massive bleeding. Diverticula remain the commonest source of massive bleeding.

115. A man aged 50 years, complaining of rectal bleeding, is found to have a pedunculated polyp of 1 cm diameter situated 10 cm from the anal verge. Which of the following procedures would you carry out?

A Take a biopsy of the polyp for histological examination.
B Arrange for a polypectomy via sigmoidoscope.
C Examine the rest of the colon by air contrast barium enema X-ray or colonoscopy.
D Leave the polyp alone and request sigmoidoscopy in 6 months' time; then remove the polyp if it has increased in size.
E Biopsy the rectal mucosa to exclude ulcerative colitis.

116. **An asymptomatic man aged 50 years on a meat-free high residue diet, has a positive guaiac-impregnated slide test on one faecal sample tested by his practitioner.**
Which of the following statement is/are correct?

A The test result has a 2% chance of being falsely positive for blood.
B The test should be repeated daily over 6 consecutive days.
C The test should be repeated if he was taking large amounts of vitamin C.
D A barium enema examination should be undertaken rather than colonoscopy.
E If he has a colorectal cancer, it is likely to be at an earlier stage than if he were symptomatic.

117. **A man aged 61 years is admitted to hospital because of bright red rectal bleeding and requires five units of blood. He is not shocked and gastroduodenoscopy is normal. His bleeding ceases and an air contrast barium enema and a small bowel X-ray series are normal. No coagulation defects are discovered. The patient has mild aortic stenosis. A surgical consultant suggests a diagnosis of angiodysplasia.**
If this condition is present, which of the following statements is/are correct?

A The most likely site for angiodysplasia in the patient is the right colon.
B Since bleeding has ceased, selective mesenteric angiography is not indicated.
C Colonoscopy might be a therapeutic as well as a diagnostic procedure.
D Even if angiodysplasia is demonstrated, this is not necessarily the site of bleeding.
E The lesion is usually not visible at laparotomy.

118. **Concerning the irritable bowel syndrome, which of the following statements is/are correct?**

A Symptoms of the irritable bowel syndrome may occur in up to 15% of the general population.
B Epigastric pain is rare in affected persons.
C It is known to cause pain in the lumbar region.
D It may present as proctalgia fugax.
E It responds to antispasmodic medication in over 50% of patients.

119. In patients with alcoholic hepatitis, which of the following statements is/are correct?

A Underlying cirrhosis is always present.
B This condition, rather than alcoholic fatty liver, is considered to be a precursor of cirrhosis.
C If they have fever and leucocytosis, overt or occult infection is likely to be present in about 95% of them.
D Their symptoms may mimic acute pancreatitis.
E If they have a liver biopsy, the presence of Mallory hyaline bodies is pathognomonic of the condition.

120. A woman aged 28 years, who lives in a city and has never left Australia, develops a sudden onset of severe pain in the right hypochondrium which radiates into her back. She has enjoyed excellent health previously, and her only medication has been an oral contraceptive which she has taken regularly for six years. On examination, there is generalised abdominal guarding and rebound tenderness. Over several hours she becomes hypotensive and febrile and she requires blood transfusion. Her serum levels are found to be: bilirubin 16 μmol/ℓ(N: 2–22); alkaline phosphatase 90 U/ℓ (N: 20–80); aspartate amino transferase (AST) 200 U/ℓ (N: 10–40) and alanine amino-transferase (ALT) 160 U/ℓ (N: 8–30). A liver scan shows a large filling defect in the right lobe and an ultrasound scan suggests this to be cystic. Serological tests for hepatitis B surface antigen, alpha-fetoprotein, and amoebiasis are negative. The most likely diagnosis is

A amoebic abscess of the liver.
B angiosarcoma of the liver.
C focal nodular hyperplasia with intrahepatic haemorrhage.
D intrahepatic endometriosis.
E cholangiocarcinoma.

121. Concerning patients with idiopathic haemochromatosis, which of the following statements is/are correct?

A This disease is inherited as an autosomal recessive trait.
B The preferred screening tests for all relatives are estimation of serum iron and percentage saturation of transferrin.
C A fluctuating serum ferritin level of less than 1000 μg/ℓ in association with elevation of transaminase enzymes, is strongly suggestive of alcoholic liver disease, with or without haemochromatosis.
D Phlebotomy therapy does not prolong life in symptomatic patients with established idiopathic haemochromatosis.
E Phlebotomy lowers the incidence of supervening hepatoma.

122. Concerning extra hepatic cholestasis, which of the following statements is/are correct?

A Serum bile acids are commonly elevated in this disorder.
B Biliary ultrasound is a reliable way of diagnosing common bile duct stones.
C The biliary tree can be well visualised by newer isotopic scanning agents.
D Percutaneous transhepatic cholangiography should not be performed if a mechanical cause is suspected.
E Sclerosing cholangitis is as frequent a complication of Crohn's disease as it is of ulcerative colitis.

123. A man aged 32 years presents with progressive fatigue of 6 weeks duration. He is found to have numerous spider naevi and liver enlargement (span 15 cm).
Biochemical tests include alanine amino transferase (ALT) 1800 U/ℓ (N: 8–30), serum bilirubin 13 μmol/ℓ(N: 1–20) and serum albumin 41 g/ℓ (N: 35–55). Liver biopsy shows marked portal tract inflammation, peri-portal necrosis (piecemeal necrosis) and extensive fibrotic septa.
Which of the following statements is/are correct?

A A history of recurrent urinary tract infection may be relevant.
B Wilson's disease is excluded by the age and histological findings.
C Prednisolone 40 mg daily should be started immediately, as hepatic failure is imminent.
D A positive HBsAg test contraindicates corticosteroid therapy.
E Upon treatment with prednisolone, improvement of symptoms and ALT level indicate control of the disease and progression to cirrhosis will not occur.

124. Concerning fatty change in the liver, which of the following statements is/are correct?

A The morphology and distribution of fatty change found in the alcoholic patient is a bad prognostic indicator of cirrhosis.
B Imaging procedures can distinguish fatty change from other storage disorders in the liver.
C When fibrosis, focal hepatocellular necrosis and inflammation are also present, the histological pattern is consistent with alcoholic liver disease.
D Fatty change does not occur in any form of viral hepatitis.
E Acute fatty liver in pregnancy has no prognostic significance.

125. A man aged 60 years presents with abdominal pain, weight loss, increasing fatigue and jaundice. He is found to have palmar erythema, ascites, hepatosplenomegaly, testicular atrophy, glycosuria and a bruit over the liver.

Laboratory results include serum ferritin 1200 μg/ℓ (N: 25–250) and alpha-fetoprotein 6 μg/ℓ (N: below 12).

Which of the following statements is/are correct?

A Despite the normal alpha-fetoprotein level, the most likely diagnosis is hepatocellular carcinoma.
B Isotopic liver scanning would be unlikely to distinguish between cirrhosis and hepatocellular carcinoma complicating chronic liver disease.
C Since hepatic bruit may occur in alcoholic hepatitis, this diagnosis could also explain the high serum ferritin values.
D If he has this hepatitis B serology — HBsAg negative, anti-HBsAg negative, anti-HBc positive — hepatocellular carcinoma could be regarded as a result of hepatitis B infection.
E If a liver biopsy shows hepatocellular carcinoma, surgical resection together with adriamycin chemotherapy is likely to produce a worthwhile prolongation in survival.

126. An alcoholic with clinical evidence of cirrhosis was admitted to hospital with acute upper gastrointestinal bleeding. Endoscopy confirmed that the bleeding was from oesophageal varices. With conservative management it stopped after 48 hours.

In this patient, injection sclerotherapy

A would reduce significantly the risk of re-bleeding.
B should be performed under general anaesthesia using a rigid oesophagoscope.
C if repeated, may eradicate the oesophageal varices.
D may precipitate hepatic encephalopathy.
E could not be employed after the use of a Sengstaken-Blakemore tube.

127. With regard to the use of chenodeoxycholic acid in the treatment of cholelithiasis, which of the following statements is/are correct?

A It is a secondary bile acid formed by the action of intestinal bacteria on the primary bile acid, cholic acid.
B In man it decreases cholesterol secretion in bile.
C There is histological evidence of liver damage in 5% of patients who have been treated for more than 6 months.
D It is most effective in patients who have small radiolucent calculi in a functioning gall bladder.
E Gallstones shown to float at oral cholecystography usually dissolve well with this therapy.

128. A man aged 30 years with a chronic duodenal ulcer, proven at endoscopy, had periodic epigastric pain for 4 years.
Concerning treatment of patients such as this, which of the following statements is/are correct?

- **A** A 6-week course of cimetidine will definitely result in endoscopic resolution of the ulcer in more than 90% of such patients.
- **B** Once the ulcer is healed, and patients are kept on a maintenance daily dosage of 400 mg cimetidine taken at bed-time, they have a 20% chance of recurrence over a 1-year period.
- **C** If long-term maintenance cimetidine therapy is stopped, the rate of recurrence will be about the same as if it had not been used.
- **D** The ulcer recurrence rate with highly selective vagotomy is about 10%.
- **E** A course of high-dose antacids is less effective than cimetidine in healing the ulcer.

129. Concerning cystic fibrosis (mucoviscidosis), which of the following statements is/are correct?

- **A** It is one of the commonest autosomal recessive inherited conditions in Australia.
- **B** A history of meconium ileus relates to more severe disease and to a relatively decreased survival rate.
- **C** Sweat sodium and chloride levels of more than 60 mmol/ℓ are required for a positive diagnosis in childhood.
- **D** Female patients with cystic fibrosis are sterile.
- **E** The most common persisting organism in the sputum of these patients is *Haemophilus influenzae*.

130. In the treatment of pulmonary tuberculosis, which of the following statements is/are correct?

- **A** Isoniazid is more likely to cause serious hepatotoxicity in patients who are slow acetylators.
- **B** Chemoprophylaxis of small pulmonary lesions, with daily isoniazid for 6 months, is effective in reducing the development of active tuberculosis.
- **C** A child aged 4 years with a recent Mantoux conversion should be treated with isoniazid.
- **D** Patients with active cavitating disease should be treated with isoniazid and rifampicin for 12 months.
- **E** In a patient receiving isoniazid or rifampicin, a 50% rise in the blood level of gamma glutamyl transpeptidase indicates that the drug should be withdrawn.

131. With regard to pneumococcal vaccine, which of the following statements is/are correct?

- **A** It has been shown to prevent pneumococcal pneumonia in high-risk groups.
- **B** It provides protection against only the 14 serotypes whose polysaccharides are included in the vaccine.
- **C** It is justified for routine administration to adults over the age of 45 years.
- **D** It is administered in 3 doses 1 month apart.
- **E** Antibody levels remain elevated for up to 8 years after immunisation of adults.

132. Concerning influenza, which of the following statements is/are correct?

- **A** Worldwide pandemics of influenza A only follow a complete shift of the H or N viral antigen.
- **B** Influenza B viruses undergo antigenic drift, but not shift, and do not cause pandemic infection.
- **C** The pattern of past influenza pandemics allows prediction of the time of the next pandemic within 1–2 years.
- **D** The pattern of past antigenic shifts allows prediction of the next shift, to assist in preparing an appropriate vaccine.
- **E** A vaccine containing the specific antigens carried by the infecting virus will have an efficacy of around 70% if administered early in a pandemic.

133. In the treatment of asthma with metered dose aerosols of beta-adrenoceptor agonists, regular and continued medication for months or years

- **A** does not cause tachyphylaxis (i.e. diminished response).
- **B** should be reserved for moderately severely affected patients who are rarely free of symptoms.
- **C** is not contraindicated in patients taking monoamine oxidase inhibitors.
- **D** increases bronchoconstriction induced by non-specific airway irritants such as histamine.
- **E** can lead to myocardial damage caused by Freon propellant.

134. A woman aged 25 years has a history of mild asthma since the age of 4 years and has had four episodes regarded as pneumonia. For the last 2 weeks she has had low grade fever with a cough and mucopurulent sputum which has contained occasional brownish pellets. A Mantoux test is 7 mm positive but she has had BCG vaccination. A chest X-ray shows an irregularly rounded lesion in the right upper lobe and a diffuse opacity in the left upper lobe. She has a blood and sputum eosinophilia but no acid-fast bacilli are found in the sputum. The most likely diagnosis is

A pulmonary tuberculosis.
B specific pneumonia.
C allergic bronchopulmonary aspergillosis.
D a lung abscess.
E actinomycosis.

135. With regard to the clinical use of disodium cromoglycate (cromolyn sodium, Intal), which of the following statements is/are correct?

A It is of value only in 'immunologically induced' asthma.
B It has been found effective clinically in children with some types of gastrointestinal allergy to food.
C It acts by inhibiting the release of toxic mediators from the membranes of tissue mast cells.
D Its action is similar to that of corticosteroids.
E It is ineffective in the treatment of acute episodes of asthma.

136. A man aged 50 years presents with malaise, fever and chills, followed by a dry cough (occasionally producing small amounts of mucoid sputum). He also has pleuritic pain, increasing dyspnoea and then develops prostration with an unremitting fever. Legionnaire's disease is suspected. In this disease,

A the causative organism has been identified as an aerobic Gram-negative bacillus.
B the organism, *Legionella pneumophilia*, can be isolated readily by culturing the sputum and tracheal aspirates.
C more often the diagnosis is made on clinical grounds and confirmed later serologically by the finding of a rise in the indirect immunoflourescent antibody titre.
D hyponatraemia does not occur as it sometimes does in other types of pneumonia.
E based on current clinical and laboratory data, the therapeutic drug of choice is erythromycin alone or with rifampicin.

137. An unconscious man in his mid-50s is brought by ambulance to a hospital emergency department. Several possible causes for his condition are excluded and blood gases, measured promptly with no supplemental oxygen, yield the following results:

Po_2 — 66 mmHg
Pco_2 — 60 mmHg
pH — 7.32
Base excess + 2 meq/ℓ.

Which of the following statements is/are correct?

A The blood sample is probably venous.
B The values are consistent neither with a diagnosis of chronic bronchitis nor with acute on chronic respiratory acidosis induced by 100% oxygen given in the ambulance.
C Intubation and ventilation are contraindicated, since the results indicate that the patient has severe chronic lung disease.
D The results are consistent with central ventilatory depression from barbiturate overdosage and normal lungs.
E The results are consistent with acute pulmonary oedema.

138. An obese man aged 45 years with a heavy alcohol intake presents with a year-long history of daytime sleepiness at work. His wife comments on his noisy snoring and his short episodes of apnoea, which cause her to wake him periodically.
Which of the following statements is/are correct?

A His daytime sleepiness is most probably due to narcolepsy.
B A detailed investigation of his sleep pattern, including EEG monitoring, would be expected to show abnormal breathing only in REM sleep.
C During sleep apnoea, EMG monitoring would show attempts at muscle activities in the absence of air flow at the nose.
D Weight restriction and diminution in his alcohol intake should solve the problem completely.
E If symptoms are severe, tracheostomy becomes essential for many such patients.

139. A middle-aged man presents with weakness, bronchospasm, malaise, fever and weight loss. He has a white blood cell count of 12 × 10^9/ℓ (N: 4 – 11 × 10^9) with 80% eosinophils, and this persists over an 8-week period of observation.
Which of the following statements is/are correct?

A The most likely diagnosis is acute allergic asthma.
B The presence of pulmonary infiltrates on chest X-ray would suggest the diagnosis of Loeffler's syndrome.
C Eosinophilia of this magnitude is invariably associated with elevated serum IgE.
D If no cause can be found, the persistence of the patient's eosinophilia is likely to be fatal.
E The hypereosinophilic syndrome responds readily to a combination of corticosteroids and cytotoxics.

140. A man aged 52 years (a non-smoker) with rheumatoid arthritis has been treated with gold injections for 9 months. For the week before presentation he has been troubled by nocturnal cough, lethargy and exertional dyspnoea, preceded by rhinorrhoea and headaches which were relieved by an aspirin preparation. He had a previous history of a nasal polypectomy for nasal obstruction 6 months ago.
His chest X-ray shows no evidence of pulmonary infiltrates or increased lung markings. His FEV_1:VC is 1.1:2.3, with no significant change after aerosol bronchodilator.
Which of the following statements is/are correct?

A The most likely diagnosis is allergic lung disease due to gold therapy.
B The most likely diagnosis is aspirin-sensitive asthma.
C He is unlikely to have asthma because his spirometry measurements did not improve significantly after aerosol bronchodilator.
D If he has allergic lung disease due to gold, pulmonary infiltrates would have been expected on the chest X-ray.
E If he has aspirin-sensitive asthma, it is likely to recur with exposure to other non-steroidal anti-inflammatory drugs such as indomethacin and ibuprofen.

141. **A woman aged 25 years first presented with a 3-week history of recurring fever and cough as well as progressive dyspnoea. She admitted to a weight loss of 3 kg over this period. Antibiotics including amoxycillin, co-trimoxazole and tetracycline were given, all with no effect. Physical examination revealed that she was severely dyspnoeic and cyanosed at rest and with a temperature of 38.6°C. There were generalised inspiratory and expiratory crackles. Chest X-ray showed an infiltrate throughout both lung fields.**

Measurement of arterial blood gases (room air) revealed: $Pa\text{O}_2$ 55 mmHg (7.3 kPa), $Pa\text{CO}_2$ 28 mmHg (3.7 kPa) and pH 7.51. Spirometry revealed on FEV1:VC of 1.05:1.1 and her diffusing capacity was 66% of predicted normal.

Whilst in hospital she improved both clinically and radiologically, being given supplemental oxygen and no other therapy. She was discharged after 10 days but reported back within 8 hours, complaining again of severe dyspnoea. Her clinical picture, blood gas measurements and chest X-ray resemble those found at her first admission.

The most likely diagnosis is

A severe asthma.
B *Mycoplasma pneumoniae* infection.
C cryptogenic fibrosing alveolitis.
D hypersensitivity pneumonitis.
E Legionnaire's disease.

142. **Concerning extrinsic allergic alveolitis, which of the following statements is/are correct?**

A The diagnosis should be suspected in any patient presenting with recurrent 'flu-like' illness.
B Demonstration of precipitating antibodies against the suspected antigen suggests active disease.
C It is a classic example of type III hypersensitivity reaction in which there is peripheral blood eosinophilia.
D The disease is usually distinguishable from sarcoidosis both radiologically and histologically.
E Face masks provide adequate protection.

143. **With regard to asbestosis, which of the following statements is/are correct?**

A If an asbestos worker has a clear chest X-ray at the time he ceases to be engaged in this employment, he will not develop asbestosis subsequently.
B The presence of fine crepitations occurring towards the end of inspiration is the most characteristic physical sign.
C Clubbing of the fingers occurs early in the disease.
D The finding of asbestos bodies in the sputum confirms a diagnosis of asbestosis.
E There is an increased incidence of carcinoma of the lung.

144. A man aged 62 years has suffered increasing shortness of breath for 1 year. He had been a jack-hammer operator for many years and until recently had smoked 40 cigarettes per day. He has a cough with scanty sputum, and no history of asthma. He is found to have marked finger clubbing and bilateral basal crepitations, and his chest X-ray shows reticulonodular opacities.

Respiratory function tests shows:

Pa_{O_2} — 56 mmHg (7.5 kPa)
P_{CO_2} — 40 mmHg (5.4 kPa)
FEV_1 — 1.771 (60%)
VC — 2.31 (59%)
DLCO (diffusing capacity) — 40% of predicted normal

Bronchoscopy is normal but examination of bronchial lavage fluid shows polymorphs 43%, lymphocytes 2.8% and macrophages 54%.

Which of the following is the most likely diagnosis?

A silicosis
B sarcoidosis
C fibrosing alveolitis
D allergic alveolitis
E carcinomatosis.

145. Concerning obstruction of small airways (less than 2 mm diameter), which of the following statements is/are correct?

A When air-flow resistance increases by 20%, FEV_1 is altered.
B It occurs in young smokers as a result of diffuse bronchiolitis associated with increased bronchial mucus goblet cells.
C Frequency-dependent dynamic compliance is the most sensitive test for it.
D Increased closing volume is the most specific test for it.
E It is present in less than 50% of emphysematous patients.

146. A man aged 24 years presents with a life-long history of recurrent chest infections characterised by daily cough and sputum. Examination and investigation reveal the presence of bronchiectasis and nasal polyposis. Electron microscopy on bronchial and nasal mucosal biopsies reveals an absence of dynein arms in the ultrastructure of the cilia.

Which of the following statements is/are correct?

A The majority of such patients have situs inversus.
B The features described are diagnostic of Kartagener's syndrome.
C Infertility is to be expected in this patient.
D Despite normal levels of sweat electrolytes, a diagnosis of cystic fibrosis is likely.
E The characteristic pathophysiological disturbance in this patient would be chronic airways obstruction.

147. After resuscitation from shock due to Gram-negative septicaemia, a man aged 60 years continues to have dyspnoea and signs of hypoxia. His chest X-ray shows widespread infiltrations.

With regard to this pulmonary complication of shock, which of the following statements is/are correct?

- **A** The underlying disorder involves damage to the alveolar-capillary membrane.
- **B** The hypoxia is caused by mucoid plugging of the small bronchioles.
- **C** Optimal treatment includes maximum hydration to correct capillary losses of fluid.
- **D** Positive end-expiratory pressure (PEEP) should be instituted to correct the hypoxia.
- **E** Corticosteroids are of proven value in treatment.

148. Regarding the diffusing capacity of the lung (transfer factor), which of the following statements is/are correct?

- **A** It measures the ability of the lungs to transfer carbon dioxide across the alveolar-capillary membrane.
- **B** It increases during exercise in normal people.
- **C** It is usually abnormal in patients with chronic asthma.
- **D** It is usually decreased following severe pulmonary embolism.
- **E** It is decreased proportionately to the arterial oxygen tension in patients with emphysema.

149. A woman aged 45 years develops a deep venous thrombosis in her leg 4 days post-cholecystectomy. She is commenced on 30 000 units of heparin by infusion over 24 hours. Two days later she has a large pulmonary embolism, at which time her coagulation profile reveals: thrombin time 11 s (control 10), partial thromboplastin time with kaolin (PTTK) 34 s (control 45), prothrombin time 14 s (control 14). The lung scan confirms a 2/3 defect in the left lung. In this situation

- **A** the PTTK and thrombin time correlate well with blood heparin levels.
- **B** the antithrombin III level will probably be reduced.
- **C** the chest X-ray may be normal.
- **D** heparin dosage should be increased until a therapeutic range is achieved.
- **E** streptokinase therapy is definitely indicated.

150. A man aged 59 years presents with mild jaundice, peripheral cyanosis and cold hands. He has marked hepatosplenomegaly and small lymph nodes in his axillae and his inguinal regions. Laboratory results reveal: a haemoglobin concentration of 105 g/ℓ (N: 135 – 180, males), a white cell count of 6.7×10^9/ℓ (N: 4–11 $\times 10^9$) and a platelet count of 210×10^9/ℓ (N: 150 – 350 $\times 10^9$). Blood film shows autoagglutination and polychromasia with occasional spherocytes present. In this case

A the patient probably has a non-Hodgkin's lymphoma.
B the direct Coombs' test is likely to be positive with complement only on the red cell surface.
C a monoclonal IgM is likely to be found in the serum.
D splenectomy is indicted.
E the Donath-Landsteiner test will be positive.

151. With respect to Hodgkin's disease and its management, which of the following statements is/are correct?

A At initial assessment, splenic involvement can be predicted reliably on clinical grounds.
B Relapse is unlikely in those patients who have had 3 years disease-free survival following initial therapy.
C Complicating second malignancy is most commonly non-Hodgkin's lymphoma.
D With 'MOPP' chemotherapy, complete remission should be achieved in up to 80% of patients with stage IIIB and stage IV disease.
E The highest rate of relapse occurs in nodular sclerosing Hodgkin's disease.

152. With regard to malignant lymphomas of diffuse (large-cell) histiocyctic type, which of the following statements is/are correct?

A Untreated patients have a poor prognosis (i.e. survive for less than 1 year).
B Chemotherapy with a single agent is optimal.
C Of patients with advanced stage disease who achieve complete remission, more than 60% have disease-free survival for more than 2 years.
D There is a significant association between bone marrow and meningeal involvement.
E Most primary gastrointestinal lymphomas are of this histological type.

153. Iron deficiency anaemia is associated with

A low serum ferritin.
B decreased total iron binding capacity.
C prolonged plasma iron clearance.
D increased numbers of sideroblasts in the bone marrow.
E increased red cell protoporphyrin levels.

154. Abnormal Schilling's test, observed both with and without the administration of intrinsic factor

A is found in patients with post-gastrectomy megaloblastic anaemia.
B is found in patients with multiple jejunal diverticula.
C is found in patients with simple atrophic gastritis.
D excludes the presence of folate deficiency.
E may be due to severe renal failure alone.

155. A mildly icteric, anaemic patient has a red cell half-life (^{51}CrT½) of 10 days (N: 20–27 days) together with absent serum haptoglobins and absent marrow iron stores.
These findings could all be explained by

A acute haemolysis associated with infectious mononucleosis.
B systemic lupus erythematosus with autoimmune haemolytic anaemia.
C microangiopathic haemolytic anaemia following aortic valve replacement.
D hereditary spherocytosis.
E paroxysmal nocturnal haemoglobinuria.

156. A man aged 63 years presents with several attacks of disorientation and amnesia, each lasting about 2 minutes. He has no other complaints. On examination, his blood pressure is 200/110 but there is no evidence of cardiomegaly or cardiac failure. Although he looks plethoric, he has no other abnormal physical signs.
His blood count reveals haemoglobin of 186 g/ℓ, MCV 83, MCH 28, a white cell count of 9.5 × 10^9/ℓ with a normal distribution and a platelet count of 430 × 10^9/ℓ. His red cell mass is 34 ml/kg body weight (N: 28–35) and his plasma volume 30 ml/kg body weight (N: 40–60). Blood urea is 6 mmol/ℓ and serum creatinine 0.09 mmol/ℓ.
Which of the following statements is/are correct?

A These findings exclude the diagnosis of polycythaemia rubra vera.
B Thiazide therapy is an appropriate means of reducing his blood pressure.
C Venesection will improve his cerebral blood flow.
D Search to exclude a low affinity haemoglobin is warranted.
E If iron deficiency is present, it may lead to an increase in blood viscosity and reduction in oxygen delivery in this man.

157. A man aged 68 years presents with a pathological fracture of the neck of the femur due to a plasmacytoma. X-rays of the remainder of the skeleton fail to disclose other lytic lesions. A full blood count is normal and erythrocyte sedimentation rate (Westergren) is 2 mm/h (N: 1–13, males). Serum protein analysis shows no paraprotein on the electrophoretogram but marked reduction in levels of all normal immunoglobulins. No Bence-Jones proteinuria is detected. Bone marrow aspiration reveals 15% plasma cells with some morphologically abnormal forms.

Which of the following statements is/are correct?

- **A** The patient has a solitary plasmacytoma of bone.
- **B** There is insufficient evidence to diagnose multiple myeloma.
- **C** The most likely diagnosis is that of non-secretory multiple myeloma.
- **D** The absence of other lytic bone lesions excludes the diagnosis of multiple myeloma.
- **E** The treatment of choice is chemotherapy with melphalan after appropriate surgical repair.

158. A woman aged 25 years, 2 weeks post-partum, is admitted to hospital because of extensive bruising and epistaxis. The following laboratory findings are reported.

Haemoglobin	**— 108 g/ℓ**
White cell count	**— 12.2 × 10^9/ℓ**
Platelet count	**— 370 × 10^9/ℓ**
Hess test	**— Negative**
Partial thromboplastin time with kaolin (PTTK)	**— 70 seconds (control 38)**
Prothrombin time	**— 12 seconds (control 13)**
Plasma fibrinogen	**— 4.9 g/ℓ (N: 1.5–3.5)**

Which of the following investigations is/are indicated to further elucidate the haemostatic defect?

- **A** bone marrow aspiration
- **B** bleeding time
- **C** factor V assay
- **D** antinuclear antibody
- **E** factor VIII assay on a mixture of normal plasma and the patient's plasma.

159. A woman aged 32 years presents with bruising and purpura for 10 days. Clinical examination reveals extensive lower limb purpura and a few palatal haemorrhages but no other abnormalities. She is currently taking no medications.

Full blood count reveals haemoglobin 142 g/ℓ, white cell count 8.2 × 10^9/ℓ and platelets 18 × 10^9/ℓ. Bone marrow examination reveals normal haemopoiesis with slightly increased megakaryocytes. Antinuclear antibodies are not demonstrated.

Which of the following statements is/are correct?

A Absence of splenomegaly is consistent with the diagnosis of immune thrombocytopenic purpura.
B She should be given immediate platelet transfusions.
C Splenectomy has at least an 80% chance of inducing remission.
D Should she become pregnant, even after splenectomy there is a risk of neonatal thrombocytopenia.
E Vinblastine-loaded platelets may have a place in future therapy.

160. Concerning acute lymphoblastic leukaemia (ALL), which of the following statements is/are correct?

A If the cell type carries B cell markers, the patient has a 5-year median survival rate of 50%.
B T cell markers are present in approximately 50% of cases that occur in children, i.e. aged less than 15 years.
C The anti-ALL antigen recognises a cell type seen only in patients with leukaemia.
D Central nervous system prophylaxis should be offered to patients as soon as remission is achieved.
E A white cell count of greater than 20 × 10^9/ℓ at the time of presentation carries an increased risk of relapse after remission.

161. Concerning acute lymphoblastic leukaemia of childhood, which of the following statements is/are correct?

A Remission can be achieved in approximately 90% of cases.
B A high white cell count at presentation has been proven to indicate a poor prognosis.
C Immunological cell markers have important prognostic significance.
D Relapse is common in the central nervous system and the testis.
E Patients in remission should receive maintenance therapy for at least 5 years.

162. A man aged 30 years, with a 2-year history of chronic granulocytic leukaemia, presents with symptoms of anaemia, abdominal discomfort and purpura.

Full blood count reveals haemoglobin 79 g/ℓ, white cell count 85×10^0/ℓ (35% blast cells) and platelets 15×10^9/ℓ.

Which of the following statements is/are correct?

A Blast transformation is probably myeloblastic in type.
B Chromosomal analysis probably will show doubling of the Ph chromosome.
C Acute lymphoid blast crisis may be confirmed by using anti-ALL antisera.
D About one-third of patients in blast crisis have blast cells which have high levels of terminal deoxynucleotidyl transferase (TdT).
E Intensive chemotherapy (as given for adult non-lymphoblastic leukaemia) induces a brief complete remission in up to 25% of patients.

163. A man aged 57 years, with manic depressive psychosis and controlled cardiac failure, is referred by a psychiatrist to determine whether the patient has any medical contraindications to the use of lithium carbonate therapy.

Which of the following statements is/are correct?

A The presence of neutropenia would prevent the initiation of lithium therapy.
B The concomitant use of diuretic therapy makes lithium intoxication more likely.
C Lithium is known to cause electrocardiographic changes.
D Hyperthyroidism is a contraindication.
E Lithium induces a diuresis.

164. In relation to cytotoxic drugs used in cancer chemotherapy, which of the following toxicities is/are both dose-dependant and usually reversible?

A myelosuppression
B nausea and vomiting
C pulmonary fibrosis
D mucosal and gastrointestinal ulceration
E cardiomyopathy.

165. Which of the following cancer chemotherapeutic agents may cause toxic pulmonary complications?

A cytosine arabinoside
B busulphan
C cyclophosphamide
D bleomycin
E methotrexate.

166. Major elevations of serum alpha-fetoprotein level (at least 10 times above normal) are frequently found in

A metastatic carcinoma of the liver.
B embryonal cell carcinoma of the testis.
C heavy smokers.
D normal pregnancy.
E adenocarcinoma of the colon.

167. A woman aged 65 years has metastatic breast cancer. Previously she had responded to the anti-oestrogen tamoxifen and combination cytotoxic chemotherapy (initially doxorubicin and cyclophosphamide and then vincristine, methotrexate and fluorouracil). The disease has now relapsed and her main problem is multiple bone metastases with pain.

Which of the following therapies would you now regard as most appropriate for this patient?

A hypophysectomy with selected hormone replacement
B medical adrenalectomy (aminoglutethamide) with cortisone replacement
C surgical adrenalectomy with cortisone replacement
D local radiotherapy
E Oophorectomy.

168. In the treatment of adenocarcinoma of the breast

A the number of axillary lymph nodes involved at mastectomy is of prognostic significance.
B the presence of high levels of oestrogen receptors in tumour tissue is a reliable predictor of a more favourable response to hormones.
C when hepatic metastases are present, cytotoxic chemotherapy is the treatment of choice.
D cerebral metastases can be expected to respond to doxorubicin (adriamycin) in about 20% of cases.
E post-surgical adjuvant chemotherapy is of benefit in pre-menopausal women.

169. In primary malignant melanoma of the skin, which of the following indicate(s) a poor prognosis?

A A lesion on the lower leg in a female.
B Melanoma arising in an area of lentigo maligna (Hutchinson's freckle).
C Invasion of subcutaneous fat by the primary lesion.
D Nodular melanoma on the trunk.
E The presence of a pre-exising naevus.

170. Cancer screening programmes of the general population have proven effective in reducing mortality in which of the following conditions?

A carcinoma of the breast
B carcinoma of the cervix
C carcinoma of the lung
D carcinoma of the colon
E carcinoma of the pancreas.

171. Concerning adriamycin (doxorubicin), which of the following statements is/are correct?

A It acts as an intercalating agent.
B Doses of adriamycin need to be modified in the presence of biliary obstruction.
C The intramuscular route is a safe alternative method of administration.
D It is proven benefit in the treatment of osteogenic sarcoma.
E Cardiotoxicity may be prevented by the concomitant use of cardiac glycosides.

172. In the management of small cell anaplastic carcinoma of the lung

A mediastinoscopy is an important staging procedure.
B bone marrow involvement adversely influences the prognosis.
C the treatment of choice includes combination chemotherapy.
D prophylactic cranial irradiation is of value in preventing cerebral metastases.
E the presence of hyponatraemia is an indication of cerebral involvement.

173. In patients with acute Guillain-Barré syndrome, which of the following statements is/are correct?

A Muscle wasting is seen early in the course of the disease.
B The cranial nerves are often affected.
C The autonomic nerves are often affected.
D The presence of a normal concentration of protein in the CSF and of nerve conduction velocities within the normal range within the first three weeks does not exclude the diagnosis.
E Corticosteroid therapy is of proven value.

174. A man aged 29 years presents with acute severe pain around the right shoulder and within 24 hours is unable to elevate the shoulder or flex his elbow. 2 weeks later muscle wasting about the shoulder and of biceps is evident. The biceps and supinator reflexes are reduced. There is vague sensory loss within the right C5 and 6 dermatomes.

These signs and symptoms are consistent with which of the following?

A cervical disc prolapse
B syringomyelia
C neuralgic amyotrophy
D poliomyelitis
E Guillain-Barré syndrome.

175. An accountant aged 54 years is suddenly noticed by his associates to be unaware of what he has been doing recently. He becomes extremely concerned by his memory loss. Closer questioning by his doctor reveals a marked loss of recent and past memory although his conversation and orientation are normal.

He is taken to hospital where his memory loss recedes spontaneously over 6 hours. Neurological examination is normal apart from transient mild asymmetry of deep tendon reflexes.

Which of the following statements is/are correct?

A As the most likely diagnosis is a temporal lobe seizure; immediate electroencephalography and anticonvulsant treatment is indicated.
B As the patient has suffered a left carotid transient ischaemic attack, he requires anticoagulant therapy to prevent recurrence.
C The patient has had a transient global amnesic episode.
D The symptoms may be due to a lesion involving the hippocampus.
E In the absence of significant neurological signs, a psychogenic cause for the amnesia is most likely.

176. A concert pianist aged 62 years notices that, when playing sustained rapid pieces of music with his left hand, he develops vertigo and diplopia.

After an attack subsides, his physical signs are likely to include

A persistent nystagmus
B visible retinal emboli on fundal examination
C absent left radial pulse
D unequal brachial blood pressure
E a bruit beneath the left clavicle.

177. A man aged 54 years has complained of steadily increasing intermittent headache for 3 months and of slight but progressive clumsiness of the left hand for 1 month. He was found one morning to be difficult to rouse after 2 days in bed with a respiratory tract infection accompanied by a productive cough.

He has bilateral papilloedema, upper motor neurone signs affecting the left face, arm and leg. The pupil of the right eye is dilated and sluggish in reacting to light. He will just rouse to pain.

Concerning this patient, which of the following statements is/are correct?

A He is very likely to have a cerebral tumour.
B If a cerebral tumour is present, it is more likely to be in the posterior fossa than above the tentorium cerebelli.
C The impairment of consciousness is due to extensive pathological changes in the right cerebral hemisphere.
D The mid-brain is likely to be displaced to the left and caudally.
E The rapid deterioration over the course of 2 days may be due to the effect of a raised $P\text{CO}_2$ on intracranial pressure.

178. In Huntington's disease

A disorders of ocular movement are most unusual.
B CT scanning will show cortical atrophy and ventricular dilatation prior to the development of clinical signs.
C grand mal seizures are uncommon except in the juvenile form.
D endogenous gamma aminobutyric acid (GABA) is depleted in the brain.
E glutamic acid decarboxylase is increased in the brain.

179. Concerning dementing illnesses, which of the following statements is/are correct?

A Multiple brain softenings, so called multi-infarct dementia, is the most common organic cause of intellectual deterioration of those over 65 years.
B Patients with Parkinson's disease are more likely to develop dementia than the general population.
C The improvement rate after ventricular shunting in patients with normal-pressure hydrocephalus exceeds 80%.
D In Alzheimer's disease, there is evidence of a marked decline in the hippocampal concentration of enzymes necessary for acetylcholine synthesis.
E Symptomatic chronic subdural haematoma is usually accompanied by fundoscopic evidence of raised intracranial pressure.

180. In the unconscious patient, which of the following statements is/are correct?

A A CT head scan is likely to establish the diagnosis in more than 50% of cases.
B Cheyne-Stokes respiration usually signifies a brain stem rather than a cerebral (supratentorial) cause.
C The absence of oculocephalic reflexes (doll's eyes movement) indicates a primary cerebral (supratentorial) cause.
D Apneustic breathing (brief end-respiratory pauses lasting 2–3 seconds often alternating with end-expiratory pauses) is a reliable sign of a pontine lesion.
E In deeply comatose patients, preservation of pupillary light reflexes suggests a metabolic cause.

181. A woman aged 26 years with a recent history of a generalised seizure disorder (grand mal) was commenced on phenytoin 300 mg daily. After 3 weeks on this dosage she had two further seizures; her plasma phenytoin level was 30 µmol/ (therapeutic range: 40–100).

Her phenytoin dose was then increased to 400 mg daily. Several days later she has developed ataxia and dysarthria. Which of the following statements is/are correct?

A Phenytoin is not the drug of first choice for grand mal epilepsy.
B Grand mal epilepsy is usually better controlled with two drugs than a single drug.
C The assay result was probably unreliable because phenytoin assays are difficult to perform.
D Because glucuronidation of phenytoin by hepatic enzymes is saturable, blood levels of phenytoin are high.
E The symptoms have occurred because the saturation of hepatic hydroxylation of phenytoin allows for an acute rise in plasma phenytoin levels as dosage is increased.

182. Concerning the management of epilepsy in pregnancy, which of the following statements is/are correct?

A Seizure frequency increases during pregnancy so anticonvulsant dosage should be increased.
B Anticonvulsant drug requirements return to the pre-pregnancy levels within one week of delivery.
C There is an increased risk of fetal perinatal haemorrhage due to anticonvulsant inhibition of vitamin K-dependent clotting factors.
D The risk of fetal malformations of lip, palate and heart is increased in infants born to mothers taking anticonvulsant drugs.
E The risk of fetal malformation is increased when the father takes anticonvulsants for epilepsy.

183. In multiple sclerosis, which of the following statements is/are correct?

A A delay in the visual-evoked potential is rare in patients with clinically normal optic discs or vision.
B Raised antibodies to measles and the presence of histocompatibility antigens (HLA-A3 and HLA-B7) are useful diagnostic tests.
C Paroxysmal symptoms frequently respond to carbamazepine.
D Elevation of body temperature can exacerbate neurological deficits.
E Oligoclonal IgG in the CSF is found in approximately 80% of established cases.

184. A man aged 42 years complains of complete visual loss following an occipital head injury at work in which he lost consciousness for 15 minutes. A skull X-ray shows no evidence of fracture and a CT head scan is within normal limits.
In cases such as this, which of the following statements is/are correct?

A The presence of a consensual and direct pupillary response to light indicates that the visual pathway is intact.
B The presence of symmetrical optokinetic nystagmus indicates that vision is still present.
C Pupillary constriction on accommodation and convergence testing indicates that vision is still present.
D The finding of bilateral posterior slow-wave activity on the electroencephalogram confirms that the patient has a significant lesion of the occipital cortex.
E An absent visual-evoked potential indicates that the patient has lost central vision.

185. In considering the problem of nephrotoxicity in relation to antibiotic therapy, which of the following statements is/are correct?

A Because tetracyclines probably have very little direct nephrotoxicity, they can be safely prescribed for patients with renal impairment.
B Cephaloridine, cephalothin and the aminoglycosides accumulate in the proximal renal tubules and are all potentially nephrotoxic.
C Antibiotic renal damage with an allergic basis, as in acute interstitial nephritis, may occur with the use of rifampicin, sulphonamides and the penicillins.
D Concomitant use of potent loop diuretics exacerbates the nephrotoxicity of gentamicin and kanamycin.
E When renal failure is present, doxycycline does not accumulate in the body, as it is largely eliminated by a non-hepatic gastrointestinal pathway.

186. Significant changes in serum potassium (K) levels may be life-threatening. Which of the following statements is/are correct?

- **A** Elevated serum K levels may be reduced by the administration of intravenous sodium bicarbonate without any significant rise in blood pH.
- **B** Peritoneal dialysis therapy lowers elevated serum K levels mainly by removal of K from the body stores.
- **C** K supplements and/or K-sparing diuretics are indicated in most non-oedematous patients treated with diuretic therapy over a long period.
- **D** One gram of potassium chloride contains approximately 13 mmol of K.
- **E** Hyperkalaemia is relatively uncommon in patients with stable chronic renal failure.

187. Hyperkalaemia may occur without marked impairment of renal function. In which of the following situations is this likely to arise?

- **A** in the elderly, due to selective deficiency of aldosterone production
- **B** in diabetics with hyperosmotic hyperglycaemia
- **C** following renal transplantation, associated with refractoriness to diuretic-induced hypokalaemia
- **D** in patients taking loop diuretics
- **E** As a result of renal tubular refractoriness to the action of aldosterone.

188. In 'moderate to severe' hyponatraemia, i.e. a serum sodium level less than 125 mmol/ℓ, which of the following statements is/are correct?

- **A** In more than 80% of patients it is due to sodium depletion.
- **B** It may be caused by administration of carbamazepine (Tegretol), chlorpropamide or amitryptiline.
- **C** When it occurs in oedematous patients during diuretic therapy, it may be corrected by potassium administration.
- **D** It may be due to hyperlipidaemia.
- **E** It may be caused by lithium carbonate administration.

189. A young woman aged 18 years presents with her first attack of loin pain, fever and pyuria. Culture of a mid-stream urine specimen shows greater than 100 000 *Proteus* organisms/ml.
In this patient, which of the following statements is/are correct?

A A positive urinary fluorescent bacterial antibody test is a reliable indicator of an upper urinary tract infection.
B Single high-dose treatment with amoxycillin (3 g orally) is preferable to a standard 5-day course.
C Even if a subsequent intravenous pyelogram is normal, a micturating cystourethrogram should be performed to exclude ureteric reflux.
D The presence of *Proteus* in the urine makes upper urinary tract infection likely.
E If the patient is pregnant, there is an increased risk of pre-eclampsia, fetal mortality and congenital defects.

190. Concerning recurrent urinary tract infections, which of the following statements is/are correct?

A Relapse due to bacterial persistence usually occurs within 6 weeks of discontinuation of therapy.
B When infection stones occur, they are most frequently caused by Gram-positive organisms embedded within struvite calculi.
C Recurrences are unlikely after pyelolithotomy for renal calculi.
D In men, chronic bacterial prostatitis is the most common cause of recurrences.
E In women, most recurrences are caused by re-infections with different organisms rather than bacterial persistence.

191. A woman aged 24 years presents with hypertension and is found on intravenous urography to have a shrunken, scarred left kidney, and a normal right kidney.
Which of the following statements is/are correct?

A The likely diagnosis is unilateral reflux nephropathy.
B A history of urinary tract infection is obtained in over 90% of such patients.
C If a micturating cystourethrogram shows gross vesicoureteric reflux on the left side, ureteric reimplantation is indicated.
D In this patient there is a 90% probability that the hypertension would be cured by removal of the left kidney.
E Hypersecretion of renin from the left kidney is not likely to be responsible for maintaining hypertension in this patient.

192. A man aged 18 years is found to have polycystic kidneys. Which of the following statements is/are correct?

A One of his parents almost certainly has polycystic kidney disease.
B He has a 30% chance of having multiple liver cysts.
C If his renal function is found to be normal, he is not likely to develop end-stage chronic renal failure.
D Treatment of complicating hypertension is not usually indicated.
E Patients with polycystic kidneys are usually good candidates for haemodialysis or renal transplantation.

193. A woman aged 42 years is admitted to hospital after a 2-weeks illness characterised by fever, generalised aching, pain in the renal angles, reddish urine, some frequency, but no dysuria. She was treated at the onset with co-trimoxazole for 5 days. There is a history of considerable analgesic abuse for 10 years. The blood pressure is 160/100 mmHg, the heart is not enlarged and the fundi are normal. The urine output is about 1.5 ℓ/day. The urine contains blood +++ and protein + and the microurine shows many distorted red cells, 2–4 leukocytes per high power field and occasional red cell casts and granular casts.

Plain X-ray of the abdomen shows the right and left kidneys to be smooth and they measure 16 and 15 cm long respectively. The haemoglobin is 110 g/ℓ and serum electrolytes show a potassium level of 5.5 mmol/ℓ and a mild hyperchloraemic acidosis. ASOT and ANF levels in the serum are normal. The serum creatinine is 0.46 mmol/ℓ (N: 0.06–0.09), but was normal 3 months ago.

Which of the following statements is/are correct?

A An intravenous pyelogram is contraindicated because of the elevated serum creatinine level.
B The most likely diagnosis is analgesic nephropathy with ureteric obstruction.
C An early renal biopsy is strongly indicated.
D The most appropriate immediate investigative procedure is aortography.
E The finding of 950 eosinophils per cmm in the peripheral blood would support a diagnosis of drug-induced interstitial nephritis.

194. With regard to bone disease in patients with chronic renal failure, which of the following statements is/are correct?

- **A** Clinical evidence of bone disease is found in about 80% of patients.
- **B** Osteomalacia is the usual histological diagnosis.
- **C** Plasma levels of 1,25-dihydroxyvitamin D are low.
- **D** Most forms of vitamin D improve renal bone disease by enhancing gastrointestinal absorption of calcium.
- **E** Patients with normal or high serum calcium levels in whom bone biopsy shows osteomalacia usually do not respond to vitamin D.

195. An otherwise asymptomatic man aged 48 years passes a calcium oxalate stone after a bout of typical renal colic. He has no previous history of stones. An adequate plain abdominal X-ray shows no other calculi, and serum creatinine, calcium and urate levels are all normal. A single random 24-hour urine collection shows elevated levels of calcium, 10.5 mmol/day (N: 2.5–6.3), and uric acid, 4.5 mmol/day (N: 3.6–4.2).
Which of the following statements is/are correct?

- **A** A bone scan is indicated to exclude lytic bone lesions.
- **B** Allopurinol should be prescribed to reduce the likelihood of further stone formation.
- **C** If given, a thiazide diuretic would be expected to reduce urinary calcium excretion.
- **D** Dietary restriction of both calcium and oxalate is necessary.
- **E** The increased fluid intake recommended during the day is not necessary at night, as polyuria due to hypercalciuria will maintain adequate nocturnal urine flow.

196. Idiopathic cyclical oedema

- **A** occurs equally in males and females.
- **B** often is associated with an awareness of weight and configuration and with difficulty in weight control.
- **C** is best controlled in the long-term with loop-acting diuretics.
- **D** may be aggravated by potassium depletion associated with diuretic therapy.
- **E** has been treated with bromocriptine.

197. Hypertension

A is common in patients with polycystic kidney disease.
B is usually caused by increased renin production in chronic renal failure.
C in chronic renal failure commonly responds to fluid removal by diuretics or dialysis.
D in kidney transplant recipients is usually due to donor renal artery stenosis.
E does not require treatment in patients with chronic renal disease.

198. Minimal change glomerulopathy may occur as a complication of, or in association with, which of the following?

A Hodgkin's disease
B bronchogenic carcinoma
C captopril therapy
D bee-stings
E therapy with non-steroidal anti-inflammatory agents.

199. A man aged 60 years, previously in good health, presents with the nephrotic syndrome. Renal biopsy demonstrates a membranous glomerulonephritis.
Which of the following statements is/are correct?

A Steroid treatment will be curative in 50% of cases.
B He should be investigated for an underlying malignancy.
C The most probable cause of his disease is systemic lupus erythematosus.
D Macroscopic haematuria suggests renal vein thrombosis.
E He is likely to require dialysis for chronic renal failure within three years.

200. Blood transfusions in patients on maintenance haemodialysis have been shown to result in

A improvement in subsequent cadaveric renal allograft survival.
B a decrease in mortality after subsequent cadaveric renal transplantation.
C a high prevalence of cytotoxic antibodies against random panels of T-lymphocytes.
D iron overload.
E aluminium intoxication.

PART II: ANSWERS AND CRITIQUES

1. Items B and C correct.

In persons with a heavy alcohol intake who do not necessarily have other evidence of physical disease, the serum GGTP level and mean corpuscular volume are most commonly found to be increased. Although not specific, these tests are valuable in screening. Serum alkaline phosphatase, serum AST and serum uric acid levels are less commonly elevated and less specific.

References

1. Wu A, et al. Macrocytosis of chronic alcoholism. *Lancet* 1974; 1: 829–830.
2. Spencer-Peet J, et al. Screening tests for alcoholism. *Lancet* 1973; 2: 1089–1090.
3. Whitfield JB, et al. Some laboratory correlates of drinking habits. *Ann Clin Biochem* 1978; 15: 297–303.

2. Items A, B and C correct.

Many of the non-barbiturate sedative-hypnotic drugs have the same addictive effects as barbiturates, and abstinence symptoms occur on withdrawal of the drug. These include hallucinations, seizures and delirium. The symptoms occur within 3–10 days after stopping long-acting drugs (chlordiazepoxide, diazepam) and within 24 hours after short-acting drugs (temazepam, oxazepam, lorazepam). This can occur even after short courses of benzodiazepines in therapeutic dosages.

Cocaine and marihuana are habit-forming, but no consistent abstinence symptoms follow their discontinuation. However, some treatment of emotional disturbances associated with their withdrawal may be necessary.

References

1. Thorn GW, et al (eds). Harrison's principles of internal medicine, 8th Edn. New York: McGraw-Hill, 1977: 721–730.
2. Khantzian EJ, McKenna GJ. Acute toxic and withdrawal reactions associated with drug use and abuse. *Ann Intern Med* 1979; 90: 361–372.
3. Greenblatt DJ, et al. Drug therapy: current status of benzodiazepines. *N Engl J Med* 1983; 309: 354, 410.

3. Items A, C and D correct.

Anticipating and preventing pain in terminal disease is preferable to treating it, and thus regular administration of appropriate amounts of analgesics such as the 'Brompton' mixture is preferable to p.r.n. administration. The anticipation of perpetual pain leads to anxiety and depression which in turn accentuates the physical component of pain.

The serum half-life of morphine taken orally is about 4 hours, and doses should be given 4-hourly around the clock. Oral analgesics allow the patients more independence and are less painful than parenteral analgesics.

An accompanying dose of a phenothiazine acts as an anti-emetic as well as potentiating the narcotic analgesia. Careful regulation of dosage of both drugs should allow a pain-free state without excessive sedation.

Dependence is not a problem when narcotics are used for the pain of malignant disease, and a change in dosage requirements usually signifies a change in disease status rather than tolerance.

References

1. Mount BM, et al. Use of the brompton mixture in treating chronic pain of malignant disease. *Can Med Assoc* 1976; 115: 122–124.
2. Twycross RG. Clinical experience with diamorphine in advanced malignant disease. *Int J Clin Pharmacol* 1974; 9: 184–198.

4. Items C, D and E correct.

Although paracetamol metabolism occurs relatively early, it produces a highly reactive metabolite which normally is detoxified in the liver by conjugation with glutathione. When protective stores of glutathione become depleted, liver cell damage occurs. After some delay this results in hepatic cell failure. This can occur after as little as 10 g of paracetamol taken as a single dose. Thus, in view of the potential delayed hepatic toxicity, it is not safe to discontinue observation 24 hours after a 15 g dose. In fact, clinical detection of liver damage may be delayed for up to 5–6 days.

The only reliable way to assess the severity of paracetamol overdose is to measure the plasma paracetamol concentration in the first 12 hours after overdose. Hepatic damage is likely if the 4-hour concentration exceeds 800 μmol/l (120 mg/l) or if the 12-hour concentration exceeds 330 μmol/l (50 mg/l).

After gastric lavage and activated charcoal to reduce paracetamol absorption, the essential aim is to replace amino acid SH groups which help to replenish glutathione levels. N-acetylcysteine given intravenously is currently the treatment of choice provided it is given within 10 hours of overdose.

References

1. Prescott LF, et al. Intravenous N-acetylcysteine: the treatment of choice for paracetamol poisoning. *Br Med J* 1979; 2: 1097–1100.
2. Oh TE. Intravenous N-acetylcysteine for paracetamol poisoning. *Med J Aust* 1980; 1: 664–665.

3. Forrest JAH, et al. Clinical pharmacokinetics of paracetamol. *Clin Pharmacokinetics* 1982; 7: 93–107.

5. Items A, B, C and D correct.

In a detailed review of hypothermia covering clinical features, pathophysiology and therapy, many associated factors are identified including ethanol excess, anorexia nervosa, diffuse erythroderma, hypothyroidism, hypopituitarism, phenothiazine drugs and exposure.

Blood volume depletion is common and needs to be corrected. One must beware of excessive medication while the patient is cold, as rewarming may lead to toxic drug levels when normal metabolism is restored.

The characteristic ECG finding is illustrated in the reference article. Its presence may be helpful when a low recording thermometer is not easily available. However, this abnormality is not always observed.

Because of the profound depression of metabolic processes, very cold tissue may survive long periods of anoxia such as that caused by cardiac arrest. Generally, resuscitative attempts should persist until rewarming is achieved. Core heating is more effective and safer than external reheating. Peritoneal dialysis is a useful technique to achieve this in adults.

Reference

1. Reuler JB. Hypothermia: pathophysiology, clinical settings and management. *Ann Intern Med* 1978; 89: 519–527.

6. Items A, B, D and E correct.

The girl's problem illustrates an anaphylactic reaction to bee-sting proteins mediated by IgE antibody directed against proteins in the bee venom. Nearly all patients with such histories have positive immediate hypersensitivity skin tests. The few patients without an elevated IgE to bee venom may be accounted for by a long interval between the last exposure to the antigen (i.e. the sting) and time of assessment. These individuals may still react in a systemic way to a bee-sting, presumably because they have such IgE bound to their basophils and mast cells. Conversely, some individuals, in particular bee-keepers, may have elevated levels of IgE anti-bee venom without any clinical disease. Compared to skin-prick tests with bee venom, IgE measurements show a 20% false-negative and 20% false-positive rate. The total serum IgE may be normal, as these patients do not necessarily have an ectopic background. The patient may also have severe reactions to other hymenoptera venoms — wasps, ants and hornets.

The pathophysiology of anaphylaxis secondary to hymenoptera stings is not well understood, but clearly adrenaline given subcutaneously is the most effective emergency drug. The sooner it is given the better, hence many allergists instruct their patients and those close to them in the use of a prepacked adrenaline syringe or an 'Anakit'. The patient may also require supplemental oxygen and fluid therapy. If the laryngeal oedema does not settle promptly, the airway must be secured with intubation and, as a last resort, tracheotomy undertaken. Corticosteroids are of dubious value in management.

Hyposensitisation therapy with pure bee venom extract has been shown to be valuable in controlled trials. Suitable patients for therapy are those who have a severe systemic reaction and a positive skin-prick test. If the latter is negative, the indication for hyposenitisation is controversial, but careful follow-up is advisable, just as it is for less severe reactions.

References

1. Leading article. Next year's bee and wasp stings. *Lancet* 1980; 2: 956.
2. Hunt KJ, et al. A controlled trial of immunotherapy in insect hypersensitivity. *N Engl J Med* 1978; 299: 157–161.
3. Austen KF. The anaphylactic syndrome. In: Samter M, et al (eds). Immunological diseases, 3rd Edn. Boston: Little Brown and Company, 1978; 2: 885–899.
4. Lichtenstein LM, et al. Insect allergy: the state of the art. *J Allergy Clin Immunol* 1979; 64: 5–12.

7. Items A, B and D correct.

Porphyria cutanea tarda is a photocutaneous syndrome characterised by bullous lesions, increased skin fragility, hypertrichosis, pigmentation and sclerodermoid plaques. These cutaneous lesions may be indistinguishable from those of porphyria variegata which may be differentiated by a positive family history and a history of acute attacks of a neurologic-visceral symptom complex.

The porphyrin excretion pattern in these two diseases is particularly valuable in distinguishing between them. Porphyria cutanea tarda is characterised by an increase in urinary uroporphyrins with a lesser rise in urinary coproporphyrins — the ratio of uroporphyrins to coproporphyrins in urine is usually greater than 5:1. In variegate porphyria the total urinary porphyrin excretion is usually much less and the uroporphyrin to coproporphyrin ratio is usually less than 1:1. In contrast, faecal porphyrin excretion is usually much less in the cutanea tarda form.

While alcohol is a major aetiological factor in porphyria cutanea tarda, oestrogen therapy, including oral contraceptives, is of increasing importance. Although the disease was previously recognised more frequently in men, the proportion of women with this disorder is increasing so that the sex ratio now approaches unity.

Some histological abnormality is present in the liver of most patients with porphyria cutanea tarda. The degree of liver damage is quite variable, with less than 10% having frank cirrhosis. Hepatic siderosis, associated with greater than 50% saturation of the total serum iron-binding capacity, occurs as a secondary event in most patients, yet porphyria cutanea tarda does not commonly develop in diseases of iron overload such as haemochromatosis and haemosiderosis. However, phlebotomy is the treatment of choice in porphria cutanea tarda and it may result in prolonged remission.

References
1. Grossman ME, et al. Porphyria cutanea tarda: clinical features and laboratory findings in 40 patients. *Am J Med* 1979; 67: 277–286.
2. Bloomer JR. The hepatic porphyrias: pathogenesis, manifestations and management. *Gastroenterology* 1976; 71: 689–704.

8. Items A, C, D and E correct.

Marfan's syndrome occurs in approximately 1.5 per 100 000 people. It is inherited as an autosomal dominant trait. However, expressivity is variable. The classic form of the syndrome is unmistakable and includes lens dislocation, aneurysm of the ascending aorta and aortic valve regurgitation, inappropriately long limbs, arachnodactyly, pectus deformity and mild joint laxity. Many affected persons do not manifest the typical features and diagnosis becomes correspondingly difficult. At least 2 of the 4 major criteria suggested should be present; these are a positive family history, ocular, cardiac and skeletal manifestations.

Life expectancy in classic Marfan's syndrome is approximately halved. Cardiovascular problems are the major cause of death. Dilatation of the ascending aorta, which is the most common cardiovascular abnormality, cannot be detected reliably by a chest X-ray. It is usually progressive and precedes the occurrence of life-threatening complications such as dissection or rupture as well as aortic valve regurgitation.

Management is complex. Ocular care includes correction of refractive errors, detection of incipient retinal detachment and rarely extirpation of the lens. Cardiovascular management depends on the specific abnormalities present. Prophylaxis against endocarditis is of prime importance and should be given whether or not there is evidence of valvular lesions. Regular assessment including ultrasonography is important to allow elective prophylactic surgery to the ascending aorta to be considered. Scoliosis will need careful assessment and treatment with bracing or spinal fusion when necessary. Genetic counselling and family investigation are of major importance.

References
1. Pyeritz RE, McCusick VA. The Marfan syndrome: diagnosis and management. *N Engl J Med* 1979; 300: 772–777.
2. Donaldson RM, et al. Management of cardiovascular complications in Marfan syndrome. *Lancet* 1980; 2: 1178–1180.

9. Item D correct.

Ionic gallium rapidly binds to the plasma protein transferrin and is distributed generally within the body. Approximately 20–30% is excreted through the kidneys within 24 hours. Subsequently the liver and biliary tract become the excretory route. Activity appears in the bowel by 24 hours and accumulates in the stool, often causing confusion in delayed studies.

The uptake of gallium in abnormal tissue is non-specific. It occurs in Hodgkin's disease tissue to a greater extent than in other lymphomas, and in several carcinomas including hepatoma, testicular tumours, mesothelioma and carcinoma of the lung. However, uptake in these conditions does not always occur. The overall sensitivity of the scan in the detection of affected nodal regions in Hodgkin's disease is 70%. Thus a negative scan cannot exclude disease, but the scan is useful is staging and follow-up. As most of the published studies were performed using low-dose techniques on equipment inferior to that currently available, it is expected that sensitivity today would exceed that reported in most published series.

Gallium citrate is also useful in the detection of inflammatory disease. In abdominal abscess detection, CT scanning or ultrasound are preferred if the site of the abscess is suspected but gallium scanning is recommended when the infection is occult. While the imaging time in inflammatory diseases is optimal at 48–72 hours post-injection, as in neoplastic disease, early scanning at 4–6 hours , if clinically necessary, can give the same information in the majority of cases.

In many patients, pyrexia of unknown origin is due to infection or drug reactions and the gallium scan should be undertaken only after these conditions have been excluded or identified and more simple attempts at disease localisation have been undertaken. However the gallium scan is helpful in demonstrating the site of the disease in many cases of focal inflammatory disease or malignancy.

References

1. Hoffer P. Status of gallium-67 in tumour detection. *J Nucl Med* 1980; 21: 394–398.
2. Turner DA, et al. Gallium-67 imaging in the management of Hodgkin's disease and other malignant lymphomas. *Semin Nucl Med* 1978; 8: 205–218.

10. Item E correct.

The value of screening a population for a given disease is influenced by many factors including the prevalence of the disease in the population to be screened, the sensitivity (i.e. true-positive rate) and the specificity (i.e. true-negative rate) of the test to be used.

In the example given, only one of the 1000 people will have the disease but 5% of the others (i.e. 5% of 999 or roughly 50 persons), will yield false-positive results. Thus, only one of 51 positive results will be truly positive and the chance that any one positive result will represent a person who actually has the disease is 1 in 51, or roughly 2%.

Reference

1. Casscells W, et al. Interpretation by physicians of clinical laboratory results. *N Engl J Med* 1978; 299: 999–1001.

11. Item D correct.

The true laboratory values for a small proportion of healthy persons will be reported consistently as abnormal because normal biological variation often overlaps with the values for persons with the given disease.

The cut-off point for normal values is usually set at 2 standard deviations from the mean, i.e. approximately 95% of persons in the population will register values in the normal range. Thus, if a healthy person undergoes a battery of 20 screening tests, the chance of registering 20 'normal' values would be $(0.95)^{20} = 0.36$, i.e. only 36%.

Reference

1. Casscells W, et al. Interpretation by physicians of clinical laboratory results. *N Engl J Med* 1978; 299: 999–1001.

12. Items B, C, D and E correct.

Modifications in the quality rather than quantity of sleep with age run parallel to an increase in complaints of insomnia. In the past, it was assumed that elderly people need less sleep than the young, the presumed diminished need for sleep being attributed to the reduced physical and mental demands made on the old. On average, sleep duration decreases little with age; what does change is individual variability. In old age there are more subjects with particularly brief or particularly long sleep times.

Ageing is accompanied by a decreased stage 4 (deep arousal, slow wave sleep), and wake periods of varying duration become more frequent. Thus 'sleep efficiency' drops significantly; older people have to spend more time in bed in order to attain the same net sleep time as young individuals. The non-REM(rapid eye movement)–REM cyclical structure of sleep, which begins the night with increasing and concludes with decreasing cycle durations, is retained into advanced age.

Objective measures show that the sleep-modifying effect of available hypnotics are slowly lost when used continually over a period of several weeks.

References

1. Soldatos CR, et al. Management of insomnia. *Annu Rev Med* 1979; 30: 301–312.
2. Kales A, et at. Chronic hypnotic-drug use. *JAMA* 1974; 227: 513–517.
3. Kales A, et al. Measurement of all-night sleep in normal elderly persons: effects of ageing. *J Am Geriatric Soc* 1967; 15: 405–414.

13. Items B, C, D and E correct.

Postural hypotension is one of the most important disorders encountered in geriatric medicine. While common in old-age, it cannot be considered a normal finding. In a survey of persons over 65 years living at home, Caird et al (1973) found the following: fall in systolic blood pressure of 20 mm or more in 24%, 30 mm or more in 9%, 40 mm or more in 5%; falls of 20 mm or more were found in 30% of subjects over 75 years of age.

Many causes have been described. Postural hypotension may occasionally be the predominant or presenting symptom/sign in diabetes mellitus or Parkinsonism. A large number of drugs have also been implicated, diuretics being amongst the most common.

Plasma expansion with 9α-fluorohydrocortisone is the most effective treatment currently available in cases requiring pharmacological intervention.

References

1. Overstall PW. Falls in the elderly. In: Isaacs B (ed). Recent advances in geriatric medicine. Edinburgh: Churchill Livingstone, 1978: 61–72.
2. Exton-Smith AN. Disturbance of autonomic regulation. In: Isaacs B (ed). Recent advances in geriatric medicine. Edinburgh: Churchill Livingstone 1978: 85–100.
3. Leading article. Management of orthostatic hypotension. *Lancet* 1981; 2: 963–964.
4. Schatz IJ. Current management concepts in orthostatic hypotension. *Arch Intern Med* 1980; 140: 1152–1154.
5. Caird FI, et al. Effect of posture on blood pressure in the elderly. *Br Heart J* 1973; 35: 527–530.

14. Item C and D correct.

Depression is common amongst the elderly but often presents with atypical symptoms. The aged have a tendency to present with physical complaints and may not complain openly of feelings of depression though other associated symptoms such as loss of concentration and interest will usually be present. In very depressed elderly people, the clinical picture may be confused with senile dementia.

The patient is often very agitated and the administration of phenothiazines alone to control the agitation is a common error. This is likely to aggravate the depressive state.

Elderly depressives, particularly males, have the highest suicide rate in the population and the condition must be considered life-threatening. It is often difficult to categorise the depressive state into endogenous or reactive conditions. The aged patient may have many losses to cope with but it cannot be automatically assumed that his depression is 'normal', inevitable or reactive.

Irrespective of apparent causes, antidepressant treatment is often efficacious and should be tried.

References

1. Pitt B. Psychogeriatrics. Edinburgh: Churchill Livingstone, 1974.
2. Whitlock FA, Evans LEJ. Drugs and depression. *Curr Ther* 1978; April: 97–99.
3. Isaacs AD, Post F (eds). Studies in geriatric psychiatry. New York: Wiley, 1978: 77–94.
4. Kiloh LG. Pseudo-dementia. *Acta Psychiatr Scand* 1961; 37: 336.
5. Butler RN. Psychiatry and the elderly: an overview. *Am J Psychiatry* 1975; 132: 893–900.

15. Items B, C and D correct.

Incontinence of urine is a very common problem in geriatric practice. It is not a diagnosis in itself but is symptomatic of some underlying condition. In this patient the previous history of cerebrovascular disease and the typical symptoms are strongly suggestive of an uninhibited neurogenic bladder — the most common cause of incontinence in the elderly.

The cystometrographic findings are characteristic, showing a small capacity, uninhibited contractions and a short interval between the first desire to micturate and the onset of voiding. Incontinence research centres use a system of simultaneous cystourethrography, flow measurement and cystography.

The neurological condition predisposes the patient to incontinence, but a search must also be made for precipitating factors. Infection is the most common of these.

The uninhibited bladder responds to retraining and this should always be attempted as a first step, or, in association with any other treatment that is undertaken. Many patients also respond to anticholinergic drugs. Long-term catheterisation of the elderly female presents a number of practical difficulties and should be reserved only for the most difficult cases.

References

1. Willington FL (ed). Incontinence in the elderly. New York: Academic Press, 1976.
2. Brocklehurst JC. The investigation and management of incontinence. In: Isaacs B (ed). Recent advances in geriatric medicine. Edinburgh: Churchill Livingstone, 1978: 21–40.

16. Item C correct.

The patient is likely to have thyrotoxicosis; her description corresponds with that of 'apathetic thyrotoxicosis' first reported by Lahey in 1931. In the elderly, atypical presentations are common with less marked nervous system signs and predominant circulatory manifestations.

The diagnosis could be established by measuring serum T_4 and T_3 concentrations. TSH would be low, not elevated.

In general, surgical treatment in the aged is restricted to patients with large goitres or with nodules suspected to harbour malignancy. Antithyroid drugs should be given in the first instance and administration of a therapeutic dose of radioactive iodine as definitive treatment should be deferred until the patient has been rendered euthyroid.

Reference

1. Exton-Smith AN, Caird FL (eds). Metabolic and nutritional disorders in the elderly. Bristol: Wright, 1980: 211.

17. All items correct.

In patients with Paget's disease, two independent groups using electron-microscopy have observed inclusion bodies in the nuclei of osteoclasts; the appearances are consistent with virus particles and they may be significant in the aetiology.

Elevated serum alkaline phosphatase and increased urinary secretion of hydroxyproline are diagnostic along with typical X-ray changes. Bone scans are sensitive to the extent of disease activity. Serum acid phosphatase may be elevated.

Pain in Paget's disease is frequently caused by secondary arthritis, in which case anti-inflammatory drugs are more appropriate than calcitonin. If this is not successful, and if there is doubt as to the mechanism, a therapeutic trial of calcitonin is sometimes used.

With drug treatment with calcitonin, a drop in urinary hydroxyproline levels and serum alkaline phosphatase occurring in the first weeks indicates that pain relief will probably follow within 3 months.

Reference

1. Martin TJ. The treatment of paget's disease with the calcitonins. *Aust NZ J Med* 1979; 9: 36–43.

18. Item E correct.

In digoxin therapy, absorption following the intramuscular route is unpredictable, especially in the shocked patient. The time taken to achieve maximum plasma concentration is no earlier than following the oral route and the overall bioavailability is about the same, i.e. about 75%. Furthermore, the intramuscular injection is painful.

The plasma concentration-time profile is most conveniently represented by a 2-compartment model. The first phase, the distribution phase, lasts about 6–8 hours and it is currently accepted that plasma digoxin concentrations during this phase do not correlate with concentrations in the myocardium. Thus, plasma concentrations measured during this phase overestimate the tissue concentration of the drug. However, during the second or elimination phase, the half-life of which is about 24–36 hours in patients with normal renal function, the plasma concentration is a good guide to tissue concentration. Thus for correct interpretation a knowledge of timing of blood sampling in relation to dosing time is important.

Whilst it is true that digoxin is cleared from the body predominantly by the kidneys (approximately 75%) and renal function is an important determinant of digoxin dose, serum creatinine estimation is an insensitive index of renal function. Thus a patient, especially an elderly one, may have a normal serum creatinine level but only about 50% of normal function, with resulting reduced digoxin clearance.

It takes 4–5 half-lives to achieve steady-state plasma concentrations of a drug. Thus plasma digoxin concentration interpretations must be made in the light of knowledge of when the last dosage change occurred.

References

1. Doherty JE et al. Clinical pharmacokinetics of digitalis glycosides. *Progr Cardiovasc Dis* 1978; 21: 141–158.
2. Smith TW, Haber E. Digitalis: medical progress. *N Engl J Med* 1973; 289: 945–952, 1010–1015, 1063–1072, 1125–1129.
3. Marcus FL. Digitalis: pharmacokinetics and metabolism. *Am J Med* 1975; 58: 452–459.

19. Items A, C, D and E correct.

In a study on quinidine-digoxin interaction, all patients on maintenance digoxin, even those on very low maintenance doses, developed a rise in serum digoxin when given quinidine 1 g daily. The rise in serum digoxin depended on the dose and duration of quinidine therapy and was not seen at quinidine doses of less than 500 mg daily. The rise in serum digoxin level reaches a plateau at about the fifth day of concomitant therapy and falls to pre-quinidine therapy levels about 4–6 days after cessation of quinidine administration.

The rise in serum digoxin level is often accompanied by systemic side-effects of nausea, vomiting, etc. These symptoms are suggestive of digoxin toxicity and the rise in serum digoxin level may be a factor in the production of ventricular arrhythmias. It has been suggested that, when quinidine is added to the therapy of a patient already receiving digoxin, the daily dose of digoxin should be halved prior to commencing quinidine therapy.

Although there are several possible explanations, there is evidence that one cause of the rise in serum digoxin is a fall in renal digoxin clearance. However there is also evidence that quinidine reduces the volume of distribution of digoxin, suggesting displacement from tissue binding sites.

References

1. Doering W. Quinidine-digoxin interaction. *N Engl J Med* 1979; 301: 400–404.
2. Editorial. Digitalis and quinidine. *Lancet* 1980; 2: 1064–1065.
3. Manolas EG, et al. Effects of quinidine and disopyramide on serum digoxin concentrations. *Aust NZ J Med* 1980; 10: 426–429.
4. Mungall DR, et al. Effects of quinidine on serum digoxin concentration. *Ann Intern Med* 1980; 93: 689–693.
5. Hager WD, et al. Digoxin-quinidine interaction: pharmacokinetic evaluation. *N Engl J Med* 1979; 300: 1238–1241.

20. Items C and E correct.

Prazosin is an important addition to the list of agents available to treat hypertension. It has significant side-effects which can be minimised by appropriate timing and size of dose and by combination with other drugs.

Prazosin does not act by a direct relaxing effect on vascular smooth muscle or by a presynaptic alpha 2 adrenergic blockade effect. It acts by blocking postsynaptic alpha 1 (vascular) adrenergic receptors. Thus it has different effects from hydralazine or phentolamine.

It is important to avoid excessive early side-effects, such as postural hypotension. Low initial doses are important and even then postural hypotension may occur in some cases. It is therefore advisable to prescribe the first dose at bedtime. Prazosin is the only specific alpha 1-blocking drug currently available.

The relative lack of reflex tachycardia (unlike the effect of hydralazine) is an important advantage and may be due to lack of effects of prazosin on the alpha 2 adrenergic receptor and a dual dilator action on both capacitance (venous) and resistance (arteriolar) vascular loads which prevents massive increases in cardiac venous return.

Prazosin has little effect on glomerular filtration rate or tubular function and its use is not contraindicated in patients with renal disease.

The use of vasoactive substances such as prazosin to modify cardiac after-load and pre-load has been an important therapeutic advance in the treatment of heart failure.

References

1. Graham RM, Pettinger WA. Drug therapy: prazosin. *N Engl J Med* 1979; 300: 232–236.
2. Hoffman BB, Lefkowitz RJ. Alpha-adrenergic receptor sub-types. *N Engl J Med* 1980; 302: 1390–1396.

21. Items B, C and E correct.

The intramuscular route for phenytoin administration is not recommended because the bioavailability following this route is incomplete and unpredictable. Phenytoin tends to crystallize out of solution in muscle. The oral bioavailability is close to 100%.

The absorption phase following oral phenytoin is relatively long (3–10 hours). The elimination half-life is about 24 hours. Therefore, the interdosing fluctuation during a once daily regimen is small and clinically unimportant in most epileptics who are controlled with phenytoin.

Up to puberty, children have rapid liver metabolism and therefore require about twice as much phenytoin as adults to produce a comparable plasma concentration. The average adult maintenance dose is 5–6 mg/kg/day whilst children require 10–12 mg/kg/day.

The metabolism of phenytoin approaches saturation at plasma concentrations of phenytoin within the therapeutic range (10–20 μg/ml or 40–80 μmol/l). As a result increments in dosage often result in disproportionate increases in plasma concentrations. The elimination time becomes longer as the plasma concentration rises. The kidney plays an insignificant part (approximately 5%) in phenytoin clearance.

In pregnancy, protein binding of phenytoin is substantially reduced from about 90% to 80%. At present, most laboratories measure total (bound and unbound) drug. Thus, in pregnancy, attempts to achieve the optimal therapeutic concentration range may result in clinical toxicity and it may be necessary to assay free (unbound) phenytoin. Similar problems may arise in renal disease.

References

1. Hooper WD, et al. Plasma protein binding of diphenylhydantoine: effects of sex hormones, renal and hepatic disease. *Clin Pharm Ther* 1974; 15: 276–282.
2. Richens A. Drug level monitoring — quality and quantity. *Br J Clin Pharmacol* 1978; 5: 285–288.
3. Richens A, Dunlop A. Serum phenytoin levels in the management of epilepsy. *Lancet* 1975; 2: 247–248.

22. Items A, D and E correct.

Lithium carbonate is used in the management of persons with manic depressive psychosis. Its major actions are on the central nervous system at both therapeutic (0.6–1.4 mmol/l) and toxic blood levels.

The sensitivity of individual patients to lithium neurotoxicity does not appear to be clearly related to dose or serum levels. The effects of lithium are potentiated by any condition which causes increased sodium loss from the body or by impaired renal function.

Lithium has an antithyroid effect and a goitre or nodule may appear even with normal thyroid function. These abnormalities are reversible on cessation of lithium but can also be treated quickly by thyroxine without lowering the lithium dosage. On the other hand, hyperthyroidism or thyroiditis can also develop during lithium treatment. Thyroid function tests are usually checked before commencing therapy and at regular intervals during therapy.

Patients taking diuretics are more prone to the toxic effects of lithium. Tremor is a frequent side-effect which responds to propranolol but not to anti-Parkinsonian agents.

References

1. Williams WO, Gyory AZ. Aspects of the use of lithium for the non psychiatrist. *Aust NZ J Med* 1976; 6: 233–242.
2. Amidsen A. Serum lithium estimations. *Br Med J* 1973; 2: 240–242.

23. Items A, C, D and E correct.

Enteric-coated aspirin or sustained-release salicylate preparations significantly reduce the incidence of gastric blood loss as measured by chromium-51 labelling. A reduced incidence of dyspepsia has also been shown in clinical trials.

High-dose aspirin is uricosuric. It blocks both the resorption of uric acid in the proximal tubule of the kidney and resecretion in the distal tubule, whereas low-dose aspirin blocks only distal resecretion and hence retains uric acid.

Aspirin irreversibly acetylates platelet membrane proteins including membrane-bound cyclo-oxygenase. Once a platelet has been exposed to aspirin it loses aggregating properties for its life-span.

In low and moderate doses, aspirin has been shown to reduce the plasma levels of naproxen, flurbiprofen, fenoprofen and ibuprofen. The clinical relevance of these interactions is unclear.

Aspirin exhibits linear pharmacokinetics at low and moderate doses; however, with high doses, metabolic pathways are saturated and small increases in dose can result in a large increase in plasma level.

References

1. Levy G, et at. Rational aspirin dosage regimens. *Clin Pharmacol Ther* 1978; 23: 247–252.
2. Buchanan WW, et al. Aspirin and the salicylates. *Clin Rheum Dis* 1979; 5(2): 499–539.

24. Items A, B and D correct.

One of the signs of reduced contraceptive efficacy of the combined oestrogen and progesterone (OCP) pill is breakthrough bleeding. This occurs when the concentration of circulating oestrogen drops below a desirable level, and should always be a warning sign. If it occurs early in a cycle, the patient should be recommended to take alternative precautions for the rest of that cycle. In some cases pregnancy can occur without any warning of breakthrough bleeding in a previous cycle.

Drugs such as the anticonvulsants all induce hepatic microsomal enzymes and thereby increase the rate of metabolism of oestrogen and progesterone. The result is lower circulating levels of the active hormones and a reduction in contraceptive efficacy.

Antibiotics such as tetracycline and ampicillin interfere with the efficacy of oral contraceptive hormones, but not via the hepatic microsomal enzyme mechanism. Many antibiotics destroy those gut bacteria responsible for the hydrolysis of oestrogen conjugates. This prevents the enterohepatic recirculation of oestrogen and hence there is less unconjugated active oestrogen available for reabsorption and circulation.

The contraceptive steroids lower the threshold for epilepsy, possibly by causing cerebral fluid retention. As a result, a patient who has been previously well-controlled might have an increased frequency of seizures. To cope with this, the dose of anticonvulsant drugs may need to be increased, but great care is needed in adjusting the dose because of the hepatic interaction. Monitoring of plasma anticonvulsant levels is helpful in controlling the epilepsy.

The majority of antituberculous drugs have not been shown to impair OCP efficacy, but rifampicin, which is now a first-line antituberculous drug, has been responsible for frequently reported pregnancies in patients on contraceptive steroids. It appears to do this by enhancing the metabolism of oestrogens and progesterones. The risk is so great that treatment with rifampicin is an absolute contraindication for use of the OCP in contraception.

Oral contraceptive steroids inhibit hepatic microsomal enzymes and thus may slow the rate of metabolism of other drugs. The usual outcome is an increase in side-effects of the other compound and this problem has been reported with imipramine, barbiturates, pethidine and chlordiazepoxide.

References

1. Friedman CI, et al. The effect of ampicillin on oral contraceptive effectiveness. *Obstet Gynecol* 1980; 55: 33.
2. Shenfield GM. Drug interactions with hormonal steroid contraceptives. *Curr Ther* 1980; 21(8): 75–87.
3. Coulam CD, Annegers JF. Do anticonvulsants reduce the efficacy of oral contraceptives? *Epilepsia* 1979; 20: 519–526.

4. Buff WC. Leading article. Induction of hepatic drug metabolising enzymes and pregnancy while taking oral contraceptives. *J Antimicrob Chemother* 1979; 5: 4–5.
5. Stockley I. Interactions with oral contraceptives. *Pharm J* 1976; 216(5856): 140–143.

25. Items A, C and D correct.

Although available evidence suggests an effect of increasing age on active transport systems in the ageing gastrointestinal tract (leading to reduced absorption of calcium, iron and galactose), most drugs are absorbed by passive diffusion. No clinically significant changes due to impaired drug absorption have been shown in elderly patients.

Total body water, both in absolute terms and as a percentage of body weight, decreases with age. With regard to drugs which are distributed in body water, higher blood levels rather than lower levels would be expected.

Age and liver disease are equally important determinants of the elimination half-times of diazepam. Elderly patients take longer to reach steady blood levels. Benzodiazepines, such as oxazepam, without active hepatic metabolites, have half-times little influenced by age.

Blood flow to the liver decreases with age. Indirect measurements suggest a reduction of about 1% per year from age 25 years. This decline is partly due to a decline in cardiac output. It has been suggested that increased plasma propranolol levels reported in the elderly, compared to those achieved in younger patients receiving a comparable dose, are due to the reduced hepatic blood flow.

Both renal tubular function and glomerular filtration rate diminish significantly with age. Prolongation of half-times for drugs excreted by the glomerular or renal tubular route can be expected in the elderly.

References

1. Vestal RE. Drug use in the elderly: a review of problems and special considerations. *Drugs* 1978; 16: 358–382.
2. Crooks J, et al. Pharmacokinetics in the elderly. *Clin Pharmacokinet* 1976; 1: 280–296.
3. Richey DP, Bender AD. Pharmacokinetic consequences of aging. *Ann Rev Pharmacol Toxicol* 1977; 17: 49–65.

26. All items correct.

Amantadine probably releases dopamine in the brain. In elderly patients, mental disturbances (particularly confusion) can occur or be aggravated by amantadine, as may occur with other anti-Parkinsonian drugs. In this regard there may be additive effects when it is used concurrently with anticholinergic drugs.

The main neuropsychiatric disturbances with indomethacin are throbbing frontal headache, vertigo and a sense of 'muzziness'; and more recently mental confusion has been reported with its use.

Severe organic brain syndrome has been reported in several patients given propranolol. Agitation, confusion, anxiety and mental torpor can occur as adverse effects in addition to disturbed sleep and nightmares.

Digitalis toxicity may produce a range of symptoms from fatigue and drowsiness to euphoria, confusion and disorientation. In an outbreak of digitoxin toxicity, 65% of 179 patients manifested toxicity as psychic disturbances. Such disturbances are especially liable to occur in the elderly with impaired mental reserves.

Numerous reports in the literature confirm that confusional states are definite, albeit rare, side-effects of cimetidine therapy, especially when the drug is administered to the elderly or to patients with renal or hepatic failure.

References

1. Lely AH, Van Enter CHJ. Large-scale digoxin intoxication. *Br Med J* 1970; 3: 737–740.
2. Flind AC, Rowley-Jones D. (Correspondence). Mental confusion and cimetidine. *Lancet* 1979; 1:379.
3. Kuhr BM. Prolonged delirium with propranolol. *J Clin Psychiatry* 1979; 40(4): 198–199.
4. Dukes MNG (ed). Meyler's side effects of drugs, 9th Edn. Amsterdam: Excerpta Medica, 1980.

27. Items A and B correct.

Cimetidine is being prescribed for many patients with problems thought to relate to gastric acid secretion. It is not of proven efficacy for all these disorders and the clinician should be particularly aware of its potential side-effects and their significance. Neurological changes are fortunately transient. They are most likely to occur with large doses of the drug in elderly patients who are critically ill, particularly with renal and/or hepatic failure. Cimetidine is partially metabolised by the liver and partially excreted unchanged so that delayed excretion occurs with severe liver disease.

The inhibition of drug metabolism by cimetidine has been extensively investigated but is more than a pharmacological curiosity. The mechanism is inhibition of one pathway for mixed function oxidation of many drugs including theophylline and warfarin (cytochrome p 450). Cimetidine has been shown to inhibit metabolism and this is relevant clinically, as blood levels of these drugs have a narrow therapeutic range.

Cimetidine impairs chlordiazepoxide and diazepam metabolism since these two drugs are metabolised extensively by hepatic mixed function oxidases. On the other hand, oxazepam and lorazepam are both conjugated by the liver before excretion and this pathway is not inhibited by cimetidine. The evidence is that ranitidine does not have these effects on the liver metabolism of drugs.

There is a growing list of relatively minor side-effects of cimetidine which include gynaecomastia, headache, rash, constipation and possibly mild hepatitis, although this has been poorly documented. Cardiac arrhythmias which occur after rapid intravenous injection of cimetidine may be fatal and it would seem very unwise to administer the drug rapidly by this route.

References

1. Editorial. Cimetidine now. *Lancet* 1981; 1: 875–877.
2. Schentag JJ. Cimetidine associated mental confusion, further studies in 36 severely ill patients. *Ther Drug Monit* 1980; 2: 133–142.
3. Serlin MG, et al. Cimetidine: interaction with oral anticoagulants in man. *Lancet* 1979; 2: 317–319.
4. Roberts RK, et al. Cimetidine impairs the elimination of theophylline and antipyrine. *Gastroenterology* 1981; 81: 19–21.
5. Patwardhan RV, et al. Cimetidine spares the glucuronidation of lorazepam and oxazepam. *Gastroenterology* 1980; 79: 912–916.
6. Shaw RG, et al. Cardiac arrest after intravenous injection of cimetidine. *Med J Aust* 1980; 2: 629–630.

28. Items A, B and E correct.

Alcohol is rapidly absorbed and 75% at least is metabolised in the liver where alcohol dehydrogenase in the hepatocytes converts it to the toxic substance acetaldehyde. This is subsequently metabolised to acetate by aldehyde dehydrogenase present in the mitochondria.

Early claims that liver damage in alcoholics was predominantly due to malnutrition have been refuted. There is also a linear relationship in population studies between the incidence of cirrhosis and the amount of ethanol intake per capita.

It has been shown that a daily intake of ethanol of 40–50 g in men and 20–30 g in women causes an increased incidence of cirrhosis in a well-nourished population.

Ethanol in concentrations up to 16% does not stimulate gastric acid secretion but it does damage the gastric mucosal membrane, causing leakage of electrolytes, protein and red blood cells into the lumen.

Ethanol also has a direct toxic effect on small bowel, inhibiting the transport of water, electrolytes, folate, thiamine and other nutrients.

References

1. Geokas MC, et al. Ethanol, the liver and the gastrointestinal tract. *Ann Intern Med* 1981; 95: 198–211.
2. Sherlock S, ed. Alcohol and disease. *Br Med Bull* 1982; 38: 1–114.

29. Item C correct.

Antimuscarinic drugs have been introduced recently to treat airways obstruction.

Because of the vagal innervation of the tracheobronchial tree, drugs which antagonise the actions of acetylcholine may reduce the effect of vagal tone on the airways, resulting in bronchodilation. However, there are also cholinergic vagal fibres innervating the mucus-secreting glands within the lung, and impairment of mucociliary flow has been reported in man after administration of anticholinergic drugs such as hyoscine and atropine.

This action is less evident with the quaternary ammonium compounds such as ipratropium bromide which are also anticholinergic and can be administered as an aerosol. Ipratropium bromide has no effect on phosphodiesterase.

There is no evidence that the vagus nerve modulates the function of the purinergic (or non-cholinergic) fibres within the lungs, and interruption of vagal fibres does not alter the release of histamine within the lungs.

Antimuscarinic drugs (e.g. ipratropium bromide), delivered as nebulised solutions or aerosol, may be effective in patients who have not had complete reversal of their airflow obstruction after administration of beta-adrenoceptor agonists.

However, ipratropium bromide should not be used to replace beta-agonists, since it is not as effective a bronchodilator in the majority of patients.

References

1. Pakes GE, et al. Ipratroprium bromide: a review of its pharmacological properties and therapeutic efficacy in asthma and chronic bronchitis. *Drugs* 1980; 20: 237–66.
2. Pavia D, et al. Effect of ipratroprium bromide on mucociliary clearance and pulmonary function in reversible airways obstruction. *Thorax* 1979; 34: 501–507.
3. Ward MJ, et al. Ipratropium bromide in acute asthma. *Br Med J* 1980; 282: 598–600.

30. Item B correct.

A high potassium (K^+) level need not imply acute tubular necrosis. Acidosis causes efflux of K^+ from cells into the extracellular fluid; thus serum K^+ can be high even in the presence of a total body deficit of K^+. Treatment with insulin and correction of acidosis will lead to passage of K^+ into cells. Considerable K^+, e.g. 50–150 mmol, will be required in the first 12 hours, providing acute renal failure (which is unlikely) does not develop.

Insulin leads to rapid entry of phosphate into the cell, resulting in a dramatic fall in serum phosphate concentration to subnormal levels. Since 2,3-diphosphoglycerate levels drop due to the low phosphate, some have advocated administering phosphate during the treatment of diabetic ketoacidosis to prevent this drop and the impaired tissue oxygenation. Despite the theoretical arguments in favour of this, as yet there is no definite evidence of a practical advantage in this form of treatment.

The administration of bicarbonate in an amount equal to the deficit has been shown experimentally to greatly over-correct the acidosis and cause a metabolic alkalosis. It is appropriate to give small doses of sodium bicarbonate (100 mmol) initially to this patient to correct the severe metabolic acidosis which may threaten cardiovascular function. However, bicarbonate should be used in moderation only because it produces a fall in CSF pH due to a lowering of respiratory drive. With appropriate doses, the fall in CSF pH is unlikely to cause cerebral oedema.

References

1. Zimmet PZ, et al. Acid production in diabetic acidosis: a more rational approach to alkali replacement. *Br Med J* 1970; 3: 610–612.
2. Assal JP, et al. Metabolic effects of sodium bicarbonate in the management of diabetic ketoacidosis. *Diabetes* 1974; 23: 405–411.
3. Kreisburg RA. Diabetic ketoacidosis: new concepts and trends in pathogenesis and treatment. *Ann Intern Med* 1978; 88: 681–695.

31. Item D correct.

The retinopathy described is directly attributable to the diabetes. When hypertensive changes are superimposed, segmental arterial constriction is likely to be a feature.

No claims have been made for the usefulness of clofibrate in proliferative retinopathy, although in one report it was found to aid the resolution of lipid exudates.

Although pituitary ablation has been useful in preserving vision in proliferative retinopathy, the less radical step of photocoagulation is as effective and distinctly more free from side-effects.

New vessels arising from the disc or acute deterioration of vision may be indications for urgent photocoagulation. Controlled trials in both the USA and UK have shown that photocoagulation (both argon laser and xenon) is useful in preserving vision in this situation.

Vitrectomy is reserved for the situation in which vision is less than 6/60 in both eyes because of vitreous haemorrhage.

References

1. Cheng H. Photocoagulation and diabetic retinopathy. *Br Med J* 1979; 1: 365–366.
2. Diabetic Retinopathy Study Research Group. Preliminary reports on effects of photocoagulation therapy. *Am J Ophthalmol* 1976; 81: 383–396.
3. Multicentre Study Group. Proliferative diabetic retinopathy: treatment with xenon-arc photocoagulation. *Br Med J* 1977; 1: 739–741.

32. Item B correct.

The patient is likely to have alcoholic pseudo-Cushing's syndrome. Prolonged ingestion of alcohol leads to consistent mild hypercortisolism which may produce clinical stigmata of Cushing's syndrome. ACTH levels have been reported to be inappropriately high and have often failed to show normal circadian variation (i.e. the condition seems to be mediated via the intact pituitary), although there is some evidence for a direct stimulatory role for alcohol and its metabolites on adrenal cells. The hypercortisolaemia settles within days or weeks of alcohol withdrawal.

Episodic steroid hypersecretion in Cushing's disease is uncommon and an unlikely explanation for this clinical picture.

Alcohol does not interfere with current steroid assays which involve competitive protein binding or radioimmunoassay techniques.

Self-administration of dexamethasone could produce clinical features of Cushing's syndrome but the plasma cortisol values would be markedly suppressed.

Liver disease may produce an abnormal pattern of cortisol metabolites but plasma cortisol levels are normal or low and Cushing's syndrome does not occur in the absence of chronic alcoholism.

References

1. Elias AN, Gwinup G. Effects of some clinically encountered drugs on steroid synthesis and degradation. *Metabolism* 1980; 29: 582–595.
2. Rees LH, et al. Alcohol-induced pseudo-Cushing's syndrome. *Lancet* 1977; 1: 726–728.
3. Morgan M. Alcohol and the endocrine system. *Br Med Bull* 1982; 38: 35–42.

33. Items A, B and C correct.

Hyperosmolar, non-ketotic diabetic coma occurs most commonly in elderly patients and is often precipitated by infection, stroke, myocardial infarct, surgical conditions or operations. In contrast to ketoacidosis, after control has been achieved the patients can usually be managed by diet alone or by diet plus oral hypoglycaemic agents.

Morbidity and mortality in the condition are often caused by thromboembolic complications and, for this reason, low dose heparin prophylaxis is indicated. The key steps in management are rehydration and a low dose insulin regimen (insulin infusion or hourly intramuscular injections). These patients are usually at least as sensitive to insulin as those in ketoacidosis.

References

1. Alberti KGMM, Hockaday JDR. Diabetic coma: a reappraisal after five years. *Clin Endocrinol Metab* 1977; 6: 421–445.
2. Keller U, et al. Course and prognosis of 86 episodes of diabetic coma. *Diabetologia* 1975; 11: 93–100.

34. Items C, D and E correct.

Diabetic polyradiculopathy usually occurs in older patients with mild diabetes, frequently not requiring insulin therapy. Microvascular complications of diabetes are infrequent and usually mild in these patients.

Onset is with pain and progressive weakness which characteristically involves muscles of the pelvic girdle and thigh. Distribution is asymmetrical and signs of sensory involvement are mild, usually attributable to associated polyneuropathy.

Reduced tendon reflexes are almost invariably seen; occasional extensor plantar responses have been reported.

CSF protein concentration is usually moderately increased.

Marked improvement or complete resolution occurs over the course of several months, although recurrent episodes of polyradiculopathy are sometimes seen.

References

1. Ellenberg M. Diabetic neuropathy: clinical aspects. *Metabolism* 1976; 25: 1627–1655.
2. Bastron JA, Thomas JE. Diabetic polyradiculopathy. Clinical and electromyographic findings in 105 patients. *Mayo Clin Proc* 1981; 56: 725–732.

35. Item B correct.

Although pigmentation is consistent with Addison's disease, the electrolyte picture is not; one would expect a high normal K^+ concentration and low normal HCO_3^- in Addison's disease. In addition, the oedema and proximal myopathy are not normal components of Addison's disease. Moreover, Addison's disease is most unusual as the result of adrenal replacement by tumour secondaries.

The picture is typical of ectopic production of ACTH by tumour. Plasma ACTH is markedly raised in this condition, as is plasma cortisol. In most cases of ectopic ACTH production the disease progresses so rapidly that gross electrolyte and myopathic changes occur before the typical facies and the body habitus changes of Cushing's syndrome develop.

Squamous cell carcinoma can be associated with hypercalcaemia, not ACTH production. The usual lung cancer to produce this syndrome is small cell anaplastic carcinoma.

Although the electrolyte changes would be compatible with aldosterone excess, aldosterone secretion from lung carcinoma is not a recognised cause and it would not explain the pigmentation or myopathy.

Reference

1. Odell WD, Wolfsen AR. Hormonal syndromes associated with cancer. *Ann Rev Med* 1978; 29: 379–406.

36. Items B, D and E correct.

Hypertension above 150/90 mmHg occurs in about 80% of patients with Cushing's syndrome. Its presence does not help to distinguish the various possible types, although its frequency falls in patients with the ectopic form.

Excess plasma ACTH nocturnally is a useful finding but may be misleading in obese subjects. A more definitive test is lack of suppression of urinary 17-hydroxysteroids after low doses of dexamethasone (0.5 mg 6-hourly for 2 days).

However, higher doses of dexamethasone (2 mg 6-hourly for 2 days) do suppress urinary hydroxysteroids to less than 50% of the level found in controls, suggesting that the hypothalamic-pituitary axis is reset upwards and responds by inhibiting ACTH-release only at higher blood levels of glucocorticoids.

Refined procedures in sellar radiography now identify pituitary microadenomas in many cases of Cushing's syndrome in addition to the more demonstrable basophil and ACTH-producing chromophobe adenomas found in some patients.

External pituitary irradiation offers effective treatment (up to 80%) in children, but management in adults is more controversial. Gold mentions impressive advances in trans-sphenoidal surgery and drug therapy in recent years.

References

1. Williams RH (ed). Textbook of endocrinology, 5th Edn. Philadelphia: Saunders, 1974: 255–265.
2. Tyrrell JB, et al. Cushing's disease. *N Engl J Med* 1978; 298: 753–758.
3. Jennings AS, et al. Results of treating childhood Cushing's disease with pituitary irradiation. *N Engl J Med* 1977; 297: 957–962.
4. Gold EM. The Cushing syndromes: changing views of diagnosis and treatment. *Ann Intern Med* 1979; 90: 829–844.

37. Items A, B, D and E correct.

The 'empty sella syndrome' is being diagnosed more often as radiological techniques improve. A recent report involving 100 consecutive patients admitted for evaluation of an enlarged sella turcica indicated that at least 25% had the 'empty sella syndrome'. Endocrine abnormalities in such patients are rare, although occasionally an inadequate growth hormone response to insulin hypoglycaemia is noted. Visual field disturbances are rare and, if present, strongly suggest the presence of an underlying pituitary tumour. Elevated prolactin levels are very uncommon.

Prolactin hypersecretion is found in approximately one-third of all chromophobe adenomas, making it the most commonly hypersecreted anterior pituitary hormone. Most patients with circulating prolactin levels above 100–200 µg/ℓ, and virtually all patients with levels above 300 µg/ℓ, have a prolactin-secreting pituitary tumour.

Long-standing target organ failure can lead to pituitary hyperplasia and this has been reported in patients with primary hypothyroidism, Addison's disease and hypogonadism. It occurs most commonly with primary hypothyroidism. Treatment with thyroxine often results in a decrease in fossa size.

References

1. Weisberg LA, et al. Diagnosis and evaluation of patients with an enlarged sella turcica. *Am J Med* 1976; 61: 590–596.
2. Frantz AG. Prolactin. *N Engl J Med* 1978; 298: 201–207.

38. Items B, C, D and E correct.

Several large series have demonstrated that definite radiological abnormalities of the pituitary fossa are present in 90% or more of acromegalic patients. This contrasts with the findings in patients with prolactin-secreting adenomas where radiological abnormalities may be minor or absent.

While fasting serum growth hormone levels are usually elevated, they may not correlate with the severity of the illness and may be normal in some patients (10% or less). The oral glucose tolerance test with measurement of plasma growth hormone levels, particularly at 60 and 90 min following glucose, is the standard diagnostic test for acromegaly. In this condition growth hormone levels fail to be suppressed below 10 mU/ℓ (5 ng/ml). However, failure of suppression may be observed in other conditions (e.g. anorexia nervosa, chronic liver disease, renal failure, metastatic carcinoma).

The somatomedins are a family of circulating peptides which are believed to mediate the effects of growth hormone on cartilage and other skeletal tissue. The levels of several of these peptides are clearly elevated in acromegaly. It has been suggested recently that measurement of at least one of them may be of value in confirming the diagnosis or monitoring response to therapy.

Surgical decompression is usually recommended when there is a visual field defect or other evidence of progressive extra-fossa extension. However, the dopamine receptor agonist, bromocriptine, has been shown to be capable of inducing shrinkage of pituitary tumours with amelioration of visual field defects. This has been reported mainly with prolactin-secreting adenomas but also occurs in some acromegalic patients, particularly if the tumour also secretes prolactin. A carefully supervised trial use of bromocriptine could be considered in patients with optic nerve compression, proceeding to surgery if the tumour fails to shrink. Bromocriptine therapy may also be useful in patients who are either unfit for, or unwilling to have, surgery.

References

1. Phillips LS, Vassilopoulou-Sellin R. Somatomedins. *N Engl J Med* 1980; 302: 371–80, 438–446.
2. Wass JAH, et al. Reduction of pituitary-tumour size in patients with prolactinomas and acromegaly treated with bromocriptine with or without radiotherapy. *Lancet* 1979; 2: 66–69.
3. Daughaday WH. Editorial. New criteria for evaluation of acromegaly. *N Engl J Med* 1979; 301: 1175–1176.
4. Steinbeck K, Turtle JR. Treatment of acromegaly with bromocriptine. *Aust NZ J Med* 1979; 9: 217–224.

39. Items A, B and E correct.

Prolactin secretion with associated galactorrhoea and amenorrhoea can be stimulated by phenothiazines and also by metoclopramide, reserpine, alpha-methyldopa and oestrogens.

It is now recognised that chromophobe adenomas of the pituitary, previously regarded as functionless, often produce prolactin, which in turn may lead to amenorrhoea and galactorrhoea. Nillius and colleagues have reported fossa abnormalities due to microadenomas in 36% of affected women.

In premature menopause, galactorrhoea does not feature, serum prolactin is not raised and serum FSH and LH levels are elevated.

The prognosis for her fertility is not poor. Even if no specifc cause is demonstrated, the elevated prolactin level can often be lowered extremely effectively by the dopaminergic drug bromocriptine. This leads to restoration of ovulation and fertility.

Primary hypothyroidism can be associated with hyperprolactinaemia and galactorrhoea, perhaps due to increased secretion of the hypothalamic hormone TRH (thyrotrophin releasing hormone) which, as well as stimulating the secretion of TSH, also stimulates the secretion of prolactin.

References

1. Spark RF, et al. Galactorrhoea-amenorrhoea syndromes: etiology and treatment. *Ann Intern Med* 1976; 84: 532–537.
2. Frantz AG. Prolactin. *N Engl J Med* 1978; 298: 201–207.
3. Editorial. Hyperprolactinaemia: pituitary tumour or not? *Lancet* 1980; 1: 517–519.
4. Bergh T, et al. Hyperprolactinaemic amenorrhoea — results of treatment with bromocriptine. *Acta Endocrinol* 1978; 88: suppl 147–164.

40. Items C and D correct.

In the clinical situation presented, the most likely diagnosis is anorexia nervosa. Extreme weight loss is not a feature of hypopituitarism and there is little to suggest a pituitary tumour. Lowered LH and FSH levels reflect the depression of pituitary gonadotropin secretion which occurs in anorexia nervosa.

Protein binding is normal as reflected by the results of T_4 and T_3 resin uptake tests. In anorexia nervosa, no abnormality in binding proteins would be expected.

The picture of a low T_3 with normal T_4 can be found in cases of starvation and in severe illness of many forms including severe lobar pneumonia. It represents failure of peripheral deiodination of T_4 to T_3, with increased formation of reverse T_3.

In the failing thyroid, normal T_3 levels may be maintained while T_4 falls with a raised TSH level. Thus the $T_3 : T_4$ pattern in compensated hypothyroidism would be the reverse of that seen in this case.

In anorexia nervosa periods often resume only several months after achieving ideal body weight. The low LH and FSH indicate that it is the hypothalamus/pituitary which is at fault, not the ovary.

Reference

1. Beaumont PJV. Endocrinology of anorexia nervosa. *Med J Aust* 1979; 1: 611–613.

41. Items C and D correct.

A raised total, and especially free, plasma testosterone level is found in many subjects with hirsutism due to the polycystic ovary syndrome or to idiopathic causes. Only if it is extremely high does it suggest the very rare arrhenoblastoma.

The oral contraceptives suppress pituitary gonadotrophin secretion and reduce ovarian androgen production; therefore they may benefit the hirsutism rather than making it worse. In addition, oestrogens increase the sex hormone binding globulin, decreasing free testosterone levels.

Plasma LH is classically elevated in the polycystic ovary syndrome.

The short dexamethasone suppression test is an effective screening test for Cushing's syndrome.

Electrolysis is slow, expensive and relatively ineffective as a cosmetic measure for hirsutism. Shaving is the best cosmetic approach.

References

1. Crapo L. Cushing's syndrome: a review of diagnostic tests. *Metabolism* 1979; 28: 955–977.
2. Casey JH. Hirsutism: pathogenesis and treatment. *Aust NZ J Med* 1980; 10: 240–245.
3. Yen SSC. The polycystic ovary syndrome. *Clin Endocrinol* 1980; 12: 177–208.

42. Items B, D and E correct.

Gynaecomastia is a common disorder which is thought to result from a decrease in the ratio of circulating androgens : oestrogens. Bilateral breast tissue measuring 4 cm or less in diameter has been reported in up to one-third of normal men, and the prevalence progressively increases with advancing age.

The role of prolactin in the genesis of gynaecomastia is unclear and serum prolactin levels are normal in the vast majority of patients. Several medications have been clearly associated with gynaecomastia, and drug ingestion is the commonest cause of non-physiological gynaecomastia in adults. Drugs implicated in gynaecomastia include hormones (e.g. oestrogens, androgens, human chorionic gonadotrophin), antiandrogens (e.g. cimetidine, spironolactone, marihuana, progestogens, digitalis), and stimulators of prolactin (e.g. reserpine, phenothiazines).

Mammary carcinoma is rare and accounts for 0.2% of all cancer in male patients. The finding of bilateral breast swelling makes a diagnosis of carcinoma even less likely. Since benign breast enlargement is so common, biopsy is not recommended unless features suggestive of malignancy such as bloody nipple discharge, fixation, ulceration, asymmetry or axillary lymphadenopathy are present.

Hypogonadism from any cause, particularly hypergonadotropic hypogonadism, can induce gynaecomastica; in these situations testosterone treatment often induces at least a partial regression. However, testosterone treatment in patients with normal circulating testosterone levels is unlikely to be beneficial.

Orchitis is common in men with mumps, developing in about one-third of cases. About half of these sustain bilateral testicular atrophy irrespective of whether there was unilateral or bilateral orchitis clinically.

References

1. Carlson HE. (Current Concepts) Gynecomastia. *N Engl J Med* 1980; 303: 795–799.
2. Nuttall FQ. Gynecomastia as a physical finding in normal men. *J Clin Endocrinol Metab* 1979; 48: 338–340.
3. Aiman J, et al. Androgen and estrogen production in elderly men with gynecomastia and testicular atrophy after mumps orchitis. *J Clin Endocrinol Metab* 1980; 5: 380–386.

43. Items B, D and E correct.

There is now good evidence to indicate that patients with the above history are likely to be suffering from a generalised disorder termed the 'immotile-cilia syndrome' (Eliasson et al, 1977). In these patients there is a defect in the structure of cilia which consists of the absence of dynein arms; these are small projections passing between the adjacent doublet microtubules that compose the sperm tail and cilia. These 'arms' can only be detected by electron microscopy and are due to the absence of the protein dynein, an important component of the contractile apparatus. The defect results in absent directed cilial movement which can also be detected by techniques to measure muco-ciliary clearance in the respiratory tract (Eliasson et al, 1977; Burns 1979).

The defective ciliary function is probably the basis for bronchiectasis since secretions pool within the bronchi and lead to secondary infection. Such patients also suffer from sinusitis and a proportion have dextrocardia; the reason for the latter association is unknown but may indicate the need for directed ciliary function during embryogenesis to enable rotation of viscera.

References

1. Eliasson R, et al. The immotile-cilia syndrome. *N Engl J Med* 1977; 297: 1–6.
2. Burns MW. Fertility, immotile cilia and chronic respiratory infections. *Med J Aust* 1979; 2: 287–288.

44. Items B, D and E correct.

Thyrotoxicosis, most commonly due to Graves' disease, complicates about 2 per 1000 pregnancies. Diagnosis can be difficult since goitre, sweating and heat intolerance may be present in the euthyroid pregnant woman. Laboratory diagnosis is complicated by the increased serum protein binding of thyroid hormones resulting from increased oestrogens.

An understanding of the fate of various hormones and drugs is important in the management of the pregnant thyrotoxic patient. Studies using either radioactive-labelled or large doses of cold thyroid hormones support the concept that they cross the placenta only with difficulty. Thus, their addition to the therapeutic regimen is of doubtful value in ensuring fetal euthyroidism. Iodides and thionamides (including propylthiouracil and carbimazole) cross the placenta readily and may block the fetal thyroid, resulting in enhanced fetal TSH production and goitre. Propylthiouracil crosses the placenta to only about one-quarter of the extent of carbimazole, and is preferred over carbimazole for use in pregnancy. Carbimazole is transferred into milk extremely well but propylthiouracil crosses into the milk only one-tenth as well; nursing women should not take carbimazole, but if propylthiouracil is used the mother can be allowed to breast-feed. In Graves' disease, thyroid stimulating immunoglobulins may cross the placenta and stimulate the fetal thyroid. resulting in neonatal thyrotoxicosis. If the mother has been receiving carbimazole, the fetal thyroid may be blocked and thyrotoxicosis will be manifested in the infant only some days after birth when the effects of carbimazole are diminishing.

Choice of therapy for thyrotoxicosis in pregnancy is between antithyroid drugs and surgery. From published studies there appears to be little to choose between them. Surgery is usually undertaken in the second trimester and some advocate routine replacement with thyroxine for the duration of pregnancy. With antithyroid drugs the minimum dose to control the thyrotoxicosis should be used and maternal hypothyroidism strenuously avoided.

References

1. Burrow GN. Maternal-Fetal considerations in hyperthyroidism. *Clin Endocrinol Metab* 1978; 7(1): 115–125.
2. Cooper DS. Antithyroid drugs. *N Engl J Med* 1984; 311: 1353–1362.

45. Items A, B and D correct.

Subacute thyroiditis appears to represent a viral-related illness in genetically susceptible people (HLA-B35). The clinical picture is quite variable in mode of onset and severity. Typically a prodromal illness with malaise, fever, or an upper respiratory tract infection is followed by moderate to severe pain in the region of the thyroid which may radiate to the ear, the angle of the jaw and down to the anterior chest. Systemic symptoms are common, as are features of mild to moderate hyperthyroidism. There may however be painless thyroid swelling without tenderness or systemic symptoms, although the patients have features of thyrotoxicosis.

Laboratory tests in subacute thyroiditis typically show a markedly elevated erythocyte sedimentation rate (ESR) and a normal leukocyte count. Thyroid autoantibodies are elevated in a minority of patients and then to only a modest degree. Plasma thyroid hormone levels are raised as a result of leakage of colloid from damaged follicles. Radioactive iodine uptake is characteristically depressed.

There is no specific therapy. However, corticosteroids give rapid symptomatic relief. In many cases the administration of simple analgesics, together with propranolol to relieve the symptoms of hyperthyroidism, is adequate.

The phase of hyperthyroidism is followed by one of hypothyroidism, but this is rarely permanent.

Reference

1. Volpe R. Subacute (de Quervain's) thyroiditis. *Clin Endocrinol Metab* 1979; 8(1): 81–95.

46. Items B and D correct.

The clinical entity of painless thyroiditis and hyperthyroidism has become increasingly recognised in the past few years. It has a predilection for the post-partum period. The hallmark of the illness is the recent onset of thyrotoxicosis in a patient with a normal to moderately enlarged non-tender gland, low radioactive iodine uptake and no history of thyroid hormone or iodide exposure. The thyrotoxicosis is transient, rarely relapsing and adequately controlled by modest doses of propranolol, if any treatment is required at all. Documented permanent hypothyroidism is uncommon but relapse in subsequent pregnancies has been well described.

The aetiology of painless thyroiditis is unknown and it may in fact be a heterogeneous disorder. Although the majority of evidence points to an immunological disorder, conventional antithyroid antibodies are variable in their presence.

Recognition of the entity is of extreme importance in view of its good prognosis, the lack of need for specific antithyroid therapy, but the potential for recurrence.

References

1. Ginsberg J, Walfish PG. Post-partum transient thyrotoxicosis with painless thyroiditis. *Lancet* 1977; 1: 1125–1127.
2. Greer MA, et al. Short-term antithyroid drug therapy for the thyrotoxicosis of Graves' disease. *N Engl J Med* 1977; 297: 173–176.
3. Woolf PO. Transient painless thyroiditis with hyperthyroidism. A variant of lymphocytic thyroiditis? *Endo Rev* 1980; 1: 411.
4. Amino N, et al. High prevalence of transient post-partum thyrotoxicosis and hypothyroidism. *N Engl J Med* 1982; 306: 849–852.

47. Item D correct.

A 'hot' nodule (i.e. increased uptake of technetium compared with the remainder of the gland) is associated with a low risk of malignancy (less than 1%). A 'cold' nodule with decreased uptake has a risk of malignancy of up to 20%. A nodule with equal uptake compared with the remainder of the gland is associated with a reported risk of malignancy almost as great as a cold nodule. The relative risk of thyroid cancer is greater in male patients with single nodules, particularly at a young age, and in nodules of this size. Thus no more than a short trial of suppressive therapy for up to 3 months would be justified in this patient and surgical resection should be advised if there is not prompt resolution of the nodule.

Hashimoto's disease and thyroid cancer may coexist in the same gland and the finding of high titres of antithyroglobulin antibodies does not exclude the diagnosis of thyroid cancer. Occasionally, lymphoma may arise in the lymphoid follicles of Hashimoto's thyroiditis.

Demonstration by ultrasound of a smooth, thin-walled cyst would make the diagnosis of thyroid cancer unlikely, but thick-walled cysts are frequently associated with malignancy.

Fine needle aspiration biopsy is being used increasingly in the diagnosis of thyroid cancer. The test combines high sensitivity with a relatively high specificity. False-negatives may occur and if there is clinical suspicion of malignancy, surgery should be done despite negative cytological findings.

Serum thyroglobulin levels are elevated in a variety of thyroid diseases and are not specific for thyroid cancer. Estimation of serum thyroglobulin concentration may, however, be useful as a marker of recurrence in patients who have had total thyroid ablation for thyroid cancer.

References

1. Van Herle AJ, et al. The thyroid nodule. *Ann Intern Med* 1982; 96: 221–232.
2. Ingbar SH, Woeber KA. The thyroid gland. In: Williams RH, ed. Textbook of endocrinology, 6th Edn. Philadelphia: Saunders, 1981: 117–247.

48. Items B, D and E correct.

Steroid suppressibility of hypercalcaemia is usually absent in primary hyperparathyroidism. This contrasts with the situation in sarcoidosis, milk alkali syndrome, vitamin D intoxication, thyrotoxicosis, multiple myeloma and some cases of hypercalcaemia associated with bone secondaries, where the hypercalcaemia is steroid suppressible.

Thiazides decrease urinary calcium excretion, and tend to exacerbate hypercalcaemia (by contrast, frusemide tends to enhance urinary calcium excretion).

A patient with a strong family history of hypercalcaemia, and low urinary calcium, is likely to have familial hypocalciuric hypercalcaemia (Marx et al, 1978). It is important to be aware of this condition, which is transmitted as a Mendelian dominant trait, as parathyroid surgery is usually not indicated. Hypocalciuria is a characteristic feature of the syndrome, and together with the family history, separates it from hyperparathyroidism.

Most assays for parathyroid hormone show a significant overlap between normal subjects and patients with primary hyperparathyroidism. A normal value does not exclude primary hyperparathyroidism.

Squamous cell carcinoma of the lung is the most common type of tumour to produce hypercalcaemia in the absence of bone metastases. The mechanism is not clear, but in most cases it does not appear to be ectopic production of parathyroid hormone.

References

1. Martin TJ, Larkins RG. Hypercalcaemia including hyperparathyroidism. *Medicine International* 1981; 6: A482–A486.
2. Marx SJ, et al. Divalent cation metabolism: familial hypocalciuric hypercalcaemia versus typical hyperparathyroidism. *Am J Med* 1978; 65: 235–242.

49. Items A, D and E correct.

Proximal myopathy is a common feature of osteomalacia of most causes. Vitamin D metabolites have a direct action on muscle; hypophosphataemia, which often occurs in osteomalacia, may also contribute.

The serum phosphorus level is usually low in all forms of osteomalacia except that associated with chronic renal disease (which is excluded in this patient by the normal creatinine).

The major source of vitamin D activity in our community is exposure to sunlight rather than the diet. However, margarine is a much richer source of vitamin D than butter as it is supplemented with vitamin D_2.

A raised serum alkaline phosphatase level of skeletal origin is usually present in osteomalacia, reflecting increased (but ineffective) osteoblastic activity.

Malabsorption is a relatively common cause of osteomalacia and partial gastrectomy may well contribute to this, particularly in elderly patients who have restricted their exposure to sunlight.

References

1. Melick RA, et al. Osteomalacia due to unusual causes presenting in adults. *Aust NZ J Med* 1979; 9: 253–257.
2. Frame B, Parfitt AM. Osteomalacia: current concepts. *Ann Intern Med* 1978; 89: 966–982.

50. All items correct.

Herpes zoster is a relatively common condition and is one of the first viral diseases for which specific therapy is becoming available. It is accepted that the condition results from reactivation of a virus that has lain dormant in spinal nerves since an episode of varicella-zoster infection.

Thoracic nerves are involved in about 55% of cases, the next most common involvement being the cervical area. The 'girdle-like' rash indicates the dermatome involved and motor neuropathies, which occur in up to 30% of affected patients, are usually restricted to that area. This paralysis has a good prognosis, with about 75% complete recovery and regained strength in most others. More serious neurological complications, although less frequent, include meningitis, encephalitis and myelitis. Cranial nerve involvement can lead to ophthalmic zoster and contralateral hemiplegia.

Immune incompetence, whether due to neoplastic disease or immunosuppressive drugs, is associated with more frequent, prolonged and more widely disseminated zoster infection. In patients with lymphomas the incidence may be as high as 25%, compared with about 5% in the wider community. Irradiation can lead to localised infection, but compromised patients usually show a more scattered involvement. When withdrawal of responsible drugs is feasible, herpetic lesions sometimes improve rapidly.

Acyclovir has been shown to be more effective and less toxic than previously tried antiviral drugs. Therapy is most successful when administered early in younger patients. Pain and post-herpetic neuralgia are reduced in most patients.

References

1. Dolin R, et al. Herpes zoster-varicella infections in immunosuppressed patients. *Ann Intern Med* 1978; 89: 375–388.
2. Editorial. Antiviral treatment of varicella zoster and herpes simplex. *Lancet* 1980; 1: 1337–1339.

51. Items B, C and E correct.

Traveller's diarrhoea is usually of short duration, self-limited and now considered to be largely due to enterotoxigenic *E. coli*. Ampicillin therapy is not indicated in cases of traveller's diarrhoea.

A normal sigmoidoscopy and absence of blood in the faeces makes a diagnosis of ameobic colitis unlikely, although it does not completely exclude it. The diagnosis of ameobic dysentery is best achieved by examination of repeated very fresh stool specimens and rectal mucosal scrapings for identification of the trophozoite of *Entamoeba histolytica*.

The clinical history and a normal sigmoidoscopy make giardiasis the most likely diagnosis. Rather than looking for *Giardia* in the stool, a more reliable method of confirmation is the microscopic examination of duodenal aspirates stained with Giemsa stain (obtained either by a Crosby peroral biopsy tube or by duodenal intubation). This is preferable to duodenoscopy and duodenal biopsy, which are expensive and discomforting to the patient.

Metronidazole ('Flagyl') and tinidazole ('Fasigyn') have replaced mepacrine ('Atabrine') as treatment for giardiasis. 2g 'Flagyl' for 3 days is an effective dose in 90% of patients. Tinidazole is probably the treatment of choice and may be given as single statim dose of 2 g orally.

Reference

1. Brandborg LL. Parasitic diseases. In: Sleisenger MH, Fordran JS. (eds). Gastrointestinal disease, 2nd Edn. Philadelphia: Saunders, 1978: 1154–1181.

52. Items A, C, D and E correct.

For treatment of giardiasis, the dosage of metronidazole is 2 g single daily dose for 3 days (90% cure-rate reported) or 250 mg 3 times per day for 7–10 days (70–83% cure-rate).

Antibiotics are contraindicated in most cases of salmonella gastroenteritis. The best antibiotics (if they have to be given) are ampicillin or co-trimoxazole ('Bactrim').

Metronidazole may interact with alcohol, producing an 'Antabuse-like' effect, and patients should be warned of this. The unpleasant metallic taste can cause compliance problems, especially with children, for whom intravenous administration may be preferable. Other less common side-effects include nausea, headache, leukopenia and peripheral neuropathy.

Mutagenesis has occurred in laboratory studies (Ames test) as well as increased tumour formation in susceptible experimental animals. Metronidazole is contraindicated in pregnancy and lactation.

References

1. Knight R. Giardiasis. *Clin Gastroenterol* 1978; 7: 31–47.
2. Joiner KA, Gorbach SI. Antimicrobial therapy of digestive diseases. *Clin Gastroenterol* 1979; 8: 3–35.

53. Items A, B, C and E correct.

Campylobacter jejuni has become well recognised as a frequent cause of enterocolitis in children and adults. It can be transmitted by direct contact with animals (especially live and dressed chicken), ingestion of contaminated food, and by faecal-oral routes. Successful culture needs a special atmosphere with increased carbon dioxide and decreased oxygen.

Campylobacter enterocolitis characteristically causes a disease of rapid onset. Malaise, fever, headache, myalgia, backache and arthralgia are common, as are abdominal cramping pains. The diarrhoea may be bloody or contain occult blood in 60% or more of patients and polymorphonuclear leukocytes are demonstrated in the stools of more than 75% of patients.

Colitis with proctitis resembling that seen in ulcerative proctitis may be seen on sigmoidoscopy. Rectal biopsy shows many of the features seen with ulcerative colitis, including decreased mucus production and crypt abscesses.

About 80% of patients have a self-limiting illness lasting less than 1 week, although relapses, usually milder than the initial episode, occur in about 25%.

Antibiotic therapy is not warranted in most patients. Recent studies have not shown that erythromycin therapy is better than placebo in the treatment of campylobacter enteritis. However, there are anecdotal reports of effective treatment with erythromycin in the severely ill, or those with protracted illness, and it seems warranted to treat such patients.

References

1. Blaser MJ, Reller LB, et al. Campylobacter enteritis. *N Engl J Med* 1981; 305: 1444.
2. Lambert ME, et al. Campylobacter colitis. *Br Med J* 1979; 1: 857–859.
3. Blaser MJ, et al. Acute colitis caused by Campylobacter fetus ss, jejuni. *Gastroenterology* 1980; 78: 448–453.
4. Butzler JP, Skirrow MB. Campylobacter enteritis. *Clin Gastroenterol* 1979; 8(3): 737–765.
5. Skirrow MB. Campylobacter enteritis: The first five years. *J Hygiene* 1982; 89(2): 175.
6. Anders BJ, et al. Double-blind placebo controlled trial of erythromycin for treatment of campylobacter enteritis. *Lancet* 1982; 1: 131.

54. Items D and E are correct.

Strongyloides stercoralis infection was acquired by many prisoners of war in the endemic regions of South-East Asia. *Strongyloides* persists because it autoinfects the host. Among Australian ex-servicemen captured at the fall of Singapore in 1942, 27.5% where shown to have *Strongyloides* larvae in the faeces after thirty or more years. Individuals with this type of strongyloidiasis are often asymptomatic and generally have low worm loads. However, in many, symptoms such as urticaria, diarrhoea and indigestion have been present from time to time.

This parasite infects man when infective filariform larvae in soil penetrate the skin, enter the bloodstream and pass to the lungs, migrate up the tracheobronchial tree and are swallowed. Reaching the duodenum and proximal jejunum, they develop into adult worms. The female adults live in the mucosa. Ova produced immediately hatch out rhabditiform larvae, which may pass out in faeces to develop into filariform larvae in the soil, or differentiate into filariform larvae in the bowel lumen and can reinfect the host by penetrating the bowel wall or the perianal skin after excretion.

High eosinophil counts are found in 75% of persons with persistent strongyloidiasis, but only 10–30% of those with disseminated disease have eosinophilia.

Larvae are found in duodenal or proximal jejunal juice, or in faeces. Studies in chronically infected persons found the diagnostic yield was highest from faecal examination, although repeated examination may be required. Rhabditiform larvae are found, seldom ova. Faeces freshly passed by an infected patient usually contain active larvae; concentration and culture techniques can increase the yield of true-positives.

If the immune response (particularly the cell-mediated arm) is depressed, the worm load can greatly increase and large numbers of filariform larvae penetrate into the bloodstream to produce a disseminated infection in which any organ can be involved. Enteric bacteria often enter the bloodstream as the larvae penetrate the bowel wall; it is thought that enteric bacteria are also carried both externally and internally by the larvae. Under these conditions, *Strongyloides* larvae may be found in a variety of specimens including sputum, urine and CSF.

Thiabendazole 25 mg/kg twice daily orally is the recommended treatment. In the normal host, 2 days therapy should suffice, but in the compromised host longer courses of treatment will be required. This will usually be of the order of 5–7 days but will depend ultimately on the results of regular close monitoring of faeces and other specimens for *Strongyloides*.

References

1. Grove DI. Strongyloidiasis in Allied ex-prisoners of war in South-East Asia. *Br Med J* 1980; 280: 598–601.
2. Masur M, Jones TC. Protozoal and helminthic infections. In: Grieco MH (ed). Infections in the Abnormal Host. New York. Yorke Medical Books, 1980: 428–430.
3. Scowden EB, et al. Overwhelming strongyloidiasis: an unappreciated opportunistic infection. *Medicine* (Baltimore) 1978; 57: 527–544.

55. Items A and E correct.

Despite screening of blood donors to eliminate the risk of hepatitis B infection, post-transfusion hepatitis remains a significant problem and the majority of cases are now classified as non-A and non-B hepatitis. Testing for hepatitis B has led to a reduction of only 20% in the overall incidence of post-transfusion hepatitis.

French and Japanese workers have isolated a virus (hepatitis C) from the serum of some patients with this form of hepatitis, but most workers believe that, because of the differing incubation periods, at least two different viruses are responsible for non-A non-B hepatitis. At present there is no satisfactory test for non-A non-B hepatitis.

Up to 40% of patients with non-A non-B hepatitis progress to chronic liver injury and at least half of these will have chronic active hepatitis. Chronic active hepatitis following non-A non-B hepatitis tends to be milder than that in patients with hepatitis B.

In a recent series, non-A non-B hepatitis virus was responsible for 40–50% of fulminant hepatitis cases, although this condition occurs in less than 2% of all patients with hepatitis.

References

1. Wong DC, et al. Epidemic and endemic hepatitis in India: evidence for a non-A, non-B hepatitis virus aetiology. *Lancet* 1980; 2: 876–878.
2. Vitvitski L, et al. Detection of virus-associated antigen in serum and liver of patients with non-A non-B hepatitis. *Lancet* 1980; 2: 1263–1267.
3. Mathiesen LR, et al. The role of acute hepatitis type A, B and non A non B in the development of chronic active liver disease. *Scand J Gastroenterol* 1980; 15: 49–54.

4. Hollinger FB, et al. Transfusion-transmitted viruses study: experimental evidence for two non A, non B hepatitis agents. *J Infect Dis* 1980; 12: 400.

56. Items A and E correct.

Hepatitis A and B have now been clearly defined in epidemiological and virological terms. For hepatitis A infection the period of faecal viral excretion and infectivity relates to the incubation phase, with minimal risk for a transient period after jaundice appears. This is in contrast to patients with hepatitis B where infectivity relates to the presence of HB_sAg—whether in the acute or chronic phase, and whether in the jaundiced or non-jaundiced clinical state. In this situation blood and/or bodily secretions such as saliva constitute the infectious risk. Laboratory confirmation of viral hepatitis is best approached by excluding hepatitis B. It is also now possible to diagnose acute hepatitis A by detecting IgM anti-HAV.

HB_sAg is the first serological marker to appear after exposure to hepatitis B virus. Clinical symptoms and biochemical changes of acute hepatitis do not arise until HB_sAg has been present for 2–8 weeks. Other markers which may indicate acute infection include antibody to hepatitis B core antigen, hepatitis B e-antigen, and DNA-polymerase. However, these markers may only be helpful in this acute clinical setting, as they can persist for years in a chronic hepatitis B virus carrier state.

The presence of antibody to HB_s indicates past infection and it appears during the convalescent phase. By this time HB_sAg has usually disappeared. Most data suggest that persons with anti-HB_s no longer harbour hepatitis B virus and are immune to reinfection with this virus.

Lymphadenopathy, splenomegaly, sore throat and rash sometimes occur with viral hepatitis, especially in the pre-jaundice phase. These symptoms and signs should not deter the physician from suspecting viral hepatitis, even in the presence of atypical peripheral blood lymphocytes. Other causes (such as infectious mononucleosis, cytomegalovirus, toxoplasmosis, bacterial liver abscess, leptospirosis, hydatid disease and bacteraemia) need to be considered, as they can simulate acute viral hepatitis. Thus the Paul-Bunnell test, cytomegalovirus and perhaps toxoplasmosis tests are indicated in this circumstance.

Until the recently-developed vaccines become readily available, the indications for passive immunisation of contacts are limited to susceptible persons exposed to infectious material. Pooled gammaglobulin from blood donors in many Western countries provides little protection against hepatitis B, because the antibody titre is quite low. If the dentist had washed his hands adequately he should not have transmitted hepatitis A. The only contacts requiring immunisation with gammaglobulin are persons in constant contact with the index case, i.e. family or 'seat' contacts. Such an immunisation programme should be undertaken only when hepatitis A appears to be a likely diagnosis in the index patient. It should take only 5–7 days to exclude other causes.

References

1. Combined Medical Research Council and Public Health Laboratory Service. Report: the incidence of hepatitis B infection after accidental exposure and anti-HB_s immunoglobulin prophylaxis. *Lancet* 1980; 1: 6–8.
2. Hoofnagle JH, et al. Type B hepatitis after transfusion with blood containing antibody to hepatitis B core antigen. *N Engl J Med* 1978; 298: 1379–1383.
3. Gust ID. Recent developments in hepatitis A. *Pathology* 1978; 10: 299–306.

57. Item D correct.

Cryptococcal meningitis should always be suspected in an immunologically compromised host. It may present as a subacute or chronic form of meningitis. Headache is generally regarded as the major presenting symptom. Fever may be absent in the immunosuppressed host.

The likelihood of bacterial endocarditis is not seriously increased by long periods of steroid therapy in an asthmatic patient.

Headaches or chronic migraine are characteristically intermittent, and not long-term as in this case. The headache of subarachnoid haemorrhage is classically of abrupt onset, usually associated with alteration in levels of consciousness.

References

1. Thomson RA. Clinical features of central nervous system fungus infection. In: Thomson RA, Green JR (eds). Advances in neurology, Vol 6. New York: Raven Press, 1974: 93–100.
2. Lewis JL, Rabinovich S. The wide spectrum of cryptococcal infections. *Am J Med* 1972; 53: 315–322.
3. Allsop JL, et al. Cryptococcal meningitis. *Proc Aust Assoc Neurol* 1970; 7: 71–76.

58. Items A, B, C and D correct.

The VDRL test was the most widely used serological test for syphilis, but most laboratories now use one of the two modifications for routine screening; the RPR or the automated reagin test (ART). These tests are flocculation tests designed to show the presence of a non-specific antilipoidal antibody, reagin. Tests of specific anti-treponemal antibodies are more expensive and time-consuming and thus are not normally used for screening purposes. Such tests include the treponema pallidum immobilisation test (TPI) the fluorescent treponemal antibody absorption test (FTA-ABS) and the treponema pallidum haemagglutination test (TPHA).

The RPR is positive in 80% of primary disease, 99% of secondary and 70% of late disease or latent syphilis (untreated). CSF shows a positive VDRL in only 22–61% of patients with neurosyphilis.

False-positive serum VDRL tests are found in many conditions including the collagen disorders, pregnancy, narcotic addiction and many infectious diseases. A false-positive VDRL in CSF rarely occurs unless blood, positive for the VDRL test, has contaminated the CSF during the lumbar puncture. Most studies have suggested that the FTA test is positive more often than the VDRL in CSF from patients with clinical neurosyphilis.

Serial VDRL titres may be used to monitor the results of treatment. Successful treatment of a patient with seropositive primary syphilis results in conversion to VDRL negativity in about 75% of patients within 3–12 months and in nearly all patients by 24 months. In late syphilis the response of reagin tests with treatment is less predictable and patients may remain seropositive for many years.

References

1. Bracero L, et al. Serologic tests for syphilis: a guide to interpretation in various stages of disease. *Mt Sinai J Med* 1979; 46: 289–292.
2. Oates JK. Serological tests for syphilis and their clinical use. *Br J Hosp Med* 1979; 21: 612–617.

59. Items A, B and E correct.

Recent advances in culture techniques have allowed ready recognition of various strains of chlamydiae as causes of a variety of common diseases ranging from urethritis to conjunctivitis and pneumonia.

The term '*Chlamydia*' refers to a genus which comprises who major species — *Chlamydia trachomatis* and *Chlamydia psittaci*. The species *Chlamydia trachomatis* now includes all those micro-organisms which have previously been known as '*Bedsonia*', TRIC agents and agents of lymphogranuloma venereum (LGV) and trachoma. These organisms only infect epithelial cells, wherein they produce typical inclusions (hence inclusion conjunctivitis). Specific diagnosis therefore requires collection of epithelial (not pus) cells which can be viewed microscopically and which constitute the best specimens for culture. This means that cells must be scraped from the urethra with a wire loop or collected from sclerae after pus has been removed. The availability of monoclonal fluorescent antibody tests is increasingly making rapid diagnosis more accessible.

Chlamydia trachomatis causes most cases of 'non-specific' urethritis in males. Contact tracing indicates a high consort infection rate. Cervical carriage is common and accounts for most cases of neonatal conjunctivitis which occurs typically 8–12 days post-partum. The strains responsible for adult conjunctivitis and pneumonia differ from genital strains. All chlamydiae can be susceptible to therapy with tetracyclines, erythromycin, sulphonamides, trimethoprim and chloramphenicol. Penicillin, ampicillin and other cell-wall antibiotics are inactive — hence one may observe 'post-gonococcal' urethritis after ampicillin therapy for proven gonorrhoea. This is the basis for the suggestion that tetracycline should be the first-line treatment for gonococcal urethritis. It is recognised that at least 25% of patients who contract gonorrhoea concurrently acquire chlamydial infection.

Concurrent bacterial or viral infection with chlamydiae is well recognised not only with 'gonococcal' urethritis, but also with respiratory infections where cytomegalovirus (CMV) and chlamydiae have been shown to co-exist.

From the clinical viewpoint it is important to consider chlamydial infection in situations where penicillin (or ampicillin/cephalosporin) has failed. Typically, in chlamydial infection, in comparison with bacterial infection, the course of the disease is more protracted, with a longer incubation, period and discharges or exudates are seropurulent rather than grossly purulent. Cotrimoxazole eradicates some but not all chlamydial infections.

References

1. Komaroff AL, Frielland G. Editorial. The dysuria-pyuria syndrome. *N Engl J Med* 1980; 303: 452–454.
2. Schachter J. Chlamydial infections. *N Engl J Med* 1978; 298: 428–35, 490–495, 540–549.

60. Items A and B correct.

A great deal of recent work has been directed to the study of dental caries, the most prevalent human infectious disease. Caries is localized progressive tooth decay due to demineralisation of the hydroxyapatite enamel surface by locally produced organic acids. Clean enamel is soon coated by a thin layer of salivary substances (mainly glycoproteins), cellular debris, food particles and a few bacteria. The bacterial load, mostly streptococci, greatly increases until the tooth surface is covered by plaque, an aggregate of bacteria, salivary proteins and inorganic salts.

Adhesive extracellular polysaccharides, produced by *Streptococcus mutans* in particular, renders plaque more dense and compact, a structure in which acid accumulates. Of several species of streptococci found in plaque, *S. mutans* is much the most cariogenic. *Lactobacillus acidophilus* is often associated with caries and is probably cariogenic in some circumstances; actinomycetes too may be contributory.

Frequent presentation of sucrose produces increased caries by increasing the frequency with which plaque pH falls to demineralising levels.

Immunisation of various species of animal, including primates, has had varying success but, overall, immunisation against *S. mutans* seems to lessen plaque load and caries, whether local or systemic antibodies appear. Secretary IgA washes over plaque in saliva and serum antibodies appear in the fluid of the gingival crevice.

Fluoride administration reduces the incidence of caries. In addition, several antibiotics and antibacterial mouthwashes (including chlorhexidine and alexidine, cetylpyridinium and benzalkonium chloride) have been shown to reduce plaque formation and gingivitis. Although most of these have undesirable side-effects or risks, they may be useful in occasional patients with diseases affecting the teeth and gums.

References

1. Andlaw RJ. Diet and dental caries — a review. *J Hum Nutr* 1977; 31: 45–52.

2. Cole JA. A biochemical approach to the control of dental caries. *Biochem Soc Trans* 1977; 5: 1232–1239.
3. Johnson RH, Rozanis J. A review of chemotherapeutic plaque control. *Oral Surg* 1977; 47: 136–141.
4. Scully C. Dental caries: progress in microbiology and immunology. *J Infect* 1981; 3: 107–133.

61. Items A, B, D and E correct.

AHC has spread in pandemic fashion, involving India, Pakistan, Bangladesh, parts of Central and South America and, more recently, the islands of the South Pacific region.

The disease has very high attack rates and appears abruptly after an incubation period of about one day. Unlike most enterovirus infections, spread is probably most often via fingers or fomites contaminated with infective eye secretions; fomites include towels and shared washing water. The disease is most prevalent under crowded conditions and where there is poor sanitation.

Symptoms begin in one eye but the other is very soon involved. They include burning sensation, eye pain, photophobia, swollen eyelids, watery discharge and the outstanding feature of subconjunctival haemorrhage. Pre-auricular nodes are often enlarged. Recovery is the rule within 10 days.

In some areas, enterovirus 70 has proven difficult to isolate from the eyes and it is quite unusual to isolate it from faeces or other sites. Diagnosis can be confirmed by demonstrating a significant rise in titre of serum neutralising antibodies to enterovirus 70.

In 1 in 10 000–15 000 cases paralysis has followed AHC, usually after an interval of about 2 weeks; because of the high numbers of cases contracting AHC, the complication of CNS involvement has been a numerically significant one. In the typical case, acute hypotonic areflexic asymmetrical proximal paralysis of the lower limbs is seen, often with fever, radicular pain and paresthesiae. The second most common neurological complication has been cranial nerve palsy, usually affecting isolated nerves (principally the facial nerve). Antibodies to enterovirus 70 should be sought in the CSF. Neurological complications have not been reported after American cases but have been seen in India and Asia.

Treatment of conjunctivitis is symptomatic. There is no specific therapy and antibiotics are not indicated unless there is a bacterial superinfection.

References

1. Kono R, et al. Pandemic of new type of conjunctivitis. *Lancet* 1972; 1: 1191–1194.
2. Mirkovic RR, et al. Enterovirus type 70: the etiologic agent of pandemic acute haemorrhagic conjunctivitis. *Bull WHO* 1973; 49: 341–346.
3. Leading Article. Neurovirulence of enterovirus 70. *Lancet* 1982; 1: 373–374.

62. Items C, D and E are correct.

Since 1958 there has been a stepwise increase in resistance of *Neisseria gonorrhoeae* isolates to penicillin and this was made evident by treatment failures. By increasing doses of penicillin, successful treatment continued for some time. However, preparations giving prolonged but low plasma penicillin levels, such as benzathine penicillin, are not suitable for the treatment of gonorrhoea; doses of procaine penicillin G in excess of 3 million units with probenecid are required for success. An appropriate alternative treatment is a single dose of 3 g oral ampicillin or amoxycillin with probenecid. Tetracycline 1.5 g stat then 0.5 g four times a day for 5 days is another well established alternative treatment for penicillin-sensitive strains.

In 1976 a totally new problem emerged with the identification of beta lactamase-producing organisms highly resistant to penicillin. Therapy with penicillin G even in very large doses will result in failure. Although the most common known sources for these organisms are Bangkok, Bali, Singapore and Manila, increasing numbers are being reported around the world from patients who have never left their country of origin.

Gonococcal bacteraemia occurs in approximately 1–3% of infected patients. Of these, up to 80% of both men and women have asymptomatic local infection before dissemination, due to the propensity of a strain with unique nutritional requirements to cause both disseminated gonococcal infection and asymptomatic genital infection. This strain is characterised by its requirement for hypoxanthine and uracil and is usually penicillin-sensitive.

Erythromycin is the treatment of choice in infected women who are pregnant and allergic to penicillin. Co-trimoxazole has been used but is probably best avoided during pregnancy. Spectinomycin is the drug of choice for penicillinase-producing *Neisseria gonorrhoeae*, but has not been proven safe in pregnancy.

While it is appropriate to commence initial therapy without waiting for laboratory confirmation, it is necessary to obtain a follow-up swab 4–7 days later to ensure that the infection has cleared.

References

1. Leading Article. Penicillinase producing N. gonorrhoeae (PPNG)—1981. Communicable Diseases Intelligence 1982; 3: 2–3. (A publication of the Commonwealth Department of Health, Australia).
2. VD Control Div. CDC. Global distribution of penicillase-producing Neisseria gonorrhoeae (PPNG). US Department of Health and Human Services: Morbidity and Mortality Weekly Report 1982; 31: 1–3.
3. Crawford G, et al. Asymptomatic gonorrhoea in men: caused by gonococci with unique nutritional requirements. *Science* 1977; 196: 1352–1353.
4. Garrod LP, et al. Antibiotic and chemotherapy, 5th Edn. New York: Churchill Livingstone, 1981: 422–426.

63. Items B and D correct.

The history strongly suggests bacterial endocarditis caused by *Streptococcus faecalis*. Penicillin G and streptomycin do not show synergism in vitro against all strains of *S. faecalis*. A combination of penicillin G and gentamicin is synergistic against almost all strains. Unfortunately there are also many strains of *S. faecalis* which are highly resistant to streptomycin and these show no synergy with penicillin G. Gentamicin is now widely regarded as preferable to streptomycin for treating enterococcal endocarditis, though its suitability for each patient should be verified by in vitro testing.

It is also generally accepted that the use of ampicillin alone is not as good as the combination of penicillin G with gentamicin. Adequate serum bactericidal activity can only be achieved when ampicillin is used in combination with an aminoglycoside, and even then very large doses of ampicillin are required.

For those allergic to penicillin, vancomycin is recommended. Although in experimental rabbit endocarditis a combination of vancomycin and gentamicin has been shown to be synergistic and more effective than vancomycin alone, clinical proof of the superiority of this combination is not available. There would be some concern at the use of two ototoxins together.

Cephalosporins are not recommended for the treatment of *S. faecalis* endocarditis. *S. faecalis* is resistant to all cephalosporins.

The mortality of *S. faecalis* endocarditis is still approximately 20%. Antibiotic therapy is difficult. Laboratory estimation of the minimum bactericidal concentration of the antibiotic together with measurement of serum bactericidal activity is essential.

References

1. Ruhen RW, Darrell JH. Antibiotic synergism against Group D streptococci in the treatment of endocarditis. *Med J Aust* 1973; 2: 114–116.
2. Gutschik E, et al. Effect of combinations of penicillin and aminoglycosides on *Streptococcus faecalis*: a comparative study of seven aminoglycoside antibiotics. *J Infect Dis* 1977; 135: 832–836.
3. Mandel G, et al. Principles and practice of infectious diseases. New York: Wiley, 1979: 651.
4. Kucers A, Bennett NMck. The use of antibiotics: a comprehensive review with clinical emphasis, 3rd Edn. London: Heinemann, 1979: 34.

64. All items correct.

Amantadine is a tricyclic amine with in vitro activity against a range of RNA viruses. However the only clinical activity is against influenza A, including those with the surface antigenic markers H0N1, H1N1, H2N2, H3N2, Hsw1N1. A number of studies have demonstrated prophylactic efficacy of amantadine and the closely related rimantadine. The drug seems to provide over 60% protection against clinical influenza and about 50% protection against infection with the virus overall. A number of studies have also shown therapeutic efficacy in influenza A infection, shown by diminution in fever and shorter duration of illness.

Prophylaxis is recommended for those who have not been vaccinated or have a contraindication to influenza immunisation and who fall into the groups for whom protection against influenza is desirable: the elderly, the chronically ill (especially if in residential institutions), health care personnel. Prophylaxis is begun as soon as influenza appears in the community and should continue throughout the period of influenza risk, as the protective effect is lost on stopping the drug. As it does not interfere with the antibody response to influenza vaccine, the drug can be taken after immunisation for about two weeks to provide protection during the period before antibodies to influenza appear.

Amantadine is given in a dose of 100 mg twice daily orally for prophylaxis. 3–7% of patients develop side-effects, mainly confined to the central nervous system and including insomnia, difficulty in concentrating, nervousness and dizziness. The drug accumulates if there is renal impairment, resulting in greater toxic effects including hallucinations, convulsions and coma.

References

1. Hayden FG, Douglas RG. Antiviral agents. In: Mandell GL, et al (eds). Principles and practice of infectious diseases. New York: Wiley, 1979: 353–369.
2. Hirsch MS, Swartz MN. Antiviral agents. *N Engl J Med* 1980; 302: 903–907, 949–953.
3. Kucers A, Bennett NMcK. Amantadine. In: The use of antibiotics: a comprehensive review with clinical emphasis, 3rd Edn. London: Heinemann, 1979: 958–964.

65. Items A, B and E correct.

Chloroquine resistance was once virtually unknown in Africa, but in the last 4 or 5 years there have been an increasing number of cases reported in East Africa.

There is now a good deal of proven chloroquine resistance in the *Plasmodium falciparum* (malignant tertian) strains of malaria in Thailand, Malaysia, the Philippines, Indo-China, parts of Indonesia and Papua New Guinea. Since chloroquine is still the most effective prophylaxis against vivax malaria, most authorities now recommend it should be taken along with either 'Maloprim' (pyrimethamine and dapsone) or 'Fansidar' (pyrimethamine and sulphadoxine). Unfortunately the frequency of both neutropenia with 'Maloprim' or 'Fansidar' and the Stevens-Johnson syndrome with 'Fansidar', has been worrying. Many would advise taking chloroquine plus 'Maloprim'. Others advocate taking cholorquine alone and adding 'Fansidar' only when very high risk areas are encountered.

Prophylaxis should begin at least one week before leaving to ensure that sensitivity to any component of the tablet does not occur. This is not common, but gastric irritation can occur. Those known to be sensitive to sulphones (dapsone is a sulphone) or sulphonamides should be given something else (see below). Continuation of the drug for at least a month after leaving a malarious area is required to ensure the destruction of any forms of the parasite still developing in the liver. By the end of the month, all falciparum parasites will have been released into the blood stream, where the drugs will kill them.

When the schizont of *Pl. falciparum* have ruptured the host hepatocyte after maturation, at the end of the so-called 'exo-erythrocytic' stage, all the merozooites ('small animals') enter the blood stream. However some of the other forms of *Plasmodia*, (e.g. *Pl. vivax*) are able to re-enter hepatocytes where they are protected from the lethal effects of the prophylactic drugs. After some weeks or months (and occasionally years) they can build up in numbers to produce a febrile illness, usually of relatively mild nature initially and rarely, if ever, fatal. The liver phase of such organisms is eradicated by primaquine (an 8-aminoquinoline drug) which needs to be taken for two weeks after an initial course of chloroquine (which will eradicate the erythrocytic trophozooite forms that include the 'ring' stage). The usual dose of primaquine is one tablet twice daily, but the Papua New Guinea strains of *Pl. vivax* may require one tablet three times a day.

Chloroquine would be the best malarial prophylactic drug for his pregnant wife: two tablets once a week before leaving and continuing for a month after return. The teratogenecity of both 'Fansidar' and 'Maloprim' in man is still under investigation; manufacturers of both drugs recommend avoidance during pregnancy. However she needs to be advised to report any significant febrile episodes during and soon after her prophylaxis. The management of such episodes must exclude malaria by including one or more thick blood film examinations.

References

1. Black RH. Malaria in Australia 1980. Tropical Medicine Technical Paper No. 7. Canberra: Australian Government Publishing Service, 1981.
2. Editorial. Chemoprophylaxis of malaria. *Ann Intern Med* 1978; 89: 417–418.
3. Editorial. Continuous in-vitro cultivation of the human malaria parasite. *Ann Intern Med* 1978; 89: 418–419.
4. Black RH. Chloroquine Resistant Falciparum Malaria. *Med J Aust* 1980; 1: 493–494.

66. Items B and E correct.

The clinical picture described is typical of mixed connective tissue disease (MCTD), a variant of systemic lupus erythematosis. However, although antinuclear antibodies are present in high titre, the specificity of the antibody is not for double stranded DNA. Hence, elevation of double stranded DNA antibody is infrequent and it is present only in low titre.

Sharp et al (1982), defined the group of patients with MCTD by the presence of antibody directed aganist the ribonucleo-ptotein (RNP) component of nuclei. RNP is one of the constituents of 'extractable nuclear antigen' (ENA), a soluble nuclear component easily extractable with buffered saline.

MCTD has been regarded as having a low incidence of renal and neurological involvement, although occasional reports are now appearing of significant renal and neurological sequelae (Bennett & Spargo, 1977; Weiss et al, 1978).

Normal serum complement levels do not exclude renal disease. They may be normal with active immune complex deposition (Ruddy et al, 1972). Serum levels represent a net balance of production and consumption.

In a patient with this type of presentation, a clinical response to steroid therapy is likely.

References

1. Sharp GC, et al. Mixed connective tissue disease. *Am J Med* 1972; 52: 148–159.
2. Bennett RM, Spargo BM. Immune complex nephropathy in mixed connective tissue disease. *Am J Med* 1977; 63: 534–541.
3. Weiss TD, et al. Transverse myelitis in mixed connective tissue disease. *Arthritis Rheum* 1978; 21: 982–986.
4. Ruddy S, et al. The complement system in man. *N Engl J Med* 1972; 287: 642–646.

67. Items A, B and E correct.

Many drugs have been implicated in drug-induced lupus. Even more can cause serological abnormality, but the claims made by some authors are probably over-estimated. Good clinical reviews of drugs which definitely, probably and possibly cause a lupus-like illness, are provided by Lee & Chase (1975) and Hahn (1980).

Antinuclear antibodies, often in high titre, are always present in drug-induced lupus. Renal and central nervous system disease is very uncommon in drug-induced disease, although both have been reported and remission of the illness has been observed following the removal of the drug. Drug-induced lupus may occur in both slow and fast acetylators, although the latter probably require higher cumulative doses of the drug.

Spontaneous SLE has been associated with HLA-DR2 and 3. Hydralazine-induced lupus is associated with HLA-DR4, suggesting that pathogenesis of this disorder is not simply due to administration of the drug to someone with a lupus diathesis. Antibodies to double stranded DNA are absent in drug-induced lupus and complement components are usually normal.

References

1. Lee SL, Chase PH. Drug induced systemic lupus erythematosus: a critical review. *Semin Arthritis Rheum* 1975; 5: 83–103.
2. Hahn BH. Systemic lupus erythematosus. In: Parker CW (ed). Clinical immunology. Philadelphia: Saunders, 1980: 583–631.

3. Reinertsen JL, et al. B-lymphocyte alloantigens associated with systemic lupus erythematosus. *N Engl J Med* 1978; 299: 515–518.
4. Batchelor JR, et al. Hydralazine-induced systemic lupus erythematosus: influence of HLA-DR and sex on susceptibility. *Lancet* 1980; 1: 1107–1109.
5. Hess EV (ed). Proceedings of Kroc Foundation conference on drug-induced lupus. *Arthritis Rheum* 1981; 24: 979–1111.

68. Items C, D and E correct.

Pregnancy is not contraindicated in SLE. Patients with significant renal impairment rarely become pregnant; those with normal or only mildly impaired renal function rarely show progressive deterioration of renal function during pregnancy.

Exacerbations of non-renal manifestations of SLE may occur at any time during pregnancy but are more likely in the post-partum period. They can usually be prevented or controlled by increasing the dose of corticosteroids during labour and for a period of around two months post-partum.

During pregnancy, corticosteroids should be used in the same manner and at the same dosages used in non-pregnant women. While it is undesirable to continue immunosuppressives during pregnancy, azathioprine has not been associated with major fetal problems and its sudden withdrawal may lead to a refractory exacerbation of the disease. Thus, if the disease is well-controlled on the drug it is probably advisable to continue it or withdraw it only slowly.

Although most pregnancies do not adversely affect the mother with SLE, the fetus is at relatively high risk. The prevalence of fetal wastage in pregnant patients with SLE is about twice that for the general population and in those with impaired renal function, is almost four times the normal rate. Live infants born to mothers with SLE are at risk of a variety of neonatal complications, the most common of which is intrauterine growth retardation. One of the more serious complications is congenital heart block; it has been suggested that one in three mothers who deliver babies with congenital heart block has or will develop SLE or another connective tissue disease.

Reference

1. Fine LG, et al. Systemic lupus erythematosus in pregnancy. *Ann Intern Med* 1981; 94: 667–677.

69. All items correct.

Fauci et al (1978, 1983) provide an excellent review of vasculitis, outlining the considerable advances which have occurred in both fundamental understanding and therapy. They give a logical discussion of clinical diagnostic approaches and appropriate therapeutic regimens, although there is no mention of the possible role of plasmapheresis.

Vasculitis is considered to result from deposition of immune complexes in blood vessel walls, with initiation of inflammation through complement activation, polymorphonuclear leukocyte accumulation and resulting tissue damage, thrombosis, haemorrhage and ischaemia in the surrounding tissue. Often circulating immune complexes cannot be identified, nor are they demonstrable in the vessel wall at the time of study; they are required for initiating the process, which may then become self-perpetuating.

Hepatitis B is frequently found in association with polyarteritis nodosa. Necrotising vasculitis may be associated with any of the connective tissue disorders, but particularly with SLE and rheumatoid arthritis.

The therapeutic response to cyclophosphamide in Wegener's granulomatosis is usually excellent. Current investigations of various combinations of cytotoxic/corticosteroid drugs appear to offer improved prognosis in necrotising vasculitis.

References

1. Fauci AS, et al. The spectrum of vasculitis. *Ann Intern Med* 1978; 89: 660–676.
2. Editorial. The course of necrotising vasculitis. *Lancet* 1980; 2: 407.
3. Fauci AS, et al. Wegener's granulomatosis: prospective clinical and therapeutic experience with 85 patients for 21 years. *Ann Intern Med* 1983; 98: 76–85.

70. Item D correct.

This woman has acute accelerated hypertension and progressive systemic sclerosis (PSS). Acute renal failure is a common cause of death in PSS, which usually presents with the triad of malignant hypertension, proteinuria and oliguria. The kidneys are of normal size, as this is an acute process, and renal biopsy shows intimal proliferation with or without fibrinoid necrosis in the interlobular arteries and not glomerulonephritis.

Steroids have not proved effective in the treatment of any phase of PSS. The only effective treatment regimens have been to control the hypertension in these patients. Formerly this often required bilateral nephrectomy but recently newer agents such as captopril have been used with benefit.

References

1. Rodnan GP. Progressive systemic sclerosis (scleroderma). In: McCarty DJ (ed). Arthritis and allied conditions, 9th Edn. Philadephia: Lea & Febiger, 1979: 762–809.
2. Kahaleh MB, LeRoy EC. Progressive systemic sclerosis: kidney involvement. *Clin Rheum Dis* 1979; 5: 167–184.
3. Lopez-Ovejeto JA, et al. Reversal of vascular and renal crises of scleroderma by oral angiotensin-converting enzyme blockade. *N Engl J Med* 1979; 300: 1417–1419.

71. Items B and C correct.

Sacroiliac joint changes are infrequent in rheumatoid arthritis. When they occur they consist of small erosions without significant sclerosis. Flexor tenosynovitis of the hand causing an impaired grip of common in rheumatoid arthritis.

Although the ESR is usually elevated, a small number of patients have a normal ESR despite active disease. The finding of a normal ESR does not exclude active rheumatoid arthritis but should be taken as an indication to review the diagnosis. Conversely, while most patients in remission show a return of the ESR towards normal, some patients with inactive disease have persistently elevated ESRs. Very marked elevations, disproportionate to the activity of synovitis, may be seen in rheumatoid arthritis associated with septic arthritis, vasculitis, amyloidosis and Sjögren's syndrome.

The typical combination of villous hypertrophy, lining cell proliferation, infiltration by lymphocytes and plasma cells and fibrin deposition is consistent with rheumatoid arthritis, but is not diagnostic since the same changes may occur in any of the seronegative arthropathies. Less specific changes are found in a variety of joint diseases. The histology of the subcutaneous rheumatoid nodule is more specific but is not pathognomonic.

The white cell count in rheumatoid synovial fluid ranges from 1 to 100 000 per mm^3 and averages around 10 000 per mm^3. The neutrophil polymorph is the predominant cell and usually constitutes about 75% of the total white cell count, although there may be a wide variation in the proportion of neutrophils, lymphocytes and mononuclear cells. A differential count of over 90% neutrophil polymorphs indicates very active acute inflammation and suggests that sepsis should be excluded.

References

1. Katz W, ed. Rheumatic diseases: diagnosis and management. Philadelphia: Lippincott, 1977.
2. Bywaters EGI. Biopsies and tissue diagnosis in rheumatic diseases. *Clin Rheum Dis* 1976; 2: 179–209.

72. Item D correct.

Pruritus or a pruritic rash developing in a patient on treatment with gold must always be viewed as a manifestation of gold toxicity. Skin rashes are by far the most common side-effect and occur in up to 30% of patients receiving this therapy. Skin reactions and proteinuria are most commonly encountered when the total dose reaches 300–400 mg, but they may occur at any time, even following cessation of gold injections. Skin rashes due to gold are of variable severity, sometimes mild and rapidly resolving, sometimes severe and lasting for as long as a year.

The development of an early skin rash is not a contraindication to the cautious reintroduction of gold once the rash has settled. Most rheumatologists would use very low doses initially, gradually working up to a maintenance dose below that previously employed.

Plasma gold levels are not related to the toxic effects of the drug and are not of value in predicting their development. Although it has been suggested that plasma gold levels may be a more logical way of controlling therapy, the lack of consistent direct correlation between plasma levels and response does not support this.

References

1. Jessop JD. Gold in the treatment of rheumatoid arthritis. Why, when and how? *J Rheumatol* 1979; 6: Suppl. 1: 12–17.
2. Davis P. Undesirable effects of gold salts. *J Rheumatol* 1979; 6 (Suppl 1): 18–24.

73. Items B and D correct.

Among the several causes of anaemia in rheumatoid arthritis, the anaemia of chronic disease is the most common. This is usually normochromic and normocytic, occasionally hypochromic and rarely microcytic. Although iron stores are often increased in this type of anaemia, the serum iron and total iron binding capacity are typically reduced.

The second most common type of anaemia is iron deficiency anaemia, usually due to blood loss following drug-induced gastric erosions. The diagnosis of iron deficiency may be difficult to make on the basis of the blood film or serum iron studies. This diagnosis is supported by a low serum ferritin level and would be confirmed by finding absent iron stores on bone marrow examination.

The serum ferritin is an index of total body iron and generally correlates with bone marrow iron stores. A low serum ferritin is typically found in iron deficiency. However, the serum ferritin may rise due to inflammation, and a low normal serum ferritin level in inflammatory disease does not exclude iron deficiency.

Significant gastric mucosal erosions or ulcers may occur in the absence of symptoms in patients taking non-steroidal anti-inflammatory drugs.

Anaemia in patients with rheumatoid arthritis does not respond to oral iron unless iron deficiency is present. Parenteral iron may cause exacerbation of the arthritis.

References

1. Bennett RM. Haematological changes in rheumatoid disease. *Clin Rheum Dis* 1977; 3: 433–465.
2. Smith RJ, et al. Serum ferritin levels in the anaemia of rheumatoid arthritis. *J Rheumatol* 1977; 4: 389–392.
3. Finch CA, Huebers H. Perspective in iron metabolism. *N Engl J Med* 1982; 306: 1520–1528.
4. Caruso I, Bianchi Porro G. Gastroscopic evaluation of anti-inflammatory agents. *Br Med J* 1980; 280: 75–78.

74. Items A, B and C correct.

Polyarticular psoriatic arthritis is treated according to the same principles as rheumatoid arthritis. The non-steroidal anti-inflammatory agents, such as salicylates and indomethacin, are useful first-line drugs and sodium aurothiomalate has also been shown to be effective. Despite the recognised cutaneous toxicity of gold, there is no evidence that this occurs any more frequently in patients with psoriatic arthritis than in those with rheumatoid disease. On the other hand, antimalarial drugs such as chloroquine should be avoided since they may provoke exfoliation.

Hyperuricaemia has been reported in psoriasis and it is said to be more common in patients with extensive skin involvement. However Wright (1978), in a carefully controlled study in which all drugs which might influence the level of serum uric acid were withdrawn, did not observe any difference in serum uric acid levels between a group of patients with psoriatic arthritis and a matched group with rheumatoid arthritis. Thus, allopurinol has no prophylactic role in the management of uncomplicated polyarticular psoriatic arthritis.

Reference

1. Wright V. Psoriatic arthritis. In: Scott JT (ed). Copeman's textbook of the rheumatic diseases, 5th Edn. Edinburgh: Churchill-Livingstone, 1978: 537–48.

75. Items B and C correct.

The most likely cause of long-standing pain and swelling of the knee in a man of this age is osteoarthritis. However, examination of aspirated synovial fluid for the presence of crystals and for a differential cell count, together with an X-ray (to exclude chondrocalcinosis and other abnormalities) would be appropriate.

The finding of hyperuricaemia in a patient with rheumatic symptoms or arthritis is insufficient for the diagnosis of gout. More than 95% of attacks of gout are typical and consist of an acute synovitis precipitated by crystal deposition. In the absence of clinical or radiological evidence of tophaceous gout, chronic arthritis is more likely to be due to a cause other than gout even in the presence of moderate elevation of the serum uric acid level.

Many factors contribute to hyperuricaemia. It is well recognised that the condition may be primary, but only rarely is it associated with a specific enzyme deficiency. Sometimes it may be caused by the high purine turnover in conditions such as the myeloproliferative disorders, but most commonly it is associated with factors which reduce renal excretion of uric acid. These include a low urinary output, essential hypertension or the effects of drugs such as alcohol, low-dose aspirin and most diuretics. By mechanisms which are not understood, obesity causes hyperuricaemia which may be corrected by weight reduction.

In the patient described, unless the mild hyperuricaemia can be shown to be responsible for joint or renal abnormalities, it would be inappropriate to introduce drugs to lower the serum uric acid level. Simple measures are preferable and these include weight reduction and increasing the urinary output by increased fluid intake.

References

1. Simpkin PA. Management of gout. *Ann Intern Med* 1979; 90: 812–816.
2. Scott JT. Long-term management of gout and hyperuricaemia. Br Med J 1980; 281: 1164–1166.

76. Items C, D and E correct.

Although the patient has no history of eye involvement, the pattern of his arthritis and soft tissue involvement is typical of Reiter's syndrome. Incomplete forms of the disease are well recognised. HLA-B27 is absent in up to 25% of patients with Reiter's syndrome and the test cannot be used for diagnostic purposes. The arthritis of Reiter's syndrome may be intensely inflammatory with turbid synovial fluid which sometimes appears purulent and in which the white cell count commonly ranges from 50–100 000/cmm with a predominance of polymorphonuclear leukocytes.

The radiological characteristics of Reiter's syndrome are erosive arthritis with a predilection for the feet. Periosteal changes occur, particularly along metatarsals and phalanges adjacent to affected joints. Fluffy calcaneal spurs and sacroliitis are common, and on long-term follow-up, 10–15% of patients develop the changes of ankylosing spondylitis.

The mucocutaneous lesions include keratoderma blennorrhagica, dystrophic nail changes with subungual hyperkeratosis, circinate balanitis and small painless mouth ulcers.

While Reiter's syndrome occurs most commonly following sexually acquired non-specific urethritis, an identical syndrome may follow enteric infections, particularly those due to *Shigella flexneri*, *Yersinia enterocolitica*, *Salmonella* and *Campylobacter*. At times the syndrome appears without any recognisable precipitating event particularly in children where the male predominance is less marked than it is in adulthood.

The seriousness of Reiter's syndrome has been underestimated. Average episodes last 2–4 months, but occasionally the arthritis becomes chronic from the outset. While remissions may last for many years, recurrences occur in at least 50% of patients although only about half of these have recognisable urethritis or enteritis. The pattern of recurrence is often incomplete, but typically includes arthritis, which may be persistent. Residual disability occurs in 30–40% of patients with Reiter's syndrome. Major problems include painful deformed feet, visual impairment following recurrent uveitis, spinal involvement and cardiac lesions such as aortic valve incompetence.

Gonococcal arthritis is more common in women. In this condition, joint involvement is polyarticular without lower limb predominance and tenosynovitis occurs frequently. Skin lesions, commonly seen before or with the arthritis, consist of small erythematous macules which may develop central petechiae or necrosis.

References

1. Csonka GW. Clinical aspects of Reiter's syndrome. *Ann Rheum Dis* 1979; 38 (Suppl): 4–7.
2. Calin A, et al. Prognosis and natural history of Reiter's syndrome. *Ann Rheum Dis* 1979; 38 (Suppl): 29–31.
3. Amor B. Reiter's syndrome: long-term follow-up data. *Ann Rheum Dis* 1979; 38 (Suppl): 32–33.

77. Items A, C and D correct.

Although there are no histological distinctions, primary and secondary Sjögren's syndrome show characteristic differences in clinical features, autoantibody profiles and HLA antigen associations.

In both primary and secondary Sjögren's syndrome, the dominant clinical manifestations result from lymphocytic infiltration of exocrine glands, particularly the salivary and lacrimal glands. Other exocrine glands may also be involved, including those in the upper and lower respiratory tract, causing a dry nose,throat and trachea with resultant otitis, bronchitis and pneumonitis. In addition there may be involvement of the gastrointestinal tract, causing oesophageal mucosal atrophy and atrophic gastritis, and desiccation of the vagina and vulva, causing dyspareunia and pruritus. Involvement of the exocrine glands of the skin causes diminished secretion and a dry skin. In primary Sjögren's syndrome there is an increased frequency of recurrent parotid gland enlargement, lymphadenopathy, purpura, Raynaud's phenomenon, renal involvement and myositis.

Earlier reports indicated an increased risk of developing lymphoma in Sjögren's syndrome, particularly the primary form. More recent analysis indicates that this risk is increased 40–50 times in primary Sjögren's syndrome and in the form associated with rheumatoid arthritis. Risk factors for the development of lymphoma include recurrent parotid swelling, lymphadenopathy and splenomegaly, all of which can occur for many years before lymphoma becomes evident.

Primary Sjögren's syndrome is associated with antibodies to SS-B and SS-A but not to the rheumatoid arthritis precipitin; only 25% of patients with the primary syndrome have antisalivary duct antibodies as opposed to 70% of those with Sjögren's syndrome secondary to rheumatoid arthritis. Sjögren's syndrome with rheumatoid arthritis is also associated with increased frequency of the HLA antigen DR4, as is rheumatoid arthritis alone; in contrast, patients with a primary Sjögren's syndrome show an increased frequency of HLA B8 and DR3. Some other antigens present on the surface of B cells appear to occur with increased frequency in both primary and secondary Sjögren's syndrome.

References

1. Moutsopoulos HM, et al. Sjögren's syndrome (Sicca syndrome): current issues. *Ann Intern Med* 1980; 92: 212–226.
2. Strand V, Talal N. Advances in the diagnosis and concepts of Sjögren's syndrome (autoimmune exocrinopathy). *Bull Rheum Dis* 1979–80; 30: 1046–1052.

78. Items B, C and E correct.

Calcium pyrophosphate dehydrate deposition disease (CPPD) has been classified into three main groups:

(a) hereditary CPPD
(b) sporadic CPPD
(c) CPPD associated with metabolic disease.

Sporadic CPPD disease appears to be the most common, although it has been suggested that careful radiological study of the relatives of patients with this disease may reveal a higher than expected prevalence of hereditary cases. Metabolic conditions associated with CPPD are less common but have been identified as hyperparathyroidism, haemochromatosis, hypothyroidism and gout; less closely associated are ochronosis, Wilson's disease, diabetes mellitus and hypophosphatasia.

CPPD disease is notable for the variety of clinical patterns of arthritis associated with it. These include pseudo-gout, pseudo-rheumatoid arthritis, progressive osteoarthritis with or without superimposed acute attacks, pseudo-neuropathic arthritis and, perhaps most commonly, an asymptomatic radiological finding.

Although not as predictably effective as in urate gout, colchicine therapy occasionally may provide dramatic relief in pseudo-gout. There is no evidence however that it has a prophylactic effect. Standard treatment of pseudo-gout is joint aspiration and intra-articular steroid or full doses of one of the non-steroidal anti-inflammatory drugs. Although associated with gout, CPPD is not directly related to hyperuricaemia. It is therefore not surprising that allopurinol is ineffective in the prevention of the clinical manifestations of this disease.

Reference

1. McCarty DJ. Calcium pyrophosphate dihydrate crystal deposition disease (pseudo gout syndrome) — clinical aspects. *Clin Rheum Dis* 1977; 3: 61–89.

79. Items A, D and E correct.

D-penicillamine is effective in 70–80% of patients with rheumatoid arthritis. It is generally agreed that efficacy is maintained and toxicity considerably reduced by a 'go low, go slow' regimen. The starting dose is usually 125 mg daily with increases of 125–250 mg made at monthly intervals to a maximum dosage of 500–750 mg daily. Treatment must be monitored with urinalysis for proteinuria, a full blood count and platelet count, and a patient interview to report any pruritus, skin rashes, mouth ulcers and other adverse effects, initially at fortnightly intervals, and after about 6 months, at monthly intervals.

A past history of penicillin allergy is not a contraindication to the use of D-penicillamine and there is no evidence that the drug causes or reactivates peptic ulceration. Indeed in the rheumatoid patient the presence of peptic ulcer disease is an indication for the early introduction of an antirheumatic drug such as gold or penicillamine to reduce reliance on the non-steroidal anti-inflammatory drugs.

D-penicillamine has been associated with a wide range of side-effects, the most common of which are proteinuria, skin rashes and isolated thrombocytopenia which reverses on withdrawal of the drug. All side-effects must be viewed seriously, but cautious re-introduction of low-dose therapy is often possible.

85. Items A, B and C correct.

In the field of antinuclear antibodies there have been a number of recent developments. It was reported initially that mixed connective tissue disease (MCTD) was associated with antibodies to an extractable nuclear antigen (ENA) but it soon became apparent that ENA contained two major components — Sm antigen and nRNP. Antibodies to Sm occur particularly in systemic lupus erythematosus (SLE). Antibodies to nRNP are not restricted to MCTD but may also be found in SLE, discoid lupus erythematosus, scleroderma and other rheumatic diseases. However, in the absence of antibodies to DNA, Sm and other histones, a high titre of antibody to nRNP is typically seen in MCTD.

A remarkable association described recently is that of antibody to the centromere in patients with the progressive systemic sclerosis variant known as the 'CREST' syndrome (calcinosis, Raynaud's phenomenon, oesophageal involvement, sclerodoctyly and telangiectasia). While this uncommon disease and its serological marker are themselves of little general clinical relevance, they are one of the group of associations found in this evolving field.

The immunofluorescent test for antinuclear antibody (ANA) is non-specific but an excellent screening test. While the titre of ANA carries most diagnostic value, the pattern of staining also provides useful information. The 4 major patterns are

1. homogeneous staining, present with a variety of antinuclear specificities, particularly nucleoprotein
2. peripheral or rim, associated particularly with antibody to native DNA and therefore most commonly seen in SLE
3. speckled, generally associated with antibody to non-histone proteins and frequently positive in mixed connective tissue disease, scleroderma and SLE
4. nucleolar, generally associated with antibody to nucleolar RNA, and found most commonly in scleroderma.

Antibody to single-stranded DNA is non-specific and is found in a number of conditions but the distribution of antibodies to native DNA is much more restricted. If the test is performed with meticulous technique and pure antigen, a strongly positive test is almost specific to SLE. Despite the diagnostic value of antibodies to native DNA, the level of antibody present is a much less reliable guide to disease activity and some patients with SLE remain well over periods of months or even years with high anti-DNA antibody levels.

Reference

1. Tan EM. The biological and diagnostic significance of antinuclear antibodies. *Aust NZ J Med* 1981; 11: 193–196.

86. Items A, B, D and E correct.

Recent separation, purification and analysis of amyloid fibrils has shown that they are composed of proteins with a common structural configuration, namely a beta-pleated sheet structure which is responsible for many of the unique ultrastructural and staining characteristics of amyloid. The configuration is probably also important in creating resistance to proteolytic digestion, which allows the inert fibrils to persist in tissues, causing atrophy and death in vital organs. Recent use of dimethylsulphoxide in the treatment of reactive systemic (secondary) amyloidosis is based on the ability of this compound to denature amyloid fibrils in experimental situations.

Classification of amyloidosis is again undergoing reappraisal. The distinction between primary and secondary amyloidosis still appears to be useful, although new terminology is creeping in. There appears to be little difference between primary amyloidosis and amyloidosis associated with myeloma and other immunocyte disorders. In both situations the major fibril protein is composed of immunoglobulin light chain, often derived from Bence-Jones protein (designated AL protein). In secondary amyloidosis the fibril protein (designated AA protein) may be derived from a larger serum component (SAA).

Amyloidosis is said to occur in 6–15% of patients with myeloma and in 20–24% of patients with 'light chain' myeloma. Monoclonal proteins, particularly Bence-Jones proteins indicative of an underlying immunocytic dyscrasia, are also present in the majority of patients with primary amyloidosis. The elaboration of light chains appears to be an essential feature of both conditions. However, this is not sufficient to produce amyloidosis, and presumably some other factor that induces the beta-pleated configuration necessary for amyloid fibril formation must also be present.

Patients with primary amyloidosis commonly present with autonomic symptoms of sexual impotence, orthostatic hypotension and disturbances of gastrointestinal motility. Neuropathy of glove and stocking distribution is common, as is median nerve entrapment. Other common features are restrictive cardiomyopathy or pericarditis, sensitivity to digitalis, macroglossia, purpura and other skin lesions and a non-inflammatory polyarthropathy of rheumatoid distribution but with a predilection for large joints. Because of the many common features between primary amyloidosis and amyloidosis associated with multiple myeloma, grouping them together rationalises a common approach to treatment with cytotoxic drugs directed towards the source of the monoclonal protein.

New treatments which may be effective in reactive systemic (secondary) amyloidosis and familial amyloidosis associated with Mediterranean fever have been described. Colchicine in a dose of 1–1.5 mg/day has been shown to decrease the frequency and severity of acute symptoms of familial Mediterranean fever, but it is not yet clear what will be its long-term effect on amyloid deposition. When used in large doses, dimethylsulphoxide appears to be capable of denaturing amyloid fibrils and may be of value in secondary amyloidosis. Treatment is still in the experimental stage and the drug suffers the major disadvantage of producing an unpleasant odour in the breath which has often led to the cessation of treatment. In the absence of well-established specific therapy, supportive measures are important. Sudden death is common and may be contributed to by sensitivity to digitalis preparations. The common occurrence of debilitating postural hypotension should be recognised and diuretics used with great caution. Steroid replacement therapy may be necessary if adrenal insufficiency occurs. Elastic stockings, however uncomfortable, may be necesary to avoid debilitating postural hypotension.

Reference

1. Glenner GG. Amyloid deposits and amyloidosis: the beta-fibrilloses. *N Engl J Med* 1980; 302: 1283–1293, 1333–1343.

87. Items A, C and D correct.

The pathogenesis of chronic urticaria is ill-understood in most cases. It is rarely a manifestation of type 1 IgE-mediated allergy, although acute urticaria/angio-oedema can be seen in type 1-mediated reactions such as hymenoptera venom anaphylaxis. Skin-prick tests are rarely of any value and are very often negative to all test allergens.

Less than 1% of the patients will have hereditary angio-oedema secondary to C1 esterase inhibitor deficiency. These patients may have a positive family history of sudden death due to glottal or laryngeal oedema and they may present with severe abdominal colic. Localised swellings arise around the face, throat, trunk, limbs or genitalia, but are characteristically non-itchy and last for several days.

Another group of patients with urticarial vasculitis present with abdominal pain, fever, angio-oedema and polyarthritis. The lesions tend to be painful rather than itchy and biopsy shows leucocytoclastic vasculitis. These patients may have hypocomplementaemia with reduced total haemolytic complement (THC). Urticaria has also been associated with hereditary deficiencies of C1q and C2, in which case the THC will be zero. Measurement of the THC is therefore a useful screening test for both of these conditions.

The causal role of substances such as salicylates, benzoates, azo-dyes and penicillin within the diet is controversial. About 30% of patients with chronic recurrent urticaria may have a precipitating factor in their diet, but exclusion and provocation tests are difficult both to perform and to interpret.

References

1. Editorial. Recurrent urticaria. *Lancet* 1981; 2: 235–236.
2. Soter NA. Chronic urticaria as a manifestation of necrotizing venulitis. *N Engl J Med* 1977; 296: 1440–1442.
3. Juhlin L. Recurrent urticaria: a clinical investigation of 330 patients. *Br J Dermatol* 1981; 104: 369–381.
4. Warin RP, Champion RH. Urticaria. In: Samter M (ed). Immunological diseases. Boston: Little, Brown & Co, 1978; 929–940.

88. Items A, B, C and D correct.

Mixed (IgM-IgG) cryoglobulins are often found in association with various infections, connective tissue and lymphoproliferative diseases.

When mixed cryoglobulins are found in the absence of a defined cause, the syndrome has been designated 'essential mixed cryoglobulinaemia' and is characterised by purpura, arthralgia and weakness.

Clinical or biochemical evidence of liver involvement was detected in up to 90% of patients in one study and both chronic active hepatitis and cirrhosis have been associated with this condition. In the study by Levo et al (1977), HBsAg was detected in 12% of sera and antibody in 48%; these results are higher than the 0.5% and the 15% observed in the general population and in two control groups of patients with rheumatoid arthritis and lupus erythematosus. The incidence of positive results was increased to 28% and 52% respectively when cryoprecipitates were examined, and thus 58% of patients were positive for either antigen or antibody or both.

Renal involvement may occur in approximately half the patients with this syndrome and is the leading cause of death. Although the majority of those with renal disease progress to renal failure, remissions may occur and long-term survival of patients with and without renal disease has been observed.

Cryoglobulinaemia alone is not an indication for treatment. Treatment is directed to any underlying disorder or to alleviate symptoms arising from the immune complex disease.

References

1. Franklin EC. Cryoproteins. In: Parker CW (ed). Clinical immunology. Philadelphia: Saunders, 1980: 534–542.
2. Levo Y, et al. Liver involvement in the syndrome of mixed cryoglobulinaemia. *Ann Intern Med* 1977; 87: 287–292.

89. Items A, B and D correct.

Angioimmunoblastic lymphadenopathy is a lymphoma-like entity characterised by diffuse proliferation of immunoblasts, plasma cells, lymphocytes and small blood vessels in lymph nodes, and by systemic involvement of multiple organs. An autoimmune haemolytic anaemia with a positive Coombs' test is seen in approximately 25% of reported cases, and features of autoimmune disease may dominate the clinical picture.

Polyclonal hypergammaglobulinaemia is most common, but monoclonal gammopathy is also seen, usually in association with overt lymphoma.

Vasculitis of small dermal vessels is reported but clinical evidence of vasculitis affecting small and medium arteries is uncommon.

A high prevalence of allergy to penicillin and other drugs has been reported and in some instances such reactions appear to have precipitated the disease.

Corticosteroids have a limited role in treatment of the disorder. Approximately 25% of patients have a favourable course with or without steroid therapy, whereas the remainder have an unfavourable course. Intensive chemotherapy may induce remissions in approximately 25% of patients.

References

1. Frizzera G, et al. Angio-immonoblastic lymphadenopathy: diagnosis and clinical course. *Am J Med* 1975; 59: 803–818.
2. Flandrin G. Angioimmunoblastic lymphadenopathy: clinical, biologic and follow-up study of 14 cases. In: Mathe G, et al (eds). Recent results in cancer research. New York: Springer-Verlag, 1978; 64: 247–262.
3. Weisenberger D, et al. Immunoblastic lymphadenopathy with pulmonary infiltrates, hypocomplementemia and vasculitis. *Am J Med* 1977; 63: 849–854.
4. Weisenberger D. Immunoblastic lymphadenopathy associated with methyldopa therapy: a case report. *Cancer* 1978; 42: 2322–2327.

90. Items A, C and D correct.

Surface markers are being used to characterise various forms of lymphoproliferative diseases and surface immunoglobulin is one such marker. Normally B cells contain intracytoplasmic immunoglobulin and express this immunoglobulin on the cell surface. By immunofluorescent techniques such surface immunoglobulin can be identified. The predominant types of immunoglobulin are IgM and IgD. The light chains may be either κ or λ and are present in ratios similar to their distribution in serum immunoglobulins, i.e. between 1.5 : 1 and 3 : 1.

Malignant lymphocytic populations demonstrate their clonal origin from a common neoplastic progenitor cell by all bearing the same surface marker characteristics. The immunoglobulin light chain is identical for all the cells in the tumour population and usually the heavy chain is also monoclonal (although occasional mixtures of IgM and IgD are seen, reflecting the maturation 'switch' seen in normal cells). Whenever the malignant cells spread, the same monoclonal characteristics will be present — whether in bone marrow or other nodal tissue.

Paraproteins are not unusual in lymphoproliferative disorders and occur regularly in mature B cell disorders where the monoclonal protein is secreted (plasma cell dyscrasias). The paraprotein is usually the same as the surface monoclonal immunoglobulin, but occasional discordance has been noted.

References

1. Siegal FP, et al. Surface markers in leukaemias and lymphomas. *Am J Path* 1978; 90: 451–459.
2. Lowenthal RM, Harlow RWH. A case of IgG lymphoma occurring in a patient with previous IgG lymphoma. *Aust NZ J Med* 1981; 11: 281–284.
3. Lowenthal RM, et al. Immunological types of lymphoproliferative disorders in a cohort: a 4-year study. *Aust NZ J Med* 1982; 12: 258–262.

91. Item D correct.

Patients whose blood pressure is more labile have a risk of cardiovascular events no lower than those whose pressure is less variable. Insurance statistics show clearly that isolated elevated blood pressure recordings (both systolic and diastolic) are associated with increased morbidity and mortality. The influence of diastolic elevation on the complications of hypertension is a popular clinical myth for which there is little good evidence. Recent studies show that all complications were more closely related to systolic rather than to diastolic pressure levels.

Thiazide diuretics elevate renin levels. Their hypotensive effect is based on the blocking of sodium reabsorption. The positive relationship between blood pressure and circulating blood volume is an important concept in the management of patients with chronic renal failure, with particular reference to salt metabolism.

Even after relating to sodium excretion rates, there is no firm evidence that patients with essential hypertension display such elevated levels. Walker et al (1979), found that plasma renin substrate was the only component of the renin-angiotensin-aldosterone system displaying a positive correlation (16% of variance) with blood pressure in a population study excluding patients with renovascular hypertension.

References

1. Tarazi RC. Clinical import of systolic hypertension. *Ann Intern Med* 1978; 88: 426–427.
2. Kannel WB, Dawler TR, McGee DC. Perspectives on systolic hypertension. The Framingham study. *Circulation* 1980; 61: 1179–1182.
3. Kannel WB, Sorbie P, Gordon T. Labile hypertension: a faulty concept? The Framingham study. *Circulation* 1980; 61: 1183–1187.
4. Walker WG, et al. The relationship between blood pressure and renin levels. *Hypertension* 1979; 1: 287–291.
5. Kaplan NM. Renin profiles: the unfulfilled promises. *JAMA* 1977; 238: 611–613.

92. Items B and E correct.

Salbutamol is a b2-adrenoceptor agonist. At high doses b1-agonist effects may become evident with increase in heart rate, myocardial contractility and cardiac output. Such effects may intensify the disordered ventilation-perfusion ratio in the lungs and thereby aggravate hypoxaemia even though airways obstruction has diminished. Such hypoxaemia may result in cardiac arrhythmias; however it is unlikely to cause accelerated hypertension. This blurred vision is due to hypertensive retinopathy.

Acute transient hypertension occurs during many activities and can be induced with sympathomimetic agents. Hypertension is unlikely to cause cardiac failure unless it is chronic, is associated with persistent high levels of vasoconstrictor substances which could result in cardiac muscle damage or is associated with a disease process which could

Ventricular asystole is best treated with sympathomimetic drugs such as isoprenaline (0.2 mg diluted in 10 ml and given at 1 ml/min) or adrenaline. The intracardiac route has no advantage over intravenous injection. Atropine and calcium have not been shown to be effective in asystole and are better used for idioventricular or other bradyarrhythmias. Cardiac pacing (transthoracic) may be attempted but is not often successful.

The acidosis occurring in cardiac arrest can often be managed by hyperventilation alone and bicarbonate should not be given routinely unless the arrest is prolonged, as concentrated sodium bicarbonate can cause significant hyperosmolality. Excess bicarbonate may lead to worsening of pulmonary oedema. Administration of bicarbonate causes a rise in P_{CO_2}, which may initially aggravate intracellular acidosis.

Resistant ventricular fibrillation is usually managed by intravenous oxylocaine and repeated DC shocks. Fine ventricular fibrillation may be coarsened and made easier to revert by the use of adrenaline, but this may aggravate the ischaemia. Recently it has been shown that methoxamine, an alpha-adrenergic stimulant, may assist defibrillation by increasing coronary flow without increasing the degree of ischaemia.

References

1. Mackintosh AF, et al. Hospital resuscitation for ventricular fibrillation in Brighton. *Br Med J* 1979; 1: 511–513.
2. Livesay JJ, et al. Optimizing myocardial supply/demand balance with alpha-adrenergic drugs during cardiopulmonary resuscitaion. *J Thorac Cardiovasc Surg* 1978; 76: 244–251.
3. Hamer A. The management of cardiac arrest in hospital. *Notes Cardiovasc Dis* 1979; 15(8): 33–36.

99. Items A, C and D correct.

A loud systolic murmur developing during or soon after a myocardial infarction usually means either rupture of a papillary muscle or perforation of the interventricular septum. When the murmur is very loud, maximal at the left sternal edge and accompanied by a thrill, the diagnosis of a perforated septum is nearly certain. An echocardiogram is helpful if doubt exists. The tear in the septum occurs most commonly in the lower septum and is often large. It occurs with equal frequency in anterior and inferior locations.

The prognosis is bad, with an average survival time of only two weeks. Most patients deteriorate rapidly with either severe cardiac failure or cardiogenic shock. If cardiogenic shock develops, intra-aortic balloon support, cardiac catheterisation and cardiac surgery must be considered.

Cardiac failure is managed by routine measures including the use of vasodilators, but the patient will also require early investigation to assess the size of the shunt, the efficiency of left ventricular contraction and the state of the coronary arteries.

Because of the poor prognosis, surgery is usually undertaken urgently. New surgical techniques have improved the survival rate.

References

1. Leading article. Perforation of the interventricular septum. *Br Med J* 1980; 281: 1305–1306.
2. Gunnar RM, et al. Management of acute myocardial infarction and accelerating angina. *Prog Cardiovasc Dis* 1979; 22: 1–30.

100. Items B, D and E correct.

The risks of coronary arteriography are low (0.5%). Depending on the experience of the investigator with the techniques, there is a suggestion that the percutaneous femoral route is safer than the brachial artery 'cutdown'. Patients who die at investigation usually have severe coronary disease. Poor left ventricular function and left main coronary obstruction are additional risk factors.

Patients with left main obstruction have a poor prognosis when treated medically (5-year survival rate of around 62%). This lesion is usually associated with significant disease in other vessels and surgical treatment is superior to medical treatment alone (5-year survival rate of around 93%).

Although it is tempting to recommend surgery for high left anterior descending vessel lesions, unequivocal evidence for the advantage of surgical over medical management is not available. Patients with this lesion should not be assigned automatically to one treatment group or another. The decision for surgery on single vessel disease should be based on symptoms, size of vessel obstructed and amount of myocardium in jeopardy.

Surgery for symptomatic three-vessel disease is regarded as superior to medical therapy alone, both in symptomatic relief and in life-expectancy. The 5-year survival rate for men below 65 years of age with three-vessel disease and who have mild to moderate angina and good left ventricular function is quite good if treated medically (85%), but this can be improved (to 95%) with surgical therapy.

References

1. European Coronary Surgery Study Group. Second interim report. Prospective randomised study of coronary artery bypass surgery in stable angina pectoris. *Lancet* 1980; 2: 491–495.
2. Leading article. Risks of coronary arteriography. *Br Med J* 1980; 281: 627–628.
3. Craddock DR, et al. Coronary artery surgery in South Australia: second report. *Med J Aust* 1980; 1: 491–493.
4. Hunt D, et al. Results of coronary artery surgery. *Med J Aust* 1981; 1: 575–576.
5. Loop FD, et al. The efficacy of coronary artery surgery. *Am Heart J* 1981; 101: 86–96.

101. All items correct.

There seems to be little basis for reassuring patients with a non-transmural (subendocardial) myocardial infarction on the basis that they have had only a 'little coronary'. There is now a body of literature (e.g. Cannon et al, 1976) showing that the late mortality rate of non-transmural myocardial infarction (NTMI) may equal or be greater than that from transmural infarction. A more recent study (Hutter et al, 1981) puts these findings on a firm footing, with analysis of rigidly matched non-transmural and transmural varieties.

Patients with NTMI have a significantly lower hospital mortality rate (9%) than that of patients with transmural infarcts (20%). Late mortality increased in patients with NTMI and, at 4.5 years, mortality in the groups was comparable. Subsequent infarction was greater in patients with NTMI (50%), contrasting with 12% in transmural anterior infarcts and 22% in transmural inferior infarcts.

During hospital stay, patients with non-transmural infarcts had fewer intraventricular conduction defects than did patients with transmural anterior infarcts; they also had fewer atrial arrhythmias, less sinus bradycardia and less atrioventricular block than did patients with transmural inferior infarcts.

It would appear that NTMI is a more unstable state in the spectrum of ischaemic heart disease than is transmural infarction. Patients with NTMI may have more viable myocardium in jeopardy and (Schulze et al, 1978) have shown a similar extent of coronary disease in both non-transmural and transmural groups.

These findings lend further weight to the opinion that patients with NTMI should be treated with considerably more vigor after myocardial infarction and should be evaluated aggressively, e.g. by exercise electrocardiography, often combined with thallium-201 imaging or cardiac catheterisation.

References

1. Cannom DS, et al. A short and long-term prognosis of patients with transmural and non-transmural myocardial infarction. *Am J Med* 1976; 61: 452–458.
2. Hutter AM, et al. Non-transmural myocardial infarction: the comparison of hospital and late clinical course of patients with that of matched patients with transmural anterior and transmural inferior myocardial infarction. *Am J Cardiol* 1981; 48: 595–602.
3. Schulze RA, et al. Coronary angiography and left ventriculography in survivors of transmural and non-transmural myocardial infarction. *Am J Med* 1978; 64: 108–113.

102. Items B and E correct.

Recent post-myocardial infarction trials have shown a reduction in mortality in patients treated with beta-blockers compared to controls; the non-selective beta blockers timolol and propranolol were started 5–7 days post-infarct, whereas the selective beta blocker metoprolol was started as soon as possible after admission. Not only was mortality reduced in the treated group but also the re-infarction rate decreased.

The relatively low incidence of coronary heart disease among women in comparison with men is well known. However neither the Framingham study nor the Health Insurance Plan Group revealed any difference in overall survival after clinical infarction had occurred. Women have no protection from secondary complications.

It has been shown that lignocaine produces significant shortening of both the effective refractory period and action potential duration at all potassium concentrations. Although high concentrations of potassium may alter somewhat the electrophysiological properties of lignocaine, the properties considered vital in terms of the drugs anti-arrhythmic actions persist.

Experimental findings and case reports challenge the routine use of atropine in acute myocardial infarction and asymptomatic bradycardia. Atropine may increase size of infarction and is not indicated in uncomplicated sinus bradycardia. However if sinus node suppression is complicated by hypotension or increased ventricular irritability, a dose of atropine 0.3–0.6 mg is appropriate treatment.

References

1. The Norwegian Multicenter Study Group. Timolol-induced reduction in mortality and reinfarction in patients surviving acute myocardial infarction. *N Engl J Med* 1981; 304: 801–807.
2. Hjalmarson A, et al. Effect on mortality of metoprolol in acute myocardial infarction. *Lancet* 1981; 2: 823–826.
3. Weinblatt E, et al. Prognosis of women with newly diagnosed coronary heart disease — a comparison with course of disease among men. *Am J Public Health* 1973; 63: 577–593.
4. Schweitzer P, Mark H. The effect of atropine on cardiac arrhythmias and conduction. Part 2. *Am Heart J* 1980; 100: 255–261.

103. Items A, B and C correct.

When cardiac failure is severe there is an increased release of catecholamines by adrenergic cardiac nerves and adrenal medulla. Catecholamine release and reflex baroreceptor activity result in tachycardia and elevation of peripheral vascular resistance in order to maintain perfusion to vital organs.

The use of vasodilators to treat patients with chronic congestive heart failure has become increasingly popular. Hydralazine acts predominantly on arteriolar vessels, reducing systemic vascular resistance with a consequent increase in stroke volume and cardiac output. Heart rate and arterial pressure as well as left ventricular filling pressure may not significantly change.

Prazosin is both an arterial and venous dilator and has the potential to improve cardiac output and reduce pulmonary congestion. The reduction in peripheral resistance may cause hypotension, but in the failing heart, when arterial resistance is increased, the use of vasodilators usually results in an increase in output without great change in blood pressure.

Although hydralazine produces a tachycardia in patients with hypertension, no increase has been observed in patients with heart failure. Neither does prazosin increase heart rate. Both agents may slow the pulse in patients with heart failure and the production of tachycardia is not a limiting factor.

References

1. Conti CR. Symposium on congestive heart failure: introduction. *Am J Med* 1981; 71: 131–134.
2. Lakier JB, et al. Rationale and use of vasodilators in the management of congestive heart failure. *Am Heart J* 1979; 97: 519–526.

104. Items A and C correct.

There is an increased risk of sudden death in patients with bifascicular block. However, death is not necessarily due to the advanced heart block itself but may have other underlying mechanisms.

Left bundle branch block with right axis deviation are the electrocardiogram changes of left posterior rather than left anterior hemi-block.

Permanent cardiac pacing is advisable and this is aimed at preventing asystolic arrest as well as alleviating symptoms in this situation. However, in asymptomatic patients with bifascicular block, the associated ischaemic heart disease rather than a bradyarrhythmia is more often the cause of sudden death, and permanent cardiac pacing is not generally advisable.

Ischaemic heart disease and sclerotic degeneration are the common causes of bifascicular block. Digoxin overdose is not regarded as a common cause.

References

1. Sub-Leader. Bundle branch block. *Br Med J* 1979; 1: 436–437.
2. McAnulty JH, et al. A prospective study of sudden death in 'high risk' bundle branch block. *N Engl J Med* 1978; 299: 209–215.
3. Surawiez B. Editorial. Prognosis of patients with chronic bifascicular block. *Circulation* 1979; 60: 40–42.

105. Items A and B correct.

Thromboembolic complications in patients with prosthetic valves have been a continuing and difficult problem, even with improved valve designs and the use of anticoagulants. The risk of emboli is greater for prosthetic valves in the mitral position, and anticoagulant prophylaxis is mandatory.

The use of coumadin anticoagulants during pregnancy carries an increased risk of fetal haemorrhage and maternal problems, yet the risk of embolic phenomena is considerable if anticoagulants are withdrawn from pregnant patients with prosthetic valves. Most authorities recommend continued anticoagulation throughout pregnancy. Some recommend replacement of oral anticoagulants with heparin during the first 3 months because of the suspicion of teratogenicity. Most recommend replacement with heparin only at the onset of labour and for a short period post-partum.

The presence of a prosthetic valve increases the vulnerability of the patient to infective endocarditis and makes eradication of any infection very difficult. Whereas endocarditis occurring early after operation carries a very high mortality, endocarditis developing later has a lower mortality. To some extent this probably reflects the less virulent organisms usually involved and their greater sensitivity to antibiotics as well as a greater resistance to infection by the patient. Medical therapy alone should be curative in over 30% of such patients. Early surgical intervention is sometimes required.

Generally, long-term suppressant antibiotic therapy is not indicated as a routine prophylaxis for those with prosthetic valves, but short-term prophylaxis to cover dental and other procedures associated with potential bacteraemia is imperative for the prevention of late prosthetic valve endocarditis.

Reference

1. Murphy ES, Kloster FE. Late results of valve replacement surgery. II. Complications of prosthetic heart valves. *Mod Concepts Cardiovasc Dis* 1979; 48(11): 59–66.

106. Items A, C and D correct.

In a large group of relatively healthy old people aged 65 years or more and living at home, there was a fall of 20 mmHg or more in systolic pressure on standing in 24%; 5% had a fall of 40 mmHg or more (Caird et al, 1973). The frequency of a fall of pressure on standing increases with age. Comparisons between subjects with and without a fall of pressure showed no significant difference in the frequency of various aetiological factors taken singly, but often two or more of these factors were present in those whose blood pressure fell on standing. Aetiological factors include organic brain disease, heart disease, neuropathy, varicose veins, anaemia, urinary infection, low serum sodium concentration and drugs interfering with peripheral sympathetic activity.

Low levels of plasma noradrenaline are found in recumbent patients with orthostatic hypotension who have strictly peripheral sympathetic dysfunction, whereas normal concentrations have been measured in those with CNS disease. Conceptually this would seem useful for purposes of prognosis and therapy. At present however, data suggest a similar natural history for both disorders, and management strategies are the same.

Hypotension on standing in the absence of symptoms is not usually an indication for therapy. However, should it be necessary, the first step in treatment is the use of simple physical manoeuvres such as keeping the upper part of the body tilted upward at night and/or applying graduated pressure (by stockings, etc.) to the lower half of the body when upright. The first procedure promotes renin release and increases blood volume; the second reduces venous pooling and improves cardiac output.

There is no ideal treatment but fludrocortisone acetate 0.1 mg daily, increasing by 0.1 mg each week to 1 mg daily, is often effective, the pharmacological mechanism being uncertain. It is the best single drug for the treatment of orthostatic hypotension. There are two contraindications to usage — overt heart failure and/or significant sustained supine hypertension.

Other tried therapies are monoamine oxidase inhibitors and tyramine (often from cheese), indomethacin and beta-adrenergic blockers.

References

1. Schatz IJ Current management concepts in orthostatic hypotension. *Arch Intern Med* 1980; 140: 1152–1154.
2. Caird FI, et al. Effect of posture on blood pressure in the elderly. *Br Heart J* 1973; 35: 527–530.

107. Item D correct.

Angina of effort, dyspnoea on exertion and syncopal attacks are classical symptoms of aortic stenosis, yet severe stenosis may be asymptomatic. Frequently the aortic systolic murmur is loud, but sometimes, particularly when associated with heart failure, the murmur may become difficult to hear or inaudible (occult aortic stenosis).

In the majority of cases the ECG shows some abnormality but there are many well-documented case reports of moderate to severe aortic stenosis with normal ECGs.

On cardiac catheterisation the finding of a gradient of 50 mmHg or higher is generally regarded as indicating severe stenosis.

In severe stenosis left ventricular function may still be normal.

Reference

1. Morgan DJR, Hall, RJC. Occult aortic stenosis as cause of intractable heart failure. *Br Med J* 1979; 1: 784–787.

108. Items A, B and D correct.

Nitroglycerine dilates vascular smooth muscle throughout the body. Systemic vascular resistance falls unless reflex vasoconstriction is marked. The blood pressure usually falls slightly when the patient is supine but the fall may be considerable in the upright posture. The dominant action of nitroglycerine is venodilation, which leads to a reduction in venous return and a subsequent decrease in left ventricular end-diastolic volume.

Nitrates are still the mainstay of treatment for acute attacks of angina and of coronary vasospasm although there is increasing use of newer prophylactic agents such as the calcium antagonists, verapamil and nifedipine. There is no necessity to withhold nitroglycerine for symptomatic treatment if the patient is taking calcium antagonists, but it is likely that less nitrate therapy will be required.

As an alternative to the longer-acting nitrates such as isosorbide dinitrate, nitroglycerine ointment is highly effective in many patients. However the dosage and duration of action cannot be precisely controlled.

Reference

1. Abrams J. Current concepts: nitroglycerin and long-acting nitrates. *N Engl J Med* 1980; 302: 1234–1237.

109. Items A and C correct.

Several investigators have examined the prevalence and prognostic significance of ventricular ectopic beats in apparently healthy persons. Depending on the age of the population studied, up to 100% of individuals in some groups may have ventricular ectopics of varying frequency and complexity, including ventricular tachycardia. Bigeminal rhythm alone has been found in up to 13% of some groups studied. Coronary artery disease, cardiomyopathy, mitral valve prolapse, long Q-T syndrome and drugs, including psychotropic agents, are commonly associated with ventricular ectopics.

In the absence of evidence of organic heart disease and traditional risk factors for coronary disease, ventricular ectopics should be considered to have little prognostic meaning and should be treated only if the patient has significant symptoms.

The response of ectopics to exercise does not predict the presence or absence of underlying heart disease. Many ectopics associated with coronary artery disease disappear with exercise and have the same predictive implications as ectopics that are sustained during exercise.

Mitral valve prolapse is associated with frequent, and occasionally complex, ventricular ectopics in about 50% of patients. The diagnosis of prolapse may not be easy and echocardiography is indicated in patients with frequent ectopics without obvious cause.

Although cessation of smoking and coffee consumption and adoption of a more 'regular' lifestyle are advocated as baseline therapy, the studies which have been reported have not demonstrated any benefit after these measures have been taken.

References

1. De Backer MD, et al. Ventricular premature contractions: a randomized non-drug intervention trial in normal men. *Circulation* 1979; 59: 762–769.
2. Moss AJ. Clinical significance of ventricular arrhythmias in patients with and without coronary artery disease. *Prog Cardiovasc Dis* 1980; 23: 33–52.
3. Regan TJ. Editorial. Of beverages, cigarettes and cardiac arrhythmias. *N Engl J Med* 1979; 301: 1060–1062.

110. Items C and E correct.

The diagnosis of oesophageal stricture is very unlikely because of the lack of previous oesophageal reflux symptoms and the intermittent rather than progressive dysphagia. A lower oesophageal ring (Schatski ring) is the most common cause of intermittent dysphagia for solids with no other symptoms. Episodes are commonly associated with eating out, talking excitedly and eating steak ('steakhouse syndrome').

Scleroderma is uncommon in males of this age and does not usually present in this way.

There is usually no need to rush into urgent oesophagoscopy. It is reasonable to administer relaxants and monitor progress over the next few hours. With time and relaxation the steak may pass. If not, a proteolytic enzyme (papain or meat tenderiser) may be used or endoscopic removal may be undertaken electively.

Reference

1. Edwards DAW. Discriminatory value of symptoms in the differential diagnosis of dysphagia. *Clin Gastroenterol* 1976; 5: 49–57.

111. Items A, D and E correct.

Reflux oesophagitis has a multifactorial pathogenesis including

a. efficiency of the antireflux mechanism
b. volume of gastric fluid
c. potency of refluxed material (content of acid, pepsin and bile)
d. efficiency of oesophageal clearance of refluxed material
e. tissue resistance of the oesophageal mucosa.

Thus, symptomatic oesophageal reflux is not due to either oesophageal reflux or to lower oesophageal sphincter pressure alone.

Reflux occurs in all humans, but patients with symptoms tend to reflux more often and for more prolonged periods. As this reflux is intermittent and associated with a transient drop of lower oesophageal sphincter pressure, these episodes often are not detected by routine radiological measures. A barium meal is not a good test for gastro-oesophageal reflux or for reflux oesophagitis.

Oesophageal pH measurement, especially over a long period, is the best way of determining the presence of acid in the lower oesophagus, but radionuclide studies better demonstrate the volume of refluxed material. Reflux or reflux oesophagitis may occur in the absence of a hiatus hernia.

Isotope studies are useful for measuring transit but are not helpful for diagnosing reflux in patients who have undergone pH testing.

References

1. Dodds WJ, et al. Pathogenesis of reflux oesophagitis. *Gastroenterology* 1981; 81: 376–394.
2. Whelan G. Management of gastro-oesophageal reflux. *Aust NZ J Med* 1982; 12: 90–96.
3. Breen KJ. Diagnosis and management of reflux oesophagitis. *Med J Aust* 1977; 1: 184–186.
4. Breen KJ, Whelan G. The diagnosis of reflux oesophagitis. An evaluation of five investigative procedures. *Aust NZ J Surg* 1978; 48: 156–161.

112. Items B, C and E correct.

A flat villous architecture in the small bowel may occur in diseases other than coeliac disease, e.g. tropical sprue enteritis (Katz & Grand, 1979).

Tests of malabsorption provide no single ideal screening test for coeliac disease. Faecal fat estimations and xylose absorption tests may be normal when flat villous architecture is present. The best screening test is probably serum or red blood cell folate level. It is estimated that 1 in 10 first-degree relatives of those with coeliac disease is affected if examination of the villous architecture of their small bowel is undertaken.

It takes 5–6 days for normal cells to migrate from crypts to villous tips. It often takes months after instituting a gluten-free diet in a patient with coeliac disease for small bowel histology to revert to normal, with poor correlation between symptomatic and biochemical improvement.

A positive small bowel biopsy is an essential criterion for the diagnosis of coeliac disease. Some would even add that the diagnosis requires confirmation by a clinical and histological relapse on gluten challenge. The demand for strict diagnostic criteria is justified in the context of a life-long commitment of adherence to a strict diet if coeliac disease is diagnosed.

References

1. Katz AJ, Grand RJ. All that flattens is not 'Sprue'. *Gastroenterology* 1979; 76: 375–377.
2. Trier S. Celiac sprue disease. In: Sleisinger MH, Fortran JS (eds). Gastrointestinal disease, 2nd Edn. Philadelphia: Saunders, 1978: 1029–1051.
3. Cooke WT, Asquith P (eds). Coeliac disease. *Clin Gastroenterol* 1974; 3: 1–235.

113. Items A, C and E correct.

In such a patient with growth retardation, hypocalcaemia and diarrhoea, one must consider a possible malabsorption syndrome, of which adult coeliac disease is the most likely cause. Hypocalcaemic tetany which does not readily respond to calcium always raises the possibility of hypomagnesaemia. Magnesium deficiency potentiates tetany caused by hypocalcaemia and, in an obscure fashion, inhibits the restoration of normal levels of calcium when calcium is given. Magnesium and calcium metabolism are closely related. Magnesium is a necessary cofactor for the release of and the peripheral action of parathyroid hormone on bone, kidney and gut, and for the hepatic 25-hydroxylation of vitamin D. In chronic diarrhoeal states, with high stool losses of magnesium, severe deficiencies may occur. In coeliac disease where calcium malabsorption may also occur, hypomagnesaemia may impair the response to what otherwise would be an adequate supplementation with calcium. The intravenous administration of magnesium may have dramatic effects on the serum calcium level and the tetany.

Medullary carcinoma of the thyroid is associated with a high level of serum calcitonin, a hormone which depresses the serum calcium level. However, for obscure reasons, hypocalcaemia occurs rarely. Even in the presence of diarrhoea, a common symptom in medullary carcinoma, this diagnosis is most unlikely.

If adult coeliac disease is being considered, the probability is much increased by the presence of Howell-Jolly bodies, which are a marker of 'splenectomy'. Hyposplenism has been reported in 21% of a recent series of patients with coeliac disease.

Sigmoidoscopy should be carried out in all patients with persistent diarrhoea. The procedure can be of considerable help in possible malabsorptive states because the stools can be examined for their characteristic colour, consistency and odour, quickly and effectively.

Croese et al (1980) have re-emphasised the frequency of folate deficiency in adult coeliac disease; it was present in two-thirds of their patients.

References

1. Foy A. Magnesium: the neglected cation. *Med J Aust* 1980; 1: 305–306.
2. Croese J, et al. Coeliac disease: haematological features, and delay in diagnosis. *Med J Aust* 1979; 2: 335–338.
3. Aurbach GD. Calcitonin and medullary carcinoma of the thyroid. In: Beeson PB, et al (eds). Cecil Textbook of medicine, 15th Edn. Philadelphia: Saunders, 1979; 2223–2224.

114. Items A, B, C and E correct.

In colonic diverticular disease, 75–80% of patients with complications of diverticulitis such as haemorrhage or perforation have no previous colonic symptoms.

Besides increasing faecal fat and mineral losses, bran increases faecal weight, relaxes the gut and alters faecal bile acids. Increased volume and water content reflect a mild osmotic diarrhoea. Studies are not yet sufficiently long-term to have established the significance of faecal mineral losses.

Analgesic treatment with morphine is contraindicated in patients with colonic diverticular disease, since morphine and its derivatives have been shown to increase intrasigmoidal pressure.

Complications due to diverticulitis should be treated by absorbable antibiotics. Diverticulitis implies micro- or macroparacolic abscess formation, and the critical site of antibiotic effect is the pericolic tissues, not the luminal surface.

Recent angiographic studies have demonstrated the high frequency of angiodysplasia (particularly in the right colon) as a cause of rectal haemorrhage.

Reference

1. Almy TP, Howell DA. Diverticular diseases of the colon. *N Engl J Med* 1980; 302: 324–331.

115. Items B and C correct.

Biopsy of the polyps may not be representative and, if malignant changes are seen, this will not give information as to whether stalk invasion has occurred. All polyps should be removed in toto and examined histologically to establish the type of polyp and to look for malignant change.

There is a 40% chance of a second polyp being present if the removed polyp is adenomatous. In addition, the bleeding may be coming from a colorectal cancer higher in the colon, so examination of the whole colon, whether by radiology or colonoscopy, is mandatory.

After polypectomy the patient should probably have a sigmoidoscopy and air contrast barium enema every 3–5 years because of the greater risk of further polyps or colorectal carcinoma in the future for such patients compared with the general population.

Biopsy of the rectal mucosa is unnecessary as usually there is no difficulty in differentiating the pseudo-polyps of ulcerative colitis from an adenoma occurring in normal rectal mucosa.

References

1. Winawer SJ, et al. Potential of endoscopy. Biopsy and cytology in the diagnosis and management of patients with cancer. *Clin Gastroenterol* 1976; 5: 575–595.
2. Zamcheck N. The present state of Carcinoma-embryonic Antigen (CEA) in diagnosis. Detection of recurrence, prognosis and evaluation of therapy of colonic and pancreatic cancer. *Clin Gastroenterol* 1976; 5: 525–538.

116. Items A and E correct.

Any single positive faecal occult blood test in an asymptomatic person over the age of 40 years must be considered significant; therefore it is not really necessary to repeat the test daily for 6 days.

False-positive rates are 11% and 2% on a normal and meat-free diet respectively for a single slide.

Vitamin C will cause a false-negative reaction, not a false-positive one.

Bleeding from colorectal cancer is intermittent and so a positive result merits either sigmoidoscopy and air contrast barium enema examination or colonoscopy. Barium enema examinations, even with air contrast, will miss more small polypoid lesions than colonoscopy, although both are equally effective (in expert hands) in detecting lesions more than 1 cm in diameter.

Asymptomatic colorectal cancers diagnosed by faecal occult blood sceening have twice the chance of being localised to the bowel wall (Dukes A or B) than have symptomatic cancers.

References

1. Bassett ML, Goulston KJ. False positive and negative hemoccult reactions on a normal diet and effect of diet restriction. *Aust NZ J Med* 1980; 10: 1–4.
2. Sherlock P, et al. The prevention of colon cancer. *Am J Med* 1980; 68: 917–931.
3. Leading article. Large-bowel polyps and colonoscopy. *Br Med J* 1979; 1: 1587–1588.
4. Goulston KJ, Davidson P. Faecal occult blood testing in patients with colonic symptoms. *Med J Aust* 1980; 2: 667–668.

117. Items A, C, D and E correct.

Before the angiographic demonstration of angiodysplasia (AGD), haemangiomas had been implicated in gastrointestinal bleeding of obscure origin. Haemangiomas are gross lesions, located most frequently in the stomach, small bowel and rectum, but rarely in the proximal colon. However, AGD (or vascular dysplasia, vascular ectasia, arteriovenous malformations) is located most commonly in the right colon and is rarely seen macroscopically by the surgeon. Boley et al (1977) suggested that these lesions are acquired, resulting from dilatation of normal vascular structures of the colon. They suggest partial obstruction of subcommunication. They demonstrated the lesions in the resected colon in 16 patients over 60 years of age undergoing colectomy for reasons other than bleeding. Although usually in the right colon, they are often multiple and can occur anywhere else in the gastrointestinal tract. AGD may be the most common cause of significant recurrent rectal bleeding.

In series where arteriography has been used to evaluate patients who have had intestinal bleeding, AGD has been implicated in 12–70% of cases. Average age on presentation with bleeding is 60 years. AGD may be revealed by mesenteric artery angiography when active bleeding has ceased. Angiographic hallmarks are an early filling vein, a vascular tuft or a slowly emptying vein.

Diagnosis may be made by colonoscopy (and AGD can be cauterised successfully).

Patients often rebleed after apparently successful resection because AGD may be multiple. Blind right hemicolectomy may be necessary in some patients.

There seems to be an association with aortic stenosis.

References

1. Boley SJ, et al. On the nature and etiology of vascular ectasias of the colon; degenerative lesions of aging. *Gastroenterology* 1977; 72: 650–660.
2. Meyer CT, et al. Arteriovenous malformations of the bowel; an analysis of 22 cases and a review of the literature. *Medicine* (Baltimore) 1981; 60: 36–48.

118. Items A, C and D correct.

Symptoms caused by disordered gastrointestinal motility are encountered in 50–70% of patients presenting to a gastroenterologist; they may also occur in as many as 14% of normal subjects.

The pain experienced may be quite diverse and is felt not only in the lower abdomen but also in the upper abdomen, particularly the epigastrium where it has been reported in 30–40% of affected patients.

It has also been demonstrated to arise in extra-abdominal sites, especially the back. Motility studies have also shown proctalgia fugax to be part of the spectrum of the irritable bowel syndrome.

The condition is difficult to treat and, although there is theoretical justification for the use of antispasmodic medications, their effectiveness has not been established by controlled trials.

References

1. Thompson WG, Heaton KW. Functional bowel disorders in apparently healthy people. *Gastroenterology* 1980; 79: 283–288.
2. Swarbrick ET, et al. Site of pain from the irritable bowel. *Lancet* 1980; 2: 443–446.
3. Harvey RF. Colonic motility in proctalgia fugax. *Lancet* 1979; 2: 713–714.
4. Drosman DA, et al. The irritable bowel syndrome. *Gastroenterology* 1977; 73: 811–822.

119. Items B and D correct.

Alcoholic hepatitis may occur with or without cirrhosis. It is considered to be a precursor for cirrhosis whereas alcoholic fatty liver can occur in any patient after a few days drinking and does not progress to cirrhosis.

Alcoholic hepatitis itself may cause fever and leucocytosis, presumably by hepatic cell necrosis. However, infections, especially septicaemia and peritonitis, should be carefully excluded in such patients.

Vomiting, pain and upper abdominal signs may be severe enough to mimic a surgical abdominal catastrophe or acute pancreatitis.

It is now known that Mallory hyaline bodies seen in the liver biopsy may occur in many other conditions and are not pathognomonic of alcoholic hepatitis.

Reference

1. Sherlock S. Diseases of the liver and biliary system, 5th Edn. Oxford: Blackwell Scientific, 1975: 445–460.

120. Item C correct.

Focal nodular hyperplasia has been observed in patients receiving oral contraceptives (particularly over a prolonged period) and may present with bleeding into the liver and peritoneal cavity. Most women with hepatocellular carcinoma, hepatic adenoma or focal nodular hyperplasia associated with oral contraceptives have been taking the pill for more than 5 years.

Negative serology for amoebiasis makes the diagnosis of ameobic abscess very unlikely. Angiosarcoma of liver is rare, usually occurring in workers exposed to vinylchloride. Intrahepatic endometriosis with bleeding has not been reported. The clinical and biochemical picture is not cholestatic as would occur in cholangiocarcinoma.

References

1. Klatskin G. Hepatic tumours: possible relationship to use of oral contraceptives. *Gastroenterology* 1977; 73: 386–394.
2. Baum JK. et al. Possible association between benign hepatomas and oral contraceptives. *Lancet* 1973; 2: 926–929.
3. Neuberger J, et al. Oral-contraceptive associated liver tumours: occurrence of malignancy and difficulties in diagnosis. *Lancet* 1980; 1: 273–276.

121. Items A, B and C correct.

Idiopathic haemochromatosis is an inherited disease and there is an association with HLA antigens, particularly HLA-A3.

Although serum iron and transferrin saturation are elevated early in the course of the disease, their specificity is reduced by a relatively high frequency of false-positives and negatives. The best screening test is the estimation of serum ferritin level: 300–5000 μg/ℓ levels are indicative of haemochromatosis (N: 10–200). All first-degree relatives over 10 years of age should be tested for serum ferritin concentration, serum iron and percentage saturation of transferrin.

A relatively low fluctuating serum ferritin level (300–1000 μg/ℓ) associated with increased levels of transaminase enzymes does suggest alcoholic liver disease. It may still be difficult to differentiate between idiopathic haemochromatosis and alcohol liver disease with iron overload, although those with the latter disease alone are unlikely to have excess HLA-A3 or a familial tendency. However, the majority of patients suffering from alcoholic cirrhosis with gross iron deposition probably have idiopathic haemochromatosis and 25% of those with idiopathic haemochromatosis have superimposed alcoholic liver disease.

There is evidence that phlebotomy therapy does prolong life in symptomatic patients with established haemochromatosis. However there are, as yet, no controlled studies to show the effect of therapy in early precirrhotic patients. Despite adequate iron removal by phlebotomy, hepatomas occur as a late sequela in about one-third of patients. However, it is probable that the apparent increase in its incidence is related to the increased life-span after phlebotomy therapy.

References

1. Powell IW, et al. Haemochromatosis 1980 update. *Gastroenterology* 1980; 78: 374–381.
2. Bassett MI, et al. Haemochromatosis new concepts: diagnosis and management. Disease a month 1980: January.

122. Items A and C correct.

Elevated serum bile acids are common in both obstructive jaundice and in hepatocellular jaundice. Bilirubin enters the hepatocyte via a transport mechanism distinct from that used for the bile acids.

Visualisation of the biliary tree is a crucial step in the investigation of patients with obstructive jaundice. However, ultrasound examinations frequently fail to demonstrate calculi in the common bile duct. The demonstration of a dilated biliary tree is a highly reliable sign, but its absence does not exclude a mechanical cause of obstructive jaundice.

New bile-seeking agents (e.g. HIDA — a radiotracer which is becoming available) allow visualisation of the biliary tree and offer an advantage over the older agent, rose bengal, because the label is technetium. This technique is particularly useful in the diagnosis of cystic duct obstruction.

Percutaneous transhepatic cholangiography is a very reliable and safe procedure when performed by experts. Mechanical obstruction is not a contraindication to the procedure, as it is now possible to perform percutaneous drainage of the biliary tree, thereby allowing conservative management of patients until their condition improves.

Sclerosing cholangitis is a rare condition which may complicate ulcerative colitis but very rarely Crohn's disease.

References

1. Chapman RWG, et al. Primary sclerosing cholangitis: a review of its clinical features, cholangiography and hepatic histology. *Gut* 1980; 21: 870–877.
2. Schwarz W, et al. Percutaneous transhepatic drainage preoperatively for benign biliary strictures. *Surg Gynecol & Obstet* 1981; 152: 466–468.
3. Dooley JS, et al. Non surgical treatment of biliary obstruction. *Lancet* 1979; 2: 1040–1044.

123. Items A and D correct.

The illness and biopsy suggest chronic active hepatitis. This entity is a syndrome with several known and some unknown causes. Several drugs may cause chronic active hepatitis, including nitrofurantoin and sulfonamides.

Wilson's disease is always an important consideration in a younger patient; it may occasionally present at this age and with similar histological appearances. The need for urgent chelation therapy makes early recognition mandatory. The only situation in which corticosteroid is unequivocally effective is chronic active hepatitis associated with positive autoantibodies ('lupoid hepatitis') which most often occurs in young women but can occur in either sex at any age. In this patient, no features are described to suggest imminent liver failure and treatment should await a fuller diagnostic work-up including hepatitis B serology, autoantibodies, copper studies and alpha-1-antitrypsin levels.

It has been suspected for several years that patients with hepatitis B and chronic active hepatitis do not benefit from corticosteroid therapy. There are now data which show that

a. patients not only do not benefit but fare less well than untreated patients because of steroid side-effects
b. hepatitis B viral replication is facilitated by corticosteroids.

While symptomatic and biochemical improvements are encouraging, they do not always correlate with histological progression of the disease. In particular, at least 16% of patients progress to cirrhosis during corticosteroid therapy.

References

1. Editorial. Chronic active hepatitis. *Br Med J* 1980; 281: 258–259.
2. Redeker AG. Treatment of chronic active hepatitis: good news and bad news. *N Engl J Med* 1981; 304: 420–421.

3. Mistilis SP, Lam KC. Treatment of chronic active hepatitis. *Aust NZ J Med* 1980; 10: 64–68.
4. Schalm SW, et al. Contrasting features and responses to treatment of severe chronic active liver disease with and without HBs antigen. *Gut* 1980; 17: 781–786.
5. Scullard GH, et al. Effects of immunosuppressive therapy on viral markers in chronic active hepatitis B. *Gastroenterology* 1981; 81: 987–991.
6. Hatoff DE, et al. Nitrofurantoin: cause of drug induced chronic active hepatitis. *Am J Med* 1979; 67: 117–121.
7. Scott J, et al, Wilson's disease, presenting as chronic active hepatitis. *Gastroenterology* 1978; 74: 645–651.
8. Kirk AP, et al. Late results of the Royal Free Hospital prospective controlled trial of prednisolone therapy in hepatitis B surface antigen negative chronic active hepatitis. *Gut* 1980; 21: 78–83.

124. Item B and C correct.

Fatty change, either alone or with other histological features, is one of the most common findings in a liver biopsy. Fatty change due to alcohol is not nearly so serious as perivenular sclerosis which is probably a precursor of cirrhosis. Fatty liver alone is potentially reversible.

CT scans have provided a non-invasive diagnostic approach to storage diseases of the liver, at least as a screening test. Penetrance of X-rays depends on the chemical constitution of tissues; it is increased over normal values for liver replaced by fat, and decreased in liver with increased stores of iron or copper. These changes can be quantified, in relation to the CT number. Since many causes of fatty liver are obvious (e.g. obesity, diabetes mellitus), histological diagnosis is not always required on initial assessment.

The presence of fibrosis, necrosis and inflammation should always make one suspect alcoholic liver disease. However, there are other causes of this histological pattern, including jejunoileal bypass, perhexiline maleate toxicity and Indian childhood cirrhosis. More importantly, a group of allegedly non-alcoholic patients without these exotic disorders may have a pattern of liver injury that is indistinguishable from alcoholic liver disease. Such patients are most often middle-aged females, obese, diabetic and with other medical disorders; the spectrum of severity may include cirrhosis. Liver function tests are only marginally abnormal while complications of cirrhosis such as ascites, jaundice, bleeding varices and portal systemic encephalopathy are rare.

Fatty change is not a feature of hepatitis A, hepatitis B or autoimmune chronic active hepatitis, but has been described in non-A, non-B hepatitis and occurs frequently in Wilson's disease. Acute fatty liver in pregnancy is fortunately rare (it is associated with a high mortality); the histological appearance differs from that of alcoholic fatty liver and may be associated with the use of tetracycline in pregnancy.

References

1. Review by an International Group. Alcoholic liver disease: morphological manifestations. *Lancet* 1981; 1: 707–711.
2. Abrams HL, McNeill BJ. Medical implications of computed tomography ('CAT scanning'). Parts 1 and 2. *N Engl J Med* 1978; 298: 255–260, 310–318.
3. Adler N, Schaffner F. Fatty liver hepatitis and cirrhosis in obese patients. *Am J Med* 1979; 67: 811–816.
4. Sternlieb I, Scheinberg IH. Wilson's disease. In: Wright R, et al (eds). Liver and biliary disease. London: Saunders, 1979: 774–787.

125. Items A, C and D correct.

In the clinical situation described, the most likely diagnosis is haemochromatosis or some other form of chronic liver disease complicated by hepatocellular carcinoma. Although features of hepatocellular dysfunction occur in less than 10% of cases of haemochromatosis at diagnosis, liver failure is one of the three cardinal features of hepatocellular carcinoma. The others are pain and weight loss. Elevated alpha-fetoprotein levels in serum do not occur in at least 50% of cases of hepatocellular carcinoma in Western society.

Gallium scanning is extremely valuable in detecting hepatocellular carcinoma (over 90% true-positives). Conventional colloid liver scans often will not distinguish chronic liver disease from a multicentric hepatocellular carcinoma, although a large defect can suggest hepatoma.

Bruits may occur in alcoholic hepatitis due to extensive intrahepatic shunting in this disorder. An increased serum ferritin may result from hepatocellular necrosis from any cause and a value as high as the one presented here may occur with alcoholic hepatitis. Serum ferritin levels can be correctly interpreted only if the serum alanine amino transferase, serum iron and iron binding capacity are also known.

There is now convincing evidence that hepatitis B is associated with hepatocellular carcinoma. The test results are consistent with the presence of replicating virus in the liver despite the negative hepatitis B surface antigen. Recent studies have shown a high incidence of anti-HBc among patients with hepatocellular carcinoma, even in western communities.

Surgical removal would not be tolerated by this patient, who almost certainly has cirrhosis. While adriamycin is the only therapeutic agent with promising efficacy against hepatocellular carcinoma, remissions occur only in about half of the patient treated and are usually of less than 12 months duration.

References

1. Schonland MM, et al. Hepatic tumours. In: Wright R, et al (eds). Liver and biliary disease. London: Saunders, 1979: 886–925.
2. Milder MS, et al. Idiopathic haemochromatosis, an interim report. *Medicine* (Baltimore) 1980; 59: 34–49.
3. Yarrish RL, et al. Association of hepatitis B virus infection with

hepatocellular carcinoma in American patients. *Int J Cancer* 1980; 26: 711–715.
4. Johnson PJ, et al. Hepatocellular carcinoma in Great Britain: influence of age, sex, HBsAg status and aetiology of underlying cirrhosis. *Gut* 1978; 19: 1022—1026.
5. Falkson G, et al. Chemontherapy studies in primary liver cancer: a prospective randomized clinical trial. *Cancer* 1978; 42: 2149–2156.
6. Friedman MA, et al. Therapy for hepatocellular cancer with intrahepatic arterial adriamycin and 5-fluorouracil combined with whole liver irradiation: a Northern California oncology group study. *Cancer Treat Rep* 1979; 63: 1885–1888.

126. Items A and C correct.

Both rigid and flexible endoscopes have been used to inject oesophageal varices under general and local anaesthesia. Prospective randomised trials have shown that repeated injection will reduce significantly the risk of re-bleeding and improve 1-year survival rates. Varices are reduced and often eradicated.

Complications of injection sclerotherapy include ulceration and perforation but not hepatic encephalopathy. Sclerotherapy may be used electively or as an emergency procedure, often after initial control of haemorrhage using vasopressin and a Sengstaken-Blakemore tube.

References

1. Clark AW, et al, Prospective controlled trial of injection sclerotherapy in patients with cirrhosis and recent variceal haemorrhage. *Lancet* 1980; 2: 552–554.
2. Willimas KGD, Dawson JL. Fibreoptic injection of oesophageal varices. *Br Med J* 1979; 2: 766–767.
3. Terblanche J, et al. A prospective controlled trial of sclerotherapy in the long term management of patients after esophageal variceal bleeding. *Surg Gynecol Obstet* 1979; 148: 323–333.

127. Items B, D and E correct.

Chenodeoxycholic acid and cholic acid are the two primary bile acids synthesised by the liver in man. Intestinal bacterial action dehydrolyses these to the secondary bile acids, lithocholic and deoxycholic acids.

Chenodeoxycholic acid, and the related ursodeoxycholic acid, appear to be effective by decreasing cholesterol secretion in bile, probably by inhibiting the activity of the rate-limiting enzyme for cholesterol synthesis, hydroxymethylglutaryl coenzyme A reductase. Treatment with 12–15 mg/kg chenodeoxycholic acid (or 8–10 mg/kg ursodeoxycholic acid) renders bile unsaturated in cholesterol.

Lithocholic acid, formed from chenodeoxycholic acid by bacterial action, is potentially hepatotoxic. Chenodeoxycholic acid given to rhesus monkeys may result in histological liver damage, but in man efficient sulphation of lithocholic acid appears to prevent this hepatotoxicity. Although some patients develop elevated serum levels of aspartate aminotransferase, consistent histological changes in the liver have not been described.

Bile acid therapy will gradually dissolve the majority of cholesterol gallstones. Non-calcified radiolucent stones, especially small stones with a relatively large surface area, dissolve more efficiently than large solitary radio-opaque stones. One indicator of stone composition is density. During oral cholecystography the iodinated cholecystographic agent increases the density of bile. Stones which float on this dense fluid are usually composed largely of cholesterol and respond well to bile acid therapy.

References

1. Small DM. Cholesterol nucleation and growth in gallstone formation. *N Engl J Med* 1980; 302: 1305–1307.
2. Hofmann AF. The medical treatment of cholesterol gallstones: a major advance in preventive gastroenterology *Am J Med* 1980; 69: 4–7.
3. Cowen AE, Campbell CB. Bile salt metabolism. *Aust NZ J Med* 1977; 7: 579–595.
4. Leading Article. Dissolving gallstones. *Med J Aust* 1980; 1: 456–457.

128. Items B, C and D correct.

In the treatment of doudenal ulcer, the composite results of worldwide clinical trials show that, after treatment with cimetidine for 6 weeks, about 80% of patients will have 'endoscopically' healed ulcers. Recurrence rate on a nightly maintenance dosage of cimetidine is 20% over a 1-year period, compared with about 55% with placebo. Cimetidine confers no protection beyond the period in which the drug is taken.

Although side-effects are rare (about 1%), the recurrence rate of duodenal ulcer after highly selective vagotomy now appears to be about 10%.

High-dose antacids (e.g. Mylanta II taken 1 and 3 hours after meals and at bed-time) are as effective as cimetidine in healing duodenal ulcers.

References

1. Leading article. New drugs for peptic ulcer. *Br Med J* 1980; 2: 9506.
2. Grossman MI. Editorial. New medical and surgical treatments for peptic ulcer disease. *Am J Med* 1980; 69: 647–649.
3. Hetzel DJ, et al. Leading article. Cimetidine and peptic ulcer. *Med J Aust* 1980; 2: 588–589.
4. Editorial. Cimetidine now. *Lancet* 1981; 1: 875–877.
5. Leading article. Antacids for duodenal ulcer. *Br Med J* 1981; 282: 1495–1496.

129. Item A, B and C correct.

In recent years there has been an improved survival rate of patients with cystic fibrosis. With about two-thirds of patients now surviving to the age of 18 years and some going on to 30 years, knowledge of the disease is becoming increasingly important to physicians.

Cystic fibrosis is inherited as a Mendelian recessive trait. The incidence in live births in Caucasian communities is between 1:2000 and 1:2500. This incidence holds for Australia, as demonstrated in Melbourne (Danks et al, 1965).

Of those born without meconium ileus, about 75% survived to the age of 17 years whereas only 50% with meconium ileus survived to the age of 12 years.

335 young patients with cystic fibrosis were examined by Shwachman (1972). The mean sweat chloride level was 113 mmol/ℓ and the sodium 112 mmol/ℓ. The control values in healthy and other sick children were 23 mmol/ℓ for both chloride and sodium levels. Generally, a sweat chloride level greater than 60 mmol/ℓ is considered confirmatory when the patient has chronic obstructive pulmonary disease, exocrine pancreatic insufficiency or a family history of cystic fibrosis.

Females are mostly fertile whereas males are almost always sterile, 95% having a discontinuous vas deferens or epididymis.

The persistence of *Haemophilus influenzae* in the sputum is uncommon, the most common persisting organisms being *Pseudomonas aerogenes* and a penicillin-resistant *Staphylococcus*.

References

1. Phelan PD, et al. Improved survival of patients with cystic fibrosis. *Med J Aust* 1979; 261–263.
2. Brown J. Cystic fibrosis. *Med J Aust* 1972; 1: 67–70.
3. Williams HE, Phelan PD. Respiratory illness in children. Oxford; Blackwell Scientific, 1975; 216–236.
4. Danks DM, et al. A genetic study of fibrocystic disease of the pancreas. *Ann Hum Genet* 1965; 28: 323–356.
5. Shwachman H. Cystic fibrosis. In: Kendig EI (ed). Disorders of the respiratory tract in children. Philadelphia; Saunders, 1972; 524–546.
6. Wood RE, et al. Cystic fibrosis. *Am Rev Respir Dis* 1976; 113: 833–878.

130. Items B, C and D correct.

The hepatotoxicity of isoniazid does not appear to be related to acetylator status. Production and degradation of the toxic metabolite both involve acetylation, so accumulation is probably similar in slow and fast acetylators. There is a positive relationship between isoniazid hepatotoxicity and age: it is much more likely in patients over 40 years of age and rare in children.

It has been shown that the reactivation rate following 6 months prophylactic isoniazid therapy is the same as that following 12 months therapy if the lesion is around 2 cm^2. For larger lesions the success rate is 65% with 6 months and 75% with 12 months therapy. It is important to treat young children whose Mantoux reaction has become positive because they have a high risk of developing active tuberculosis.

Nine months therapy with rifampicin and isoniazid is as effective as

12 months unless there are cavities, in which case the additional three months treatment results in fewer reactivations.

Small rises in gamma glutamyl transpeptidase are common with therapy and of no significance. However a more than two-fold rise in aspartate amino transferase, especially with systemic symptoms, requires cessation of isoniazid and rifampicin.

References

1. Trelis A, et al. Five years of follow-up of the I.U.A.T. Union trial of isoniazid prophylaxis in fibrotic lesions. *Bull Int Union Tuberc* 1979; 54: 65.
2. Leading Article. Chemoprophylaxis for tuberculosis. *Tubercule* 1981; 62: 69–72.
3. Tomah K. Tuberculosis case-finding and chemotherapy: questions and answers. Geneva: World Health Organisation, 1979.

131. Items A, B, and E correct.

Polyvalent vaccines containing the capsular polysaccharides of 14 highly invasive serotypes have been available in the United States for more than two years and are now marketed in Australia. The evidence of their efficacy rests principally on trials undertaken among South African gold miners and Highland dwellers in Papua New Guinea. There is also evidence that the vaccine is effective in children with sickle cell disease. The vaccine has also been shown to be immunogenic in people of all ages over two years. In this age-group a single dose of vaccine produces long-lasting elevation in serum antibody against each of the 14 capsular polysaccharides in the majority of recipients of vaccine.

Patients with nephrosis and systemic lupus erythematosus respond satisfactorily to the vaccine, as do patients undergoing home renal dialysis. Patients with Hodgkin's disease respond poorly if immunised during, or even some years after, radiation and chemotherapy, but their response to many of the vaccine serotypes is satisfactory if they are immunised before treatment is begun, even if the spleen has been removed.

A drawback to the vaccine is its poor immunogenicity in those under the age of 2 years, especially for serotypes 1, 6, 12, 14, 19 and 23. However, in children between the ages of 6 months and 2 years there has been some evidence of benefit in prevention of otitis media.

There are reports of occasional severe local and systemic reactions to the vaccine, although it generally has wide acceptability. Reactivity is probably due to interaction between the injected antigens and circulating antibodies, so that individuals with high circulating antibodies are more likely to have a reaction. Pneumococcal vaccine is different from most killed vaccines for which a spaced course of injections is needed to establish durable immunity. In the case of the pneumococcal vaccine, a single injection seems adequate to provide prolonged antibody elevation in persons over the age of 2 years.

Some controversy surrounds the question of general indications for use of the vaccine. Mortality from pneumococcal disease is significantly higher amongst the elderly, those with pre-existing lung, liver and renal disease, and following splenectomy. Although there are expectations of substantial financial benefits from use of the vaccine in this population, hard evidence on the magnitude of this benefit is still lacking. It can be argued that the use of pneumococcal vaccine is more likely to be helpful to the elderly at risk of complications of influenza, than is the use of influenza vaccine. However, some of the groups at greatest risk of developing pneumococcal disease are incapable of mounting a response to the vaccine.

References

1. Douglas RM, Riley ID. Pneumococcal disease and its prevention with polyvalent pneumococcal polysaccharide vaccines — a review. *Aust NZ J Med* 1979; 9: 327–338.
2. Editorial. Indications for pneumococcal vaccine. *Lancet* 1981; 1: 251–253.
3. Austrian R. The assessment of pneumococcal vaccine. *N Engl J Med* 1980; 303: 578–580.
4. Austrian R. Pneumococcal vaccines: development and prospects. *Am J Med* 1979; 67: 547–549.

132. Items A, B and E correct.

Pandemic influenza (worldwide epidemic disease) is always due to influenza A virus after a sudden shift of either the haemagglutinin (H) or neuraminidase (N) antigen.

Influenza B virus does not undergo such sudden shifts; the antigens change gradually and thus cause less extensive epidemics. Gradual change in the A virus (drift) can also precipitate epidemics which can cause considerable morbidity and mortality but on a less widespread scale.

Antigenic shifts in the A virus are irregular events. In this century, they occurred in 1918, 1957 and 1968. There is no way of predicting what the next change in antigenic determinants will be.

The vaccine is 70% effective in preventing the disease only if it contains the specific antigens of the infecting organism. Preparation of the vaccine takes about 6–8 weeks from identification of the likely viruses to general availability.

References

1. Richman DD. Use of temperature-sensitive mutants for live attenuated influenza-virus vaccines. *N Engl J Med* 1979; 300: 137–138.
2. Selby P (ed). Influenza: virus, vaccine and strategy. Sandoz Institute: Academic Press, 1976: 17–21.

133. Items A and C correct.

Although there is experimental evidence showing diminished response (tachyphylaxis) after repeated administrations of adrenergic agents, there are clinical studies indicating that this does not develop in asthmatic subjects. In particular, dose-response studies have been conducted on asthmatic subjects at 3-monthly intervals over a period of regular administration of oral bronchodilator for 12 months. These studies showed that there was no change in the acute response to isoprenaline, indicating that resistance of the beta 2 receptors in the bronchi had not developed in this period of time.

In another study, both the metabolic and airways effects of salbutamol were studied for a period of 4 weeks before and after regular aerosol administration. Although there were changes in the metabolic effects of acute salbutamol, the dose-response curve obtained on the airways showed that there was no development of resistance to acute administration of beta agonists. Furthermore there had been no change in the response to histamine provocation after regular aerosol administration of salbutamol. Thus, a number of studies have failed to show tachyphylaxis with regular bronchodilator administration.

The doses of Freon required for myocardial damage are far in excess of those administered to patients. It is the current convention to give regular bronchodilators even to asthmatic subjects who have mild to moderate airflow obstruction. This is based on the premise that asthmatics frequently have a significant degree of airflow obstruction which they do not perceive readily.

References

1. Larsson S, et al. Lack of bronchial beta adrenoceptor resistance in asthmatics during long-term treatment with terbutaline. *J Allergy Clin Immunol* 1977; 59: 93–100.
2. Peel ET, Gibson GJ. Effects of long term salbutamol therapy on the provocation of asthma by histamine. *Am Rev Resp Dis* 1980; 121: 973–978.
3. Harvey JE, et al. Airway and metabolic responsiveness to intravenous salbutamol: effect of regular inhaled salbutamol. *Clin Sci* 1981; 6: 579–585.
4. Rubinfeld AR, Pain MCF. Perception of asthma. *Lancet* 1976; 1: 882–884.

134. Item C correct.

The most likely diagnosis is allergic bronchopulmonary aspergillosis. Fungi of the genus aspergillus can involve the lungs in three ways:

a. Forming an aspergilloma in an existing cavity
b. Invasion of an area of pulmonary necrosis
c. Colonisation of the bronchi with the development of an allergic reaction.

The last is the most common and is most often seen in patients who are asthmatic.

Aspergillus produces a variety of X-ray changes which may occur rapidly, taking the form of alveolar infiltrations, nodular mucoid impactions and peribronchial thickening. The condition is not infrequently misdiagnosed as tuberculosis (because of common involvement of the upper lobes), as carcinoma or probably most often as pneumonia.

The expectoration of brownish rubbery plugs is almost diagnostic and in these the fungus may be found. Both type I and type III allergic reactions can be demonstrated by a prick test with *aspergillus*. Precipitins are found in more than 70% of the cases.

In the acute phase, corticosteroid therapy is indicated and in some patients it is necessary to continue with this to prevent frequent relapses.

References

1. Henderson AH, et al. Pulmonary aspergillosis. *Thorax* 1968; 23: 513–518.
2. Campbell MJ, Clayton YM. Bronchopulmonary aspergillosis. *Am Rev Respir Dis* 1964; 89: 186–189.
3. Editorial. Diagnosing allergic bronchopulmonary aspergillosis. *Br Med J* 1977; 2: 1439–1440.
4. Rosenburg M, et al. The assessment of immunologic and clinical changes occurring during corticosteroid therapy for allergic bronchopulmonary aspergillosis. *Am J Med* 1978; 64: 599–606.
5. Patterson R, Greenberger P, et al. Allergic bronchopulmonary aspergillosis; staging as an aid to management. *Ann Intern Med* 1982; 96: 286–291.

135. Items B, C and E correct.

Initially disodium cromoglycate was thought to be of value only in 'immunologically induced' asthma. This view has been modified by further experience and evidence that this drug can inhibit non-immunological mast cell degranulation.

Several reports support the controversial observation that children with some types of gastrointestinal allergy are improved with disodium cromoglycate therapy.

The drug inhibits release of histamine, leukotrienes and serotonin, and appears to be a non-specific stabiliser of mast cell membranes. This contrasts with the action of corticosteroids, which are believed to counteract the local effects of toxic mediators at tissue sites.

Disodium cromoglycate does not antagonise released histamine, so it is ineffective in the treatment of acute episodes of asthma. In fact it may produce bronchospasm on the initiation of treatment, so is contraindicated during acute attacks. Its role is prophylactic for epidosic asthmatics and in anticipation of exercise-induced asthma.

References

1. Bernstein H, et al. Therapy with cromolyn sodium. *Ann Intern Med* 1978; 89: 228–233.
2. Dannaeus A, et al. The effect of orally administered sodium cromoglycate on symptoms of food allergy. *Clin Allergy* 1977; 7: 109–115.
3. Bernstein IL. Cromolyn sodium in the treatment of asthma: changing concepts. *J Allergy Clin Immunol* 1981; 68: 247–253.

136. Items A, C and E correct.

In 1977 the US Centre for Disease Control announced that aerobic Gram-negative bacilli had been isolated from lung tissue from patients in the Philadelphia epidemic and the organism, *Legionella pneumophilia*, appeared to be a previously unrecognised species. There are now four distinct serogroups of *L. pneumophilia*. Diagnosis is possible, but difficult, by direct culture of the organism from lung tissue, pleural fluid, or sputum.

Most often the diagnosis is established (ultimately) by serological means with the demonstration of a four-fold or greater rise in indirect fluorescent antibody titre to a level of 1:128 or convalescent titres of 1:256. Unfortunately, because of the time needed for the appearance of antibodies, seroconversion is not of much assistance in diagnosis at the stage of the acute disease. Most patients show diagnostic seroconversion at the end of 3 weeks but in some it does not occur until 6 weeks.

Hyponatraemia, probably due to the syndrome of inappropriate antidiuretic hormone secretion, occurs in Legionnaire's disease just as it does in other types of bacterial pneumonia.

Therapy with erythromycin has been found to be most effective, either alone or with the addition of rifampicin in more seriously ill patients. Most reports suggest that rifampicin should be held in reserve for those patients not responding satisfactorily to erythromycin. A dose of 0.5 g of erythromycin 6-hourly appears to have been sufficient for most cases, but the dosage recommended by American authorities is double this (1 g 6-hourly). A further current recommendation is that erythromycin should be administered for a prolonged period (as long as 3 weeks is suggested) even though most patients respond rather dramatically with subsidence of fever within 24–48 hours. However, relapses or prolonged convalescence have been reported if treatment is discontinued after less than 2 weeks.

References

1. Sanford JP. Legionnaire's disease — the first thousand days. *N Engl J Med* 1979; 300: 654–656.
2. Sanford JP. Legionnaires' disease: one person's perspective. *Ann Intern Med* 1979; 90: 699–703.
3. Swartz MN. Clinical aspects of legionnaires' disease. *Ann Intern Med* 1979; 90: 492–495.
4. Finland M. Legionnaires' disease: they came, saw & conquered. *Ann Intern Med* 1979; 90: 710–713.

137. Items B and D correct.

Central ventilatory depression, such as that which occurs after barbiturate overdosage in a person with normal lungs, could easily explain this clinical picture and the abnormality of his blood gases.

The blood sample cannot be venous because the Po_2 is greater than 60 mmHg.

If he had chronic bronchitis or 'acute on chronic' respiratory acidosis the base excess would be higher. If there were chronic lung disease, the

Po_2 should be lower than 62 mmHg with a Pco_2 of 60 mmHg. In acute pulmonary oedema the Pco_2 would not be so high and there would be obvious clinical signs without unconsciousness.

Reference

1. West JB. Ventilation, blood flow and gas exchange, 3rd Edn. Oxford: Blackwell Scientific, 1977.

138. Items C and E correct.

The clinical presentation suggests obstructive sleep apnoea as the cause of daytime sleepiness. Complete obstruction of the upper airway may occur for periods of 60–90 seconds during sleep leading to episodic severe hypoxia. Narcoleptics usually have no history of obstructive sleep apnoea.

Obstructive sleep apnoea may occur during both non-REM and REM sleep, although the periods of apnoea tend to be longer during REM sleep. The muscles of respiration make continuing attempts to function normally, but the upper airway obstruction prevents any air flow. Recently devices have been tried whereby continuous positive pressure is exerted via the nose during sleep in an attempt to prevent upper airway closure. The results thus far have been promising.

Weight reduction and reduction in alcohol intake will certainly improve the situation, but these measures do not completely solve the problem. In chronic severe snorers and in patients with mild sleep apnoea, alcohol intake before retiring may cause a marked increase in sleep apnoea and hypoxia. The same pertains to patients with true obstructive sleep apnoea where alcohol accentuates their already serious problem.

It is the degree of hypoxia in severe sleep apnoea — the Pao_2 sometimes falls to 20 mmHg (2.6 kPa) or less — which indicates the need to overcome the airways obstruction by means of tracheostomy. This leads to improvement in symptoms.

References

1. Phillipson EA. Editorial. Pickwickian, obesity-hypoventilation, or fee-fi-fo-fum syndrome? *Am Rev Respir Dis* 1980; 121: 781–782.
2. Sullivan CE, et al. Reversal of obstructive sleep apnoea by continuous positive airway pressure applied through the nares. *Lancet* 1981; 1: 862–865.
3. Coverdale SGM, et al. The importance of suspecting sleep apnoea as a common cause of excessive daytime sleepiness: further experience from the diagnosis and management of 19 patients. *Aust NZ J Med* 1980; 10: 284–288.
4. Sullivan CE, Issa FG, et al. Pathophysiology of sleep apnoea, In: Lenfant C (ed). Sleep and breathing. Lung biology in health and disease, Vol 21. New York: Dekker, 1984: 299.

139. Item D correct.

Persistence of eosinophilia of over 1500/mm^3 for longer than 6 months constitutes the hypereosinophilic syndrome. Mortality is high and death is usually caused by organ failure, presumably induced by the eosinophil infiltrate. Cardiac, neurological and pulmonary involvement are the usual causes of death.

Eosinophilia of this degree is not found in acute allergic reactions. In acute allergic asthma, the count is likely to lie between 400 and $1000/mm^3$.

Loeffler's syndrome is considered to be a minimally symptomatic condition which resolves within about 4 weeks. Generally, it is agreed to represent an allergic response to a variety of agents. Infiltrates are transient and migratory.

Elevated IgE may be a useful pointer to parasitic infestation but in the hypereosinophilic syndrome IgE levels are frequently normal.

Corticosteroids and cytotoxic drugs are often ineffective. A combination of prednisone and cyclophosphamide was beneficial only occasionally in one series; vincristine was reportedly effective as induction therapy in two patients in the same series. However, hydroxyurea has been reported to be beneficial in patients unresponsive to steroids.

References

1. Ottesen EA, Cohen SG. The eosinophil, eosinophilia and eosinophil-related disorders. In: Middleton E, et al (eds). Allergy principles and practice. St Louis: Mosby, 1978: 584–632.
2. Beeson PB, Bass DA. Major problems in internal medicine XIV: the eosinophil. Philadelphia: Saunders, 1977: 167.
3. Chusid JM, et al. The hypereosinophilic syndrome. *Medicine* 1975; 54: 1–27.
4. Parrillo JE, et al. Therapy of the hypereosinophilic syndrome. *Ann Intern Med* 1978; 89: 167–172.
5. Epstein DM, et al. The hypereosinophilic syndrome. *Radiology* 1981; 140: 59–62.

140. Items B, D and E correct.

The patient described has asthma and his current exacerbation probably has been precipitated by aspirin. The short duration of his respiratory symptoms and onset following recent administration of aspirin are important clues to the diagnosis. Furthermore, the FEV_1 : VC ratio of 48% indicates airways obstruction. The temporal relationship between removal of nasal polyps and the onset of asthma in the older age-group has been noted previously. Although there is no clear explanation of this relationship, the onset of asthma within 6–12 months of nasal polypectomy is a recognised pattern. These spirometric values together with a chest X-ray which did not show any pulmonary infiltrates would not support a diagnosis of allergic lung disease due to gold therapy.

The ability of aspirin to precipitate asthma in sensitive individuals is related to the effect of aspirin upon prostaglandin biosynthesis. The non-steroidal anti-inflammatory drugs are likely to precipitate attacks in sensitive individuals because all these compounds inhibit prostaglandin biosynthesis as an integral part of their anti-inflammatory mechanism of action.

The fact that the spirometric findings in this patient did not change significantly after a bronchodilator should not dissuade one from the diagnosis of asthma. During an acute exacerbation it is not uncommon for a patient to become relatively refractory to aerosol bronchodilator.

References

1. Samter M, Beers RF. Intolerance to aspirin; clinical studies and consideration of its pathogenesis. *Ann Intern Med* 1968; 68: 975–983.
2. Szczeklik A, et al. Relationship of inhibition of prostaglandin biosynthesis by analgesics to asthma attacks in aspirin-sensitive patients. *Br Med J* 1975; 1: 67–69.
3. Leading article. Aspirin sensitivity in asthmatics. *Br Med J* 1980; 281: 958-959.

141. Item D correct.

In the acute phase of hypersensitivity pneumonitis the characteristic features are restrictive ventilatory defect associated with hypoxia and hyperventilation. The diffusing capacity is usually reduced. Chest X-ray shows fine infiltrates involving both lungs (usually in the upper two-thirds of the lung fields predominantly), although sometimes this may not be evident. Weight loss is a very common feature of hypersensitivity pneumonitis. Prompt improvement usually follows removal from exposure to the offending antigen. The rapid recurrence on re-exposure is typical of this disease.

In asthma, the diffusing capacity is normal or increased. The lung function pattern is usually obstructive although in severe asthma the vital capacity becomes quite diminished. Cryptogenic fibrosing alveolitis is a progressive condition, not characterised by the features outlined in this case.

The dramatic speed of improvement and the rapidity of exacerbation are uncharacteristic of mycoplasma pneumonia or Legionnaire's disease.

References

1. Roberts RC, Moore VL. Immunopathogenesis of hypersensitivity pneumonitis. *Am Rev Respir Dis* 1977; 116: 1075–1090.
2. Lee JH. Hypersensitivity pneumonitis (extrinsic allergic alveolitis). *Aust NZ J Med* 1981; 11: 299–301.
3. Pepys J. Hypersensitivity diseases of the lungs due to fungi and organic dusts. In: Kallos P, et al (eds). Monographs in Allergy. Basel: Karger, 1969: Vol 4.

142. Items A and D correct.

Extrinsic allergic alveolitis (hypersensitivity pneumonitis) is an uncommon but by no means rare disorder affecting the gas exchanging tissues within the lung. Inhalation of avian antigen derived from pigeons, budgerigars and cockatoos is the most frequent cause of the disorder in Australia, but the provoking antigen may be present elsewhere in the home or work place. Recognition of the pattern of this disease is essential, because in some patients an antigen can only be suspected, and recovery follows only if home or work environment is changed. There is no definitive immunological test and the diagnosis rests upon clinical suspicion, characteristic histological findings on lung biopsy and, occasionally, challenge with suspected antigen.

The disease is commonly misdiagnosed as viral infection or mycoplasma pneumonia, neither of which is likely to be recurrent. The usual presenting symptoms are acute dyspnoea, cough and febrile illness, which are frequently recurrent and which can be accompanied by profound weight loss. An interval of 4–6 hours following exposure to the inhaled antigen is characteristic but not invariable.

Circulating precipitins only indicate contact with the antigen and do not correlate with disease activity. The allergic response in this disease combines features of both type III and IV responses and it is therefore difficult to characterise. Occasional eosinophils are seen in the lesions and peripheral eosinophilia is absent.

The appearances are usually readily distinguishable from sarcoidosis. In the acute and subacute forms the chest X-ray usually shows micronodular infiltrates which involve predominantly the lower and mid zones and which can persist for several weeks. Hilar gland enlargement does not occur. The inflammatory response consists of lymphocyte and plasma cell invasion of alveolar walls together with occasional histiocytes forming granulomata. The bronchioles are also involved.

Inhaled particles between 0.5 and 3 mm in diameter are too small to be effectively filtered by simple face masks. Acute attacks may respond to corticosteroids but the disease is reversible only by removal of, or from, the offending antigens.

References

1. Lee JH. Hypersensitivity and the lung. *Mod Med Aust* 1979; 22(8): 17–24.
2. Schatz M, et al. Immunopathogenesis of hypersensitivity pneumonitis. *J Allergy Clin Immunol* 1977; 60: 27–37.

143. Items B, C and E correct.

Asbestosis may appear for the first time and progress long after exposure to asbestos dust has ceased. Genetic factors may influence the response to exposure as indicated by a study in which the HLA-B27 was present more frequently in patients with asbestosis than in the general population.

Finger clubbing, though common and occurring early in asbestosis, does not correlate closely with the degree of fibrosis.

The finding of asbestos bodies in the sputum only indicates that there has been exposure to asbestos and does not imply the presence of asbestosis. In city dwellers, asbestos bodies can be found in most lungs at autopsy.

There is an increased incidence of carcinoma of the lung in asbestosis and although it is the cause of death in 15–20% of asbestosis cases, its occurrence does not appear to be dose-related. It rarely occurs in non-smokers. Mesothelioma, though a relatively rare tumour, is closely associated with asbestos exposure but it is also not dose-related. Low levels of exposure to asbestos for relatively brief periods are sufficient to cause mesothelioma after a long latent period, e.g. 30 years. Smoking does not play a synergistic role in its development.

References

1. Becklake MR. Asbestos-related diseases of the lung and other organs: their epidemiology and implications for clinical practice. *Am Rev Respir Dis* 1976; 114: 187–227.
2. Becklake MR. Exposure to asbestos and human disease. *N Engl J Med* 1982; 306: 1480–1482.

144. Item C correct.

A lung biopsy in this patient showed the histological features of fibrosing alveolitis which, on the basis of the information provided, is the most likely diagnosis, although the radiological picture is consistent with all of the given possibilities.

Although the patient's work history is consistent with the presence of silicosis, the respiratory function tests are not. These show a severe restrictive pattern with mild airways obstruction (probably a result of his smoking) and a marked reduction in diffusing capacity — changes not seen in silicosis but characteristic of fibrosing alveolitis.

Sarcoidosis, though unusual at this age, may occur in the seventh decade, but finger clubbing is rare. In sarcoidosis a bronchial lavage shows an excess of lymphocytes, not polymorphs. Pulmonary alveolar lavage is a relatively new technique designed to examine the alveolar cellular content, with the normal proportions being macrophages 90%, lymphocytes 7% and polymorphs and eosinophils constituting the remaining 3%. There is no universal agreement as to the various characteristics of pulmonary alveolar lavage cells in specific diseases, although there are some trends appearing in the early reports.

Allergic alveolitis could produce similar respiratory function changes but the history given is not typical of this disease and the bronchial lavage would have an excess of lymphocytes.

Carcinomatosis is an alternative but less likely diagnosis. The length of history would not exclude it. Occasionally metastases from an adenocarcinoma elsewhere might give this picture.

References

1. Bernard J, et al. Editorial. Bronchoalveolar lavage. *Thorax* 1980; 35: 1–8.
2. Haslam PL, et al. Bronchoalveolar lavage in pulmonary fibrosis: comparisons of cells obtained with lung biopsy and clinical features. *Thorax* 1980; 35: 9–18.
3. Weinberger SE, et al. Clinical significance of pulmonary function tests: use and interpretation of the single-breath diffusing capacity. *Chest* 1980; 78: 483–488.

145. Items B and C correct.

The small airways component, which represents 10–20% of the total resistance of air flow in the normal individual, has to be increased 50–100 times before any alterations occur in the standard spirometric measurements of airflow. Hence, this has been termed 'the quiet zone' because significant disease can occur before detection by spirometry.

Autopsy studies of young smokers show mural inflammatory cells, alteration of bronchiolar epithelium, surface denudation, decreased ciliated epithelial and clara cells and increased mucus-secreting cells with excess mucus within small airways. All of these changes result in bronchiolar obstruction leading to ventilation-perfusion imbalance and gas exchange disturbance.

Measurement of dynamic frequency-dependent compliance is probably the most sensitive test for small airways obstruction. However, as it requires the placement of an oesophageal balloon, it is an invasive procedure and not applicable to routine or epidemiological studies.

The closing volume of the lung is the volume of air remaining in the lung when the small airways are occluded on expiration. A high closing volume occurs in a wide variety of disorders which do not produce small airways obstruction, e.g. obesity, ascites, postoperative fluid retention and kyphoscoliosis.

All patients with emphysema will have evidence of bronchiolitis and loss of support of small airways and hence obstruction.

References

1. Niewoehner DE, et al. Pathologic changes in the peripheral airways of young cigarette smokers. *N Engl J Med* 1974; 291: 755–758.
2. Hogg JC, et al. Site and nature of airway obstruction in chronic obstructive lung disease. *N Engl J Med* 1968; 278: 1355–1360.
3. Rodarte JR, et al. New tests for the detection of obstructive pulmonary disease. *Chest* 1977; 72: 762–768.
4. Burrows B, Hasan FM. Abnormalities in small airways. *Disease a Month* 1977; 23(10): 34.
5. McCarthy D, Milic-Emili J. Closing volume in asymptomatic asthma. *Am Rev Respir Dis* 1973; 107: 559–570.

146. Items A, C and E correct.

The absence of dynein arms in the ultrastructure of the cilia from bronchial and nasal mucosa is the clue to the diagnosis of the immotile cilia syndrome. The normal rapid and incessant movements of cilia (about 20 cycles per second) are impaired or absent in this syndrome and this leads to gross abnormalities in mucociliary clearance — a very important defence mechanism in the lung.

A recent study of 14 patients revealed that 9 had evidence of situs inversus but none had signs of any other congenital malformations. Kartagener's syndrome (situs inversus — bronchiectasis — sinusitis or absent frontal sinuses) can be regarded as a sub-group within the immotile cilia syndrome. The prevalence of the immotile cilia syndrome is approximately 1 per 20 000 — about twice as common as Kartagener's syndrome.

During investigations of unexplained infertility in males, some of those with sperm immotility were found to have the sperm tail devoid of dynein arms. This led to the discovery that cilia from the respiratory tract and elsewhere in these men showed the same defect.

Mucociliary clearance is often diminished in cystic fibrosis but not completely absent as in the immotile cilia syndrome. The prognosis is much worse in cystic fibrosis. Severely impaired mucociliary transport mechanisms lead to chronic obstructive airflow limitation.

Reference

1. Afzelius BA, Mossberg B. Editorial. Immotile cilia. *Thorax* 1980; 35: 401–404.

147. Items A and D correct.

The term 'adult respiratory distress syndrome' (ARDS) has been applied to a category of disorders in which the peripheral gas exchange units are involved. Encompassed within the term 'ARDS' are such appellations as 'adult hyaline membrane disease', 'shock lung' and 'traumatic wet lung'. Despite the diverse nature of the medicosurgical disorders associated with ARDS, diffuse lung injury with damage to the alveolar-capillary (A-C) membrane appears to be the common denominator. The cardinal clinical features of the ARDS include respiratory distress, hypoxia due to intrapulmonary shunting of blood, decreased lung compliance and widespread infiltrations on the chest X-ray.

Because of the damage to the A-C membrane, vigorous fluid resuscitation may augment or produce pulmonary abnormalities leading to respiratory failure. If available, the insertion of a Swan-Ganz pulmonary artery catheter may help to balance the opposing problems of maintaining critical organ perfusion with as little effect on pulmonary wedge pressure as possible. A vigorous policy of fluid restriction needs to be followed once the syndrome has developed.

PEEP is probably the most important advance in the management of ARDS. The primary benefit is to increase the functional residual capacity with a subsequent reduction in the magnitude of intrapulmonary shunting of blood and an increase in pulmonary compliance.

The value of corticosteroids in ARDS is still highly controversial.

Reference

1. Hopewell PC, Murray JF. The adult respiratory distress syndrome. *Ann Rev Med* 1976; 27: 343–356.

148. Items B and D correct.

The diffusing capacity (transfer factor) measures the ability of the lungs to transfer carbon monoxide (in small quantities) from the alveolar gas to the blood. Carbon monoxide is used because it is avidly taken up by haemoglobin. Decreased uptake indicates reduced diffusing capacity, as occurs, for example, in emphysema, in thickening of the alveolar-capillary membrane, or in severe mismatching of ventilation and perfusion in the lungs (V/Q mismatching).

In normal people during exercise more of the lung is used, capillaries open to accommodate the increased cardiac output and the diffusing capacity increases. Asthmatics have normal alveolar capillary membranes with no disturbance of diffusing capacity, unless bad V/Q matching interferes with the measurement. However, the value is decreased in patients with interstitial lung disease, emphysema and acute pulmonary embolism. There is no close relationship between arterial oxygen tension and transfer factor, because uptake of oxygen is not diffusion-limited.

Reference

1. Weinberger SE, et al. Clinical significance of pulmonary function tests: use and interpretation of the single-breath diffusing capacity. *Chest* 1980; 78: 483–488.

149. Items B, C and D correct.

There has been much controversy over the years as to the best methods for monitoring heparin therapy. The most sensitive methods for measuring heparin levels are tedious, time-consuming and unsuitable for routine monitoring. Although the PTTK and thrombin time do not correlate particularly well with the more sensitive methods, these two tests are probably the most generally used.

Assuming that this patient has been receiving her heparin correctly there can be little doubt that she is resistant to conventional dosages. Following thrombosis it is not unusual for patients to have increased heparin requirements. There are various reasons for this, including a low anti-thrombin III level; heparin has its pharmacological action via antithrombin III. It has been well demonstrated that anti-thrombin III levels fall during heparin therapy; this may explain the tendency for rapid recurrence of thrombosis following cessation of heparin if oral anticoagulation is unsatisfactory.

The indications for streptokinase therapy remain controversial. However, many workers feel that this therapy is indicated only in massive pulmonary embolism with cardiac decompensation and where there is concern as to whether the patient is going to survive the acute episode. In any case, streptokinase is contraindicated within 10 days of major surgery because of the high risk of haemorrhage.

References

1. Wessler S, Gatel SN. Heparin: new concepts relevant to clinical use. *Blood* 1979; 53: 525–544.
2. Marder EJ. The use of thrombolytic agents: choice of patient, drug administration, laboratory monitoring. *Ann Intern Med* 1979; 90: 802–808.

150. Items A, B and C correct.

This patient almost certainly has a non-Hodgkin's lymphoma complicated by cold agglutinins. The hepatosplenomegaly and lymphadenopathy in this case point towards a non-Hodgkin's lymphoma, as these features are not found in classically cold haemagglutinin disease. The cold agglutinins are manifest clinically by cold intolerance and peripheral cyanosis. Depending on the thermal amplitude of the cold agglutinins there is likely to be a degree of haemolysis.

The Coombs' test is usually positive with complement only present on the red cell surface, as the IgM cold agglutinin elutes off at 37°C. Cold haemagglutinin disease usually has a high titre narrow thermal range cold agglutinin present but no evidence of lymphoma. However, there does appear to be a relationship between chronic cold agglutinin disease and lymphoma.

The cold IgM agglutinin found in cold agglutinin disease is monoclonal in nature although a clear monoclonal band is not usually found in the serum. Some cases of chronic cold haemagglutinin disease progress on to classical non-Hodgkin's lymphoma and some cases of non-Hodgkin's lymphoma, as illustrated by this case, may be complicated by cold agglutinins. In such situations, it is not uncommon to find a monoclonal IgM present in the patient's serum.

Classical cold haemagglutinin disease is usually managed symptomatically but, if the symptoms are severe, alkylating agents may help to control the level of the cold agglutinin. In the case illustrated, the normal approach would be to treat the non-Hodgkin's lymphoma along conventional lines with chemotherapy, which usually leads to control of the cold agglutinins. Only rarely is splenectomy indicated.

The Donath-Landsteiner test is negative in this condition, as a cold biphasic haemolysin is not present, and it is positive in paraxysmal cold haemoglobinuria.

Reference

1. Horwitz CA. Autoimmune haemolytic anaemia: 3. Cold antibody type. *Postgrad Med* 1979; 66: 189–200.

151. Items B, D and E correct.

Splenic enlargement does not necessarily imply involvement with Hodgkin's disease, nor does absence of clinical splenomegaly reliably indicate lack of involvement. Staging laparotomies have shown an error of up to 25% occurs in the clinical assessment of splenic involvement, and approximately one-third of the patients with clinical stage II disease have abdominal disease.

Although 90% of treatment failures occur during the first 3 years after therapy, late relapses in the abdomen have been reported in patients with stage IA and IIA disease. Late relapse is especially associated with nodular sclerosing Hodgkin's disease which frequently runs an indolent course and also has the highest rate of relapse after 'MOPP'-induced complete remission. 'MOPP' therapy for stage III and IV disease yields complete remission in up to 80% of patients and over 60% are free of disease at 5 years.

Complicating second malignancy occurs in long survivors with more radical therapy now being used and is most commonly acute non-lymphocytic leukaemia. A 4% actuarial probability of the development of acute leukaemia within 7 years after the diagnosis of Hodgkin's disease has been reported for patients who received both chemotherapy and extended field radiotherapy. Other second malignancies reported include non-Hodgkin's lymphoma, squamous cell carcinomas, and adenocarcinoma of various sites as well as a variety of soft tissue sarcomas.

References

1. Arseneau JC, et al. Risk of new cancers in patients with Hodgkin's disease. *Cancer* 1977; 40: 1912–1916.
2. Brody RS, et al. Multiple primary cancer risk after therapy for Hodgkin's disease. *Cancer* 1977; 40: 1917–1926.
3. Sweet DL, et al. Hodgkin's disease: problems of staging. *Cancer* 1978; 42: 957–970.
4. Young RC, et al. Patterns of relapse in advanced Hodgkin's disease treated with combination chemotherapy. *Cancer* 1978; 42: 1001–1007.
5. Krikorian JG, et al. Occurence on non-Hodgkin's lymphoma after therapy for Hodgkin's disease. *N Engl Med* 1979; 300: 452–458.
6. Coleman CN, et al. Hematologic neoplasia in patients treated for Hodgkin's disease. *N Engl J Med* 1977; 297: 1249–1252.
7. The Prince of Wales Hospital Oncology Cooperative Group (Lymphoma), Sydney. Hodgkin's disease: ten year's experience of a combined lymphoma clinic. *Med J Aust* 1980; 1: 118–121.
8. Ultman JE, DeVita VT, Jr. Hodgkin's disease and lymphomas. In: Isselbacher KJ, et al, eds. Harrison's Principles of Internal Medicine. 9th edn. New York: McGraw-Hill, 1980: 1633–1647.
9. Weller SA, et al. Initial relapse in previously-treated Hodgkin's disease. 2. Retrograde transdiaphragmatic extension. *Int J Radiat Oncol Biol Phys* 1977; 2: 863–872.

152. Items A, C, D and E correct.

Diffuse histiocytic lymphoma is associated with a poor prognosis, and in most instances requires cytotoxic chemotherapy with multiple drug regimens.

Several recent treatment protocols have achieved complete remission rates of around 60% and, though long-term follow-up is incomplete, the indications are that at least half of those achieving complete remission have prolonged disease-free survival. Patients achieving only partial remissions have survival little different from patients showing no clinical response.

Although bone marrow involvement in diffuse histiocytic lymphoma occurs in less than 10% of patients at presentation, there is correlation between meningeal disease and bone marrow and hepatic involvement.

Although most primary gastrointestinal lymphomas are diffuse histiocytic in type, the prognosis is significantly better than that in primary nodal disease, when disease is confined to the gut.

References

1. Bunn PA, et al. Central nervous system complications in patients with diffuse histiocytic and undifferentiated lymphoma: leukemia revisited. *Blood* 1976; 47: 3–10.
2. Ultmann JE. Cure of histiocytic lymphoma. *Ann Intern Med* 1982; 97: 274–275.
3. Laurence J, et al. Combination chemotherapy of advanced diffuse histiocytic lymphoma with the six-drug COP-BLAM regimen. *Ann Intern Med* 1982; 97: 190–195.

153. Items A and E correct.

Iron deficiency anaemia is associated with low serum levels of ferritin, decreased levels of serum iron, but usually increased iron binding capacity (transferrin).

The plasma iron clearance in iron deficiency states is rapid and there are no sideroblasts seen on bone marrow aspiration. Usual findings on bone marrow aspiration are erythyroid hyperplasia and absence of haemosiderin in macrophages when the marrow particles are stained for iron.

The red cell protoporphyrin levels are raised and bilirubin levels decreased as a reflection of defective haem synthesis.

Reference

1. Brown E. Hypochromic anaemias: iron deficiency anaemia. In: Beeson PB, McDermott W (eds) Cecil Loeb Textbook of medicine, 15th Edn. Philadelphia: Saunders, 1979: 1743–1751.

154. Items A, B and E correct.

The Schilling's vitamin B_{12} absorption test is one of the classic investigations used in the diagnosis of pernicious anaemia. The first part of the absorption test is carried out without intrinsic factor, and the demonstration that B_{12} is normally absorbed when intrinsic factor is added highlights the basic defects in pernicious anaemia, i.e: lack of gastric intrinsic factor.

In most patients with a post-gastrectomy state leading to vitamin B_{12} deficiency, the same correction with intrinsic factor is seen. However, there may be a second problem in post-gastrectomy patients depending on the type of gastrectomy. Where there is a blind loop, bacterial overgrowth interferes with the vitamin B_{12} intrinsic factor complex and renders the B_{12} unabsorbable in the terminal ileum. By the same mechanism, multiple jejunal diverticula can be associated with bacterial overgrowth in the small intestine. In both of these situations the abnormality can be corrected by antibiotic therapy to reduce the bacterial overgrowth.

In simple atrophic gastritis, the Schilling's test is usually normal but any mild abnormality is corrected by the addition of intrinsic factor. Folate deficiency may occur as part of the spectrum of a malabsorption syndrome secondary to primary small intestinal disorders. The Schilling's test, both with and without intrinsic factor, may be abnormal and certainly does not exclude the presence of coexistent folate deficiency.

In the classical Schilling's test the absorption of vitamin B_{12} is assessed by measurement of radioactivity in urine collected over a 24-hour period. This depends on normal renal function; spuriously low B_{12} absorption results can be seen in renal failure. The problem is usually circumvented by measuring plasma levels of radioactivity.

Reference

1. Beck WS. Vitamin B12 deficiency. In: Williams WJ, et al (eds). Hematology, 2nd Edn. New York: McGraw-Hill, 1977: 307–334.

155. Items C and E correct.

The condition described is that of a patient with haemolytic anaemia where the haemolysis is principally intravascular. The unusual finding is the absence of marrow iron stores which in most haemolytic states are increased. Where there is continuing and chronic intravascular haemolysis there can also be haemoglobinuria and with this a steady loss of iron in the form of haemosiderinuria.

The two conditions which might cause this pattern are microangiopathic haemolytic anaemia secondary to heart valve prothesis and paroxysmal nocturnal haemoglobinuria.

Acute haemolysis occurring in infectious mononucleosis is associated with the development of an IgM antibody with anti-i specificity. Though this is principally an intravascular haemolysis, the condition is usually not chronic enough to give rise to iron depletion. In systemic lupus erythematosus with an autoimmune haemolytic anaemia, the antibody is usually of the warm type and the haemolysis is principally extravascular.

In hereditary spherocytosis the abnormal shape of the red cells due to defective red cell membrane metabolism leads to sequestration in the spleen. With prolonged sequestration the red cells lyse, being unable to survive within the stressful environment of the splenic vasculature. This is also an extravascular form of haemolysis and not associated with significant haemosiderinuria.

Reference

1. Rosse WF. Paroxysmal nocturnal hemoglobinuria. In: Williams WJ, et al (eds) Hematology, 2nd Edn. New York: McGraw-Hill, 1977: 560–570.

156. Items A, C and E correct.

In a patient with raised haemoglobin and haematocrit values, red cell mass and plasma volume estimations are essential to establish whether erythrocytosis is present or whether the abnormal results are due to a reduced plasma volume. A marked reduction in plasma volume (as in this patient) is the hallmark of so-called relative or 'spurious' polycythaemia. True erythrocytosis, whether primary (polycythaemia rubra vera) or secondary (to hypoxaemia, high oxygen affinity haemoglobin, etc.) will be characterised by an increase in red cell mass and often also in plasma volume.

Thiazide diuretics, by further reducing plasma volume, may aggravate relative polycythaemia and are inappropriate as antihypertensives in this patient.

In the past venesection was thought to be illogical in relative polycythaemia, since reduced plasma volume was the underlying problem. However Humphrey et al (1979) have shown that cerebral blood flow is impaired in proportion to haematocrit elevation in these patients and improves with venesection aiming to reduce the haematocrit to 42–46%.

Iron deficient erythrocytes are less deformable and have increased intrinsic viscosity compared to normal red cells, and this increased viscosity can cause impairment of tissue oxygenation.

References

1. Golde DW, et al. Polycythaemia, mechanisms and management. *Ann Intern Med* 1981; 95: 71–87.
2. Humphrey PRD, et al. Cerebral blood flow and viscosity in relative polycythaemia. *Lancet* 1979; 2: 873–876.
3. Hutton RD. The effect of iron deficiency on whole viscosity in polycythaemic patients. *Br J Haematol* 1979; 43: 191–199.

157. Items C and E correct.

There is sufficient evidence to make a diagnosis of multiple myeloma, but the neoplastic cells are not secreting an abnormal protein which can be detected. This patient has a biopsy-proven plasmacytoma of bone, a diffuse involvement of the bone marrow with abnormal plasma cells and immunoglobulin deficiency. Non-secretory myeloma accounts for only about 1% of patients in most large series and, although prognosis was at one time considered worse than that for conventional secretory myeloma, there is little to substantiate this claim.

The finding of bone marrow infiltration with abnormal plasma cells negates the diagnosis of solitary plasmacytoma on bone. Lytic bone lesions are absent at presentation in as many as 30% of patients and their absence does not preclude the diagnosis of multiple myeloma.

Treatment is the same as for classical myeloma, with systemic chemotherapy after appropriate internal fixation.

Reference

1. Hobbs JR. Growth rates and responses to treatment in human myelomatosis. *Br J Haematol* 1969; 16: 607–617.

158. Items D and E correct.

The abnormality in coagulation is located in the so-called 'intrinsic pathway'; it is most likely that this patient has a circulating inhibitor directed against the factor VIII molecule. This is the most common circulating anticoagulant encountered and it has been described in association with chronic inflammatory disorders such as systemic lupus erythematosus, less commonly during pregnancy and in the puerperium. An initial laboratory test is a mixing experiment to show that normal plasma does not correct the abnormality in the patient's serum as would occur in a deficiency state.

In systemic lupus erythematosus, various acquired anticoagulants have been described. These include an anti-factor VIII and, in particular, a unique inhibitor that is probably directed towards phospholipid, interfering with phospholipid-dependent coagulation reactions and associated with thrombosis. The other situation in which factor VIII inhibitors are present is in patients with haemophilia A (congenital factor VIII deficiency) but this is only in about 5% of those who have received multiple plasma transfusions.

Antibodies, mainly directed against factor VIII, also occur in association with penicillin reactions and dermatitis herpetiformis, and also in normal people, especially the elderly. The majority of these antibodies are only against factor VIII clotting activity but have been described as having activity against von Willebrand factor where there is an abnormal bleeding time, low factor VIII antigen and abnormal platelet retention.

Where there is a major bleeding diathesis, the treatment of choice is immunosuppressive therapy with cyclophosphamide or azathioprine; steroids and factor VIII concentrates should not be used alone as they may boost antibody titres and should be reversed for the major haemorrhagic situations and when adequate immunosuppression is given concurrently. Immunosuppressive treatment appears to be somewhat more effective in non-haemophiliac patients with acquired inhibitors rather than in the haemophiliac population.

References

1. Shapiro SS. Acquired anticoagulants. In: Williams WJ, et al, (eds) Hematology, 2nd Edn. New York: McGraw-Hill, 1977: 1447–1454.
2. Stableforth P, et al. Acquired von Willebrand syndrome with inhibitors both to factor VIII clotting activity and ristocetin-induced platelet aggregation. *Br J Haematol* 1976; 33: 565–573.

159. Items A, C, D and E correct.

Chronic idiopathic (immune) thrombocytopenic purpura (ITP) is rarely associated with splenomegaly and its presence should raise the suspicion of an alternative diagnosis such as lymphoma or connective tissue disorder.

The platelet life-span is often measured in minutes in ITP, and though the platelet count may not rise, clinical benefit can be derived from platelet transfusion. In this patient without active bleeding, platelet transfusion would be of little benefit.

Splenectomy is considered in patients who have had a suboptimal or no response to steroids. A complete remission occurs in 80% of patients. A response to splenectomy cannot be predicted confidently but is more likely in those who have had an initial good response to steroids, who are less than 60 years old, who have had a short history and in whom the platelet count rises to more than $500 \times 10^9/\ell$ after surgery.

Although IgG antibody directed at a platelet-associated antigen is in lower titre post-splenectomy, it is detectable and can be the cause of serious neonatal thrombocytopenia, which may present for 3–4 weeks after birth.

Vincristine and vinblastine intravenously often can give a satisfactory although transient improvement in platelet count. Several groups have used vinblastine-loaded platelets with encouraging results, but the procedure should be regarded as experimental at this stage. These are thought to damage the macrophages which are destroying the platelets.

References

1. Karpatkin S. Auto-immune thrombocytopenic purpura. *Blood* 1980; 56: 329–343.
2. McMillan R. Chronic idiopathic thrombocytopenic purpura. *N Engl J Med* 1981; 304: 1135–1147.

160. Items D and E correct.

On the basis of cell surface markers, acute lymphoblastic leukaemia (ALL) can be divided into three broad groups, B, T and common, or non-T non-B cell ALL. The overall incidence of these groups is as follows:

B = 4%
T = 15–20%
Common or non-T non-B = 75%

These groupings have prognostic significance, as the overall survival of the non-T and non-B cell is best, the T cell group intermediate and the B cell group worst, most patients dying within 2 years. Common or non-T non-B ALL is recognised by the 'Greaves' antisera. These antisera recognise a cell which is not seen in normal adult marrow (less than one cell in 10^4) but is present in fetal liver and regenerating marrow post-chemotherapy.

Induction therapies should include vincristine and prednisone. L-asparaginase and cytosine arabinoside or an anthracycline are often added. Central nervous system prophylaxis has been shown to be of great benefit in preventing relapse. This consists of cranial irradiation combined with intrathecal chemotherapy. Children at increased risk of relapse include those under 2 years of age or older than 10 years and those with high white cell counts. In most studies it has been shown that boys are at greater risk than girls. Children with massive extramedullary disease also appear to be at increased risk.

References

1. Tsukimoto I, et al. Surface markers and prognostic factors in acute lymphoblastic leukaemia. *N Engl J Med* 1976; 294: 245–248.
2. Sather H, et al. Differences in prognosis for boys and girls with acute lymphoblastic leukaemia. *Lancet* 1981; 1: 739–743.
3. Green DM, et al. Comparison of three methods of central-nervous-system prophylaxis in childhood acute lymphoblastic leukaemia. *Lancet* 1980; 1: 1398–1401.

4. Greaves M, Janossy G. Patterns of gene expression and the cellular origins of human leukaemias. *Biochem Biophys Acta* 1978; 516: 193–230.
5. George SL, et al. A reappraisal of the results of stopping therapy in childhood leukaemia. *N Engl J Med* 1979; 300: 269–273.
6. Ekert H, et al. Results of cessation of treatment in childhood acute lymphoblastic leukaemia. *Med J Aust* 1981; 1: 523–525.
7. Roath S. Acute lymphoblastic leukaemia of B cell origin. *Clin Lab Haematol* 1979; 1: 87–94.

161. Items A, B, C and D correct.

Complete remission can now be obtained in 85–95% of cases of children with the common type of acute lymphoblastic leukaemia (ALL). Initial high white cell count (especially greater then $100 \times 10^9/\ell$), CNS leukaemia at presentation, age under 12 months or over 13 years, and cell markers demonstrating the leukaemic cells to be either B or T cell type are all bad prognostic features. Boys have a worse prognosis than girls, partly because of a higher incidence of T-cell disease, and because of occurrence of testicular disease.

Before 1970, remission in ALL terminated in meningeal leukaemia in more than 50% of cases. The testis in boys also appears to be a 'sanctuary' area where occult disease gives rise to relapse often after maintenance therapy is ceased.

All patients require maintenance therapy for at least 24 months; however, if continued beyond 36 months, it is accompanied with no fewer relapses and greater toxicity both short-and long-term. At the conclusion of maintenance therapy up to 20% of cases relapse in the ensuing 12 months; after this period actuarial survival curves plateau, suggesting that the 75–80% of the children who remained in remission for the first 24–30 months remain in remission over the long-term (approaching 50% of those in whom initial complete remission was achieved).

CNS prophylaxis has salvaged a significant number of children who otherwise would have had relapse in that site, as a prelude to a systemic relapse. However, there are clinical studies which demonstate short-term memory loss, frequently occurring with cranial irradiation and intrathecal methotrexate. Intelligence quotients and other cognitive tests before and after CNS prophylactic therapy also have shown a decrease in IQ score which may decrease with time. In addition, varying degrees of hypothalamic-pituitary end-organ damage have been noted in children treated for acute leukaemia.

References

1. Mauer AM. Therapy of acute lymphoblastic leukaemia in childhood. *Blood* 1980; 56: 1–10.
2. Simone JV. Outlook for acute lymphoblastic leukaemia in children in 1982. *Annu Rev Med* 1981; 32: 207–212.
3. Shalet SM, et al. Endocrine function following the treatment of acute leukaemia in childhood. *J Pediatr* 1977; 90: 920–923.

162. All items correct.

Virtually all patients with chronic granulocytic (myelogenous) leukaemia experience a change from the chronic, relatively benign course to either an accelerated period of disease or a phase known as 'blast crisis'. The accelerated phase may have many of the clinical features of blast crisis but still retaining blood and bone marrow features of the chronic phase of the disease. Fever, lymphadenopathy, basophilia (20%), additional chromosomal abnormalities to the Ph chromosome and myelofibrosis are all recognised as features of this transformation/accelerated phase. In about 60% of patients the blast crises have the features of acute myelogenous leukaemia, in 30% lymphoid crisis is seen and in 10% various acute leukaemic pictures (megakaryoblastic, erythroleukaemic myelomonocytic) are seen.

The most frequent chromosomal abnormalities in blast crisis are doubling of Ph1, trisomy 8 and isochromosome 17 (the latter two changes being also seen in acute myelogenous leukaemia).

Approximately one-third of patients experience an acute transformation which is lymphoid in type. The characteristics of the blast cells in this type of transformation are as follows: morphologically they resemble blast cells of acute lymphoblastic leukaemia; they contain high levels of terminal deoxynucleotidyl transferase and react immunologically with antisera raised to the blast cells of common childhood ALL. These patients have a 50% response rate to chemotherapy, effective in acute lymphoblastic leukaemia (e.g: vincristine and prednisone).

In blast crisis the overall response to chemotherapy as given in acute myelogenous leukaemia is disappointing. At best about 25% of patients achieve a remission, with median survivals of 2–5 months. In those selected patients with lymphoid blast crisis, where ALL-type therapy achieves remission, survival averages 5–12 months.

Reference

1. Koeffler HP, Golde DW. Chronic myelogenous leukemia — new concepts (in two parts). *N Engl J Med* 1981; 304: 1201–1209, 1269–1274.

163. Items B, C, and E correct.

Lithium carbonate is used mainly for the long-term control of mania and to prevent relapse in bipolar manic depressive illness. Its major actions are on the central nervous system at both therapeutic and toxic levels. Lithium intoxication, presenting with drowsiness, tremor, dysarthria, ataxia, anorexia, nausea, vomiting and diarrhoea, is likely to occur at therapeutic levels if the patient is taking any drug such as a diuretic which depletes body sodium.

Lithium induces a reversible leucocytosis, and its use in ameliorating the leucopenia associated with systemic chemotherapy is subject to investigation. Although it may produce reversible T wave flattening and inversion, it may be used safely in patients with cardiac disease if serum levels are monitored.

Lithium can have a mild antithyroid effect. Disturbances of thyroid function, however, are not a contraindication to its use. Thyroid function should be checked prior to commencement and at regular intervals (yearly) during therapy in all patients.

A nephrogenic diabetes insipidus with polyuria and polydipsia is produced in one-third of patients, although this is not usually a clinical problem. Lithium may impair glucose tolerance or produce frank diabetes in some patients and the possibility of carbohydrate intolerance should be considered if lithium therapy is planned.

References

1. Jefferson JW, Geist JH. Primer of lithium therapy. Baltimore: Williams & Wilkins, 1977.
2. Lyman GH, et al. The use of lithium carbonate to reduce infection and leukopenia during systemic chemotherapy. *N Engl J Med* 1980; 302: 257–260.
3. Tilkian AG, et al. The cardiovascular effects of lithium in man: a review of the literature. *Am J Med* 1976; 61: 665–670.
4. Williams WD, Gyory AZ. Aspects of the use of lithium for the non-psychiatrist. *Aust NZ J Med* 1976; 6: 233–242.
5. Russell JD, Johnson GFS. Affective disorders, diabetes mellitus and lithium. *Aust NZ J Psych* 1981; 15: 349–353.

164. Items A, B and D correct.

It is now recognised that cytotoxic drugs can cause irreversible organ damage, which is related to the cumulative dose of the drug. For instance, adriamycin can cause an irreversible cardiomyopathy, increasing in incidence after a cumulative dose of 500 mg/m^2 has been reached. Similarly, bleomycin may cause irreversible pulmonary fibrosis after a cumulative dose of 300 mg has been given.

Reversible toxicities include myelosuppression, nausea and vomiting, and mucositis. These effects are dependent on the size of dose given at any one time. Hence the severity of each toxicity limits the dosage of the cytotoxic drugs administered at each treatment.

Reference

1. Carter SK, Mathe G. Malignant diseases. In: Avery GS (ed). Drug treatment: principles and practice of clinical pharmacology and therapeutics, 2nd Edn. Sydney: Adis Press, 1980: 953–1009.

165. Items B, C, D and E correct.

Pulmonary toxicity secondary to the administration of cancer chemotherapeutic agents may take several different forms. The long-term administration of busulphan will result in the development of diffuse pulmonary fibrosis in about 5% of patients. It is a slowly evolving process and rarely observed with less than a year of chronic administration of the agent. Histologically a characteristic picture is seen. It is irreversible, although cessation of the drug may avoid further progression.

The pulmonary toxicity of cyclophosphamide is extremely uncommon and appears to be idiosyncratic, occurring after either short- or long-term administration. Onset is generally acute with a diffuse pneumonitis which may progress to pulmonary fibrosis. Cessation of the drug may result in partial or complete resolution of the pneumonitis. No other specific therapy has proven effective.

Bleomycin induces pulmonary toxicity in aobut 5% of patients. It is a dose-related phenomenon, rarely being seen until the total dose of bleomycin exceeds 300 mg. Initial presentation is generally as an acute pneumonitis with cough, dyspnoea and diffuse pulmonary infiltrate on X-ray, but occasionally it is more insidious. The majority of cases which become clinically apparent progress to chronic pulmonary fibrosis which is life-threatening and irreversible. Cessation of the drug may prevent progression but use of other agents such as steroids have no proven benefit. Limiting the total dose of bleomycin administered to 300–360 mg and regular respiratory function monitoring have been the principal means of preventing this toxicity.

A synergistic effect between prior bleomycin exposure and subsequent high dose oxygen support during anaesthesia has been suggested. The prior bleomycin administration may have been below maximum tolerated dose and have been unassociated with any evidence of pulmonary toxicity. Within 48 hours of high-dose oxygen, a rapidly progressive pulmonary infiltrate may develop which is almost invariably fatal. The histological changes in the lungs resemble hyaline membrane disease of neonates. Limitation of oxygen during anaesthesia to below 50% is advised as a preventive measure in these patients.

Pulmonary toxicity occurring in conjunction with methotrexate administration is very uncommon. It appears to be idiosyncratic and may occur after short-term or prolonged administration. It is manifested by a diffuse pneumonitis, often associated with fever but, unlike many of the other drug-induced lung toxicities, progression to fibrosis does not occur. It is usually a self-limited phenomenon and prognosis is not altered by steroid usage.

References

1. Willson JKV. Pulmonary toxicity of antineoplastic drugs. *Cancer Treat Rep* 1978; 62: 2003–2008.
2. Sostman HD, et al. Cytotoxic drug-induced lung disease. *Am J Med* 1977; 62: 608–615.
3. Goldiner PL, et al. Factors influencing postoperative morbidity and mortality in patients treated with bleomycin. *Br Med J* 1978; 1: 1664–1667.
4. Ginsberg SJ, Comis RL. The pulmonary toxicity of antineoplastic agents. *Semin Oncol* 1982; 9(1): 34–51.

166. Items B and D correct.

Biochemical markers, used to detect the presence of cancer of various types and to monitor progress of the malignancy, are a valuable clinical tool. Unfortunately those markers which have reached clinical utility are only specific for a single or small number of cancers. The search for a more generally useful marker continues. Serum alpha-fetoprotein (AFP) when first identified appeared to have potential as a marker specific for a number of cancers without overlap in non-malignant conditions. Further studies have now shown that there is considerable overlap with benign conditions and its use as a general marker is limited. However, it still has value in selected circumstances.

Two malignancies in which the level of serum AFP is consistently and markedly elevated are germ cell tumour of the testis and primary hepatoma. When other malignancies directly involve the liver, the level of AFP may rise, but rarely more than 10 times above normal.

Some elevation of serum AFP levels may occur in heavy smokers and in patients with several non-malignant conditions including severe emphysema, cirrhosis of the liver, chronic active hepatitis and ataxia telangiectasia. However, the only condition, other than malignancies, where major elevations (at least 10 times above normal) can be expected to occur is normal pregnancy. The fetus produces quite large amounts of this glycoprotein which enters the maternal circulation.

In a small proportion of cases, other primary malignancies may be associated with elevations of serum AFP; these include adenocarcinomas of the stomach, breast, lung or pancreas but major elevations are very unusual.

References

1. Sell S, Becker FF. Alpha-fetoprotein. *J Natl Cancer Inst* 1978; 60: 19–26.
2. Wespic TH, Kirkpatrick A. Alpha-fetoprotein and its relevance to human disease. *Gastroenterology* 1979; 77: 787–796.
3. Lokich JJ. Tumor markers: hormones, antigens and enzymes in malignant disease. *Oncology* 1978; 35: 54–57.

167. Item B correct.

When cytotoxic chemotherapy and simple hormone manipulation (e.g. tamoxifen) have failed in a patient with metastatic breast cancer, a second course of hormonal therapy is often attempted.

Surgical adrenalectomy is known to produce about a 30% response in such patients. Recently aminoglutethimide (which blocks adrenal steroid biosynthesis, i.e. a medical adrenalectomy) has been shown to produce similar response rates. It is generally very well tolerated and eliminates the need for surgery.

References

1. Bonadonna G, Veronesi U, eds. Breast cancer. *Semin Oncol* 1978; 5: 341–474.
2. Editorial. Aminoglutethimide. *Lancet* 1981; 1: 1194–1195.

168. Items A, B, D and E correct.

The approach to the treatment of breast cancer should depend upon knowledge of several important factors. There is a clear inverse relationship between the number of axillary lymph nodes found to be involved with carcinoma at mastectomy and subsequent disease-free and overall survival rates.

Oestrogen receptor assays of tumour tissue, either primary or a metastasis, are useful in assessing likely response to hormonal manipulation. If the levels of oestrogen receptors are high, the potential for response to hormones is about 70%.

When metastatic disease has developed, the choice of therapy depends partly on the sites of involvement. Liver metastases are associated with a low response to hormones, irrespective of the levels of oestrogen receptors. Results with cytotoxic chemotherapy are consistently superior in therapeutic response and survival.

Cerebral metastases are common in breast cancer and respond poorly to hormonal therapy. The majority of cytotoxic agents fail to cross the blood-brain barrier in therapeutic concentrations. An example is doxorubicin (adriamycin), which is otherwise a very effective drug in breast cancer. Cerebral irradiation is thus the treatment of choice.

In pre-menopausal women with positive axillary lymph nodes at mastectomy, post-surgical adjuvant chemotherapy, with either single drugs or combination chemotherapy, improves both disease-free survival and overall survival. The same is not yet true for post-menopausal women and such adjuvant therapy would not be recommended for this group at present.

References

1. Henderson IC, Cannelos GP. Cancer of the breast: the past decade. *N Engl J Med* 1980; 302: 17–30, 78–90.
2. Editorial. Breast cancer: adjuvant chemotherapy. *Lancet* 1981; 1: 761–762.
3. Carter SK. Editorial. Adjuvant chemotherapy of breast cancer. *N Engl J Med* 1981; 304: 45–47.
4. Dalley DN, et al. Combination chemotherapy with cyclophosphamide, adriamycin, and 5-fluorouracil (CAF) in advanced breast carcinoma. *Med J Aust* 1980; 1: 216–218.
5. Bonadonna G, Veronesi U (eds). Breast cancer. *Semin Oncol* 1978; 5: 341–474.

169. Items C and D correct.

Careful assessment of the various prognostic features of malignant melanoma is important in management decisions. Certain sites of presentation are of prognostic importance, with lesions of the head and neck, trunk, palms of the hands and soles of the feet having a poorer prognosis than presentation on the rest of the limbs. Generally, females with malignant melanoma have a better prognosis than males, independent of other prognostic variables; the precise reason for this is unclear.

The development of a malignant melanoma in an area of lentigo maligna is relatively common in elderly people. The developmental stages of lentigo maligna may show slow evolution over many years, but once dermal invasion has occurred and the diagnosis of malignant melanoma made, the prognosis is identical to other melanomas and is dependant on depth of invasion and extension to other sites.

The most important determinant of prognosis in malignant

melanoma is the depth of invasion of the primary lesion. The potential for development of metastatic disease is directly dependent on this, with involvement of the more superficial levels of the dermis asociated with less than a 5% potential for recurrence or metastases, progressing to a 70–80% potential when subcutaneous fat has been invaded.

Nodular melanomas have a notoriously rapid growth phase, with early invasion of the deeper layers of the dermis and subcutaneous fat. They occur more commonly in males, which may partly account for the worse prognosis in men, and frequently lack a protective host-cellular response which is manifested by a surrounding cuff of lymphocytes and macrophages.

Malignant melanoma, particularly of the superficial spreading type, commonly arises from a pre-existing naevus and in itself does not indicate a poor prognosis.

References

1. Clark WH, et al. The developmental biology of primary human malignant melanomas. *Semin Oncol* 1975; 2: 83–104.
2. Lichtenfeld J. Current concepts in the management of malignant melanoma. *Am J Med Sci* 1976; 272: 184–195.
3. Everall JD, Dowd PM. Diagnosis, prognosis and treatment of melanoma. *Lancet* 1977; 2: 286–289.

170. Item B correct.

Breast cancer screening programmes including patient education in regular breast self-examination, the use of mammography and breast ultrasound examinations have improved the potential for detecting smaller breast carcinomas. However, the biology of breast cancer is such that metastases may occur at any stage of tumour development and the size of the primary lesion is not a reliable determinant of this. Perhaps for these reasons the earlier detection of breast cancer has not yet been shown to improve the potential for cure.

Long-term follow-up of the results of routine Papanicolaou smears of the cervix in large populations of women have clearly shown improvements in detection of early stage cancers of the cervix. Local resection of the carcinoma in situ or early invasive forms have resulted in a progressive decline in mortality from this cancer over the past two decades.

A variety of screening procedures for earlier detection of lung cancer have been evaluated over the past few years. Routine chest X-ray examinations have not proven of value, as the tumour has the propensity to metastasise before it has reached a size detectable by this means. Other procedures such as segmental bronchoscopies, sputum cytology and tantalum bronchography are presently being assessed but appear to be of limited value.

Simple methods to detect the presence of occult faecal blood which may allow for an earlier diagnosis of colon cancer are presently being evaluated in large population studies. Significant levels of both false-positive and false-negative results have been demonstated which are likely to limit both the sensitivity and specificity of this procedure and thereby prevent its routine application in screening programmes.

No reliable screening programmes have yet been developed for carcinoma of the pancreas.

References

1. Biahrs OH, et al. Report of the working group to review the National Cancer Institute — American Cancer Society Breast Cancer Demonstration Projects. *J Natl Cancer Inst* 1979; 62: 641–709.
2. Carlile T. Breast cancer detection. *Cancer* 1981; 47: 1164–1169.
3. Canadian Task Force. Cervical cancer screening programs: epidemiology and natural history of carcinoma of the cervix. *Can Med Assoc J* 1976; 114: 1003–1031.
4. Richart RM, Bannon BA. Screening strategies for cervical cancer and cervical intraepithelial neoplasia. *Cancer* 1981; 47: 1176–1181.
5. Boucot KR, Weiss W. Is curable lung cancer detected by semiannual screening? *JAMA* 1973; 224: 1361–1365.
6. Taylor WF et al. Some results of screening for early lung cancer. *Cancer* 1981; 47: 1114–1120.
7. Winawer SJ. Screening for colorectal cancer: an overview. *Cancer* 1980; 45: 1093–1098.

171. Items A, B and D correct.

Adriamycin, an anthracycline antibiotic, is an important cancer chemotherapeutic agent widely used in oncological practice. Its recognised mechanism of action involves intercalation between base pairs on the DNA helix, forming an irreversible complex and subsequently inhibiting DNA-dependent RNA synthesis.

Approximately 60% of the drug is metabolised in the liver, with both unchanged drug and its metabolites being excreted by the biliary route. In the presence of disturbed liver function with elevations of serum alkaline phosphatase (SAP) and bilirubin levels, metabolism and excretion are impaired, resulting in a prolongation of serum half-life and elevated tissue levels, increasing the risks of toxicity. Doses therefore must be reduced in the presence of these disturbances. Standard dose reductions would include 50% normal dose when SAP and bilirubin levels are 2–5 times above normal, 75% reduction when SAP and bilirubin levels are more than 5 times normal.

Adriamycin is extremely irritant to skin and muscle tissues, producing severe necrosis if accidentally injected into these sites. For this reason it is mandatory that the agent be administered by the intravenous route and careful attention must be paid to avoid extravasation outside the vein. The drug is not absorbed when given orally.

Adriamycin has a broad spectrum of activity and is of potential value in the treatment of acute leukaemias; lymphoma; breast, lung, gastric, thyroid, bladder, ovarian and endometrial cancers; soft tissue and osteogenic sarcomas. In the last malignancy, it is of proven benefit as both adjuvant therapy in the early stages of disease and as a palliative therapy in metastatic disease.

One of the most severe forms of toxicity is cardiac. It is a dose-related phenomenon producing a progressive cardiomyopathy which may be irreversible. The risk is less than 1% when total doses remain below 500 mg/m^2 but rises exponentially above this dose level. Therefore total cumulative doses are limited to less than 500 mg/m^2 except in very specific circumstances. No other means have been demonstrated to be effective in preventing this toxicity; the once-proposed hypothesis that cardiac glycosides protect against the cardiotoxicity of adriamycin has been disproved.

Prior radiotherapy to the mediastinum potentiates or adds to the effects of adriamycin on the heart. Patients who have had prior mediastinal radiotherapy should probably not have a total cumulative dose greater than 400mg/m^2. Other less well defined factors which influence adriamycin cardiotoxicity include mode of administration (constant infusion may cause less damage than bolus doses with higher peak levels) and pre-existing cardiac disease, especially in those with an abnormal electrocardiogram. Incidence of cardiotoxicity seems to increase with increasing age.

References

1. Blum RH, Carter SK. Adriamycin — a new anticancer drug with significant clinical activity. *Ann Intern Med* 1974; 80: 249–259.
2. Henderson DI, Frei E. Adriamycin cardiotoxicity. *Am Heart J* 1980; 99: 671–673.
3. Minow RA, et al. Adriamycin cardiomyopathy — risk factor. *Cancer* 1977; 39: 1397–1402.
4. Merill J, et al. Adriamycin and radiation synergistic cardiotoxicity. *Ann Intern Med* 1975; 82: 122–123.
5. Von Hoff DD, et al. The cardiotoxicity of anti-cancer agents. *Semin Oncol* 1982; 9(1): 23–33.

172. Items C and D correct.

At least 70% of patients presenting with small cell anaplastic carcinoma of the lung (SCLC) have metastatic disease and in previous studies surgery has proven unsuccessful in influencing this prognosis. However, although most centres consider that surgical excision is contraindicated, there is some accumulating evidence that surgery in the early stages may improve prognosis. Therefore mediastinoscopy, a procedure primarily performed for determination of operability, is generally considered unnecessary. Evaluation of other possible metastatic sites is more important to guide therapeutic decisions.

Bone marrow involvement occurs in 25–40% of patients with SCLC and does not correlate closely with bone involvement. Recent evidence has indicated that involvement of this site does not adversely influence prognosis per se and in general it is the number of sites involved and their degree of involvement which has an adverse effect rather than specific sites.

Studies have now clearly demonstrated that this histological type of lung cancer is very sensitive to both radiotherapy and chemotherapy. The use of combination chemotherapy either alone or in conjunction with radiotherapy has significantly improved the prognosis for many patients, with median survivals of 14–18 months and 30% of patients surviving beyond 2 years compared to a median survival of 3 months without therapy or following surgery alone.

Cerebral metastases occur in 30% of patients with SCLC at some time during the course of the disease. In patients achieving remission with therapy it is the principal site of relapse in 20–25%. The use of prophylactic cranial irradiation at the time of initial treatment has now been shown to reduce the incidence of relapse in this site to less than 10%.

Hyponatraemia in this setting is most likely to be due to inappropriate secretion of ADH, which may occur either as a specific paraneoplastic syndrome due to ectopic secretion from the tumour or, less commonly, as a more general manifestation of disseminated malignancy. While it can occur in conjunction with cerebral involvement it is not a specific indication of this.

1. Bunn PA, et al. Advances in small cell bronchogenic carcinoma. *Cancer Treat Rep* 1977; 61: 333–342.
2. Hansen HH, et al. Staging and prognostic features in small cell anaplastic bronchogenic carcinoma. *Semin Oncol* 1978; 5: 280–287.
3. Weiss RB. Small cell carcinoma of the lung: therapeutic management. *Ann Intern Med* 1978; 88: 522–531.
4. Hansen M, et al. Diagnostic and therapeutic implications of ectopic hormone production in small cell carcinoma of the lung. *Thorax* 1980; 35: 101–106.
5. Cohen MH. Treatment of small cell lung cancer: progress, potential and problems. *Int J Radiat Oncol* 1980; 6: 1079–1802.
6. Ihde DC, et al. Bone marrow metastases in small cell carcinoma of the lung: frequency, description and influence on chemotherapeutic toxicity and prognosis. *Blood* 1979; 53: 677–686.
7. Shore DF, Paneth M. Survival after resection of small cell carcinoma of the bronchus. *Thorax* 1980; 35: 819–822.

173. Items B, C and D correct.

In patients with acute Guillain-Barré syndrome, early muscle wasting is unlikely. If wasting is prominent early, an alternative diagnosis of acute axonal neuropathy (e.g. nitrofurantion neuropathy) should be suspected.

The facial nerves are often affected in acute Guillain-Barré syndrome. When other cranial nerves, such as III or IV, are affected it is sometimes called the Miller-Fisher variant. Postural hypotension and a fixed tachycardia are commonly found, indicating autonomic nerve involvement.

In the study reported by McLeod et al (1976), nerve conduction velocities and CSF protein values were normal in 14% of patients during early stages of the disease. Abnormalities were noted later in some of these patients.

Steroid therapy has not been shown to be of definite value in acute Guillain-Barré type polyneuropathy. However in the chronic syndrome, the use of corticosteroids has been advocated by some.

Reference

1. McLeod JG, et al. Acute idiopathic polyneuritis. A clinical and electrophysiological follow-up study. *J Neurol Sci* 1976; 27: 145–162.

174. Item C correct.

'Neuralgic amyotrophy' is one of various terms used for the acute syndrome described. Others include 'acute brachial neuritis' and 'paralytic brachial neuritis'. Pain is usually the first symptom, rapidly followed by flaccid weakness of muscles innervated by the brachial plexus. Sensory loss is often patchy and is a minor part of the syndrome.

The incidence of neuralgic amyotrophy is variable from year to year. It may occur in epidemics or clusters and may be postoperative, post-infective or post-vaccination. About half of the cases seen are idiopathic, but some have familial associations. About 25% of patients have upper respiratory tract infections. The condition is usually treated with corticosteroids. Although early treatment with steroids may alleviate pain, it does not shorten the period of disability due to weakness.

Cervical disc prolapse is unlikely since involvement of shoulder girdle muscles, biceps and supinator muscles indicates that several dermatomes are affected. Muscle wasting is not a feature of cervical disc prolapse.

Syringomyelia does not present acutely, and muscle weakness, wasting and loss of reflexes occur later. Dissociated sensory loss is the important clinical feature of syringomyelia. Poliomyelitis does not have sensory features. The Guillain-Barré syndrome is unlikely since it does not usually affect a single limb, being classically, but not invariably, symmetrical.

References

1. Editorial. Neuralgic amyotrophy — still a clinical syndrome. *Lancet* 1980; 2: 729–730.
2. Devathasan G, Tong HI. Neuralgic amyotrophy: criteria for diagnosis and a clinical with electromyographic study of 21 cases. *Aust NZ J Med* 1980; 10: 188–191.

175. Items C and D correct.

The given history is typical of a transient global amnesic episode which is a clearly recognisable syndrome with several causes. The entity is quite common, with many patients not coming to the attention of the physician because of the transient nature of the event. The most common cause is vertebrobasilar insuffiency with ischaemia of the dominant posterior hippocampal gyrus. Other lesions, including tumours in this region, can also cause transient global amnesia.

Temporal lobe (partial complex) seizures occur very rarely as amnesic events without disturbance of consciousness, indifference to memory or aura and post-ictal state. An electroencephalogram during or immediately after a partial complex seizure is generally diagnostic.

Autopsies and arteriography or regional cerebral blood flow studies have usually demonstrated stenosis or occlusion of the dominant posterior cerebral artery or the posterior choroidal artery (supplying the posterior hippocampus). Although symptoms are generally not recurrent, exclusion of a tumour or infarction necessitates a CT head scan. Since the major risk factors for stroke are generally present, the syndrome is not entirely benign and patients warrant further medical supervision.

References

1. Shuping JR, et al. Transient global amnesia due to glioma in the dominant hemisphere. *Neurology* 1980; 30: 88–90.
2. Rollinson RD. Transient global amnesia — a review of 213 cases from the literature. *Aust NZ J Med* 1978; 8: 547–549.

176. Items C, D and E correct.

The patient described has a typical story of the 'subclavian steal syndrome'. In this condition, stenosis or occlusion of the subclavian artery proximal to the origin of the vertebral artery is present and this may result in a reversal of blood flow in the vertebral artery on that side when vasodilatation occurs in the arm during sustained exercise. This haemodynamic event is associated with symptoms of brain-stem ischaemia.

Stenosis is usually 2–3 times more common on the left than on the right (combined with the innominate artery) and is rarely bilateral (1–2% of cases). Men are more commonly affected than women.

Symptoms are generally transient, although 25% of patients may have persistent abnormal neurological signs. An absent or dimished radial pulse and reduced brachial blood pressure on the affected side is noted. Cerebral symptoms occur in about 45%, combined cerebral symptoms with arm weakness or paraesthesia occur in 40%, and arm symptoms alone occur in 10% of patients.

References

1. Patel A, Toole JF. Subclavian steal syndrome — reversal of cephalic blood flow. *Medicine* (Baltimore) 1965; 44: 289–303.
2. Fields WS, Lemak NA. Joint study of extracranial arterial occlusion. VII: Subclavian steal — a review of 168 cases. *JAMA* 1972, 222: 1139–1143.

177. Items A, D and E correct.

The combination of any two of the three ways in which a cerebral tumour presents, namely, progressive focal neurological deficit, evidence of raised intracranial pressure and epilepsy of late onset, makes the diagnosis of a cerebral tumour very likely. The patient described has the first two of these three features.

The description given is that of a supratentorial tumour, particularly with the clinical evidence of transtentorial herniation (impaired consciousness and dilated pupil). Posterior fossa neoplasms present with raised intracranial pressure, but the neurological deficit is indicative of damage to the cerebellum and brain stem.

Pathological changes in one cerebral hemisphere alone, no matter how extensive, will not cause impaired consciousness. The pathological process must involve either both cerebral hemispheres or the projection of the reticular activating system. In this patient, the impaired consciousness can be presumed to be due to shift of brain contents from the right to the left under the falx and shift of the mid-brain downwards and to the left by the herniation of the medial aspect of the right temporal lobe. This causes compression of the third cranial nerve against the edge of the tentorium and also distortion of the mid-brain. The caudal displacement of the mid-brain in these circumstances may lead to avulsion of small branches of the basilar artery and this in turn to the petechial haemorrhages in the mid-brain characteristic of tentorial herniation. When such vascular damage occurs, recovery is unlikely.

A very important factor in controlling intracranial pressure is the $P\text{CO}_2$ which in turn determines the calibre of capillaries within the central nervous system. When intracranial pressure is raised and intracranial displacements begin, these can be rapidly aggravated by a rise in $P\text{CO}_2$, which increases the cerebral blood flow and the amount of blood within the skull. This may produce a rapid deterioration in an already critical situation.

Reference

1. Plum F, Posner JB. The diagnosis of stupor and coma, 3rd Edn. Philadelphia: Davis, 1980: 142–6.

178. Items C and D correct.

Ocular movement disorders in patients with Huntington's disease have been studied recently by several authors. Disturbances of saccadic eye movement, smooth pursuit and reflex movements have been found in about one-third of cases, the abnormality probably being more common in the rigid and infantile varieties.

A number of studies have been made in an attempt to predict carriers of the disease. Unfortunately the CT scan is not reliable in this respect.

Juvenile Huntington's disease represents about 5% of all cases and in 70% the disease is transmitted from an affected male. From a clinical point of view, there are a number of differences between this form and the adult type and as many as half will have grand mal seizures often difficult to control. In the adult form epilepsy is most unusual.

A number of biochemical abnormalities have now been described in Huntington's disease. There is a marked decrease of endogenous GABA. Glutamic acid decarboxylase (GAD), the enzyme responsible for GABA synthesis, is also depleted. GABA receptors appear intact. Other abnormalities which have been described include a depletion of choline acetyltransferase (CAT) and acetylcholinesterase (ACHE). Dopamine concentration is increased and chorea may result from the unopposed action of the nigrostriatal dopamine system. Unfortunately, attempts to correct these biochemical abnormalities with drug therapy including sodium valproate and choline, have not produced especially encouraging results.

References

1. Editorial. Chemistry of Huntington's chorea. *Lancet* 1980; 1: 1119–1120.
2. Caraceni T, et al. Biochemical aspects of Huntington's chorea. *J Neurol Neurosurg Psychiatry* 1977; 40: 581–587.
3. Propert DN. The growing edge: presymptomatic detection of Huntington's disease. *Med J Aust* 1980; 1: 609–612.
4. Tyler KL, Tyler HR. Huntington's disease. In: Tyler R, Dawson D (eds). Current neurology. Boston: Houghton Mifflin, 1978; 1: 116–41.

179. Items B and D correct.

Alzheimer's disease is the most common cause of progressive dementia in later life. Pathological studies indicate that cerebrovascular disease accounts for only 20–30% of dementia cases.

Patients with Parkinson's disease appear to have a higher incidence of dementia than unaffected people matched for age, and the dementia is associated with the histological changes seen in Alzheimer's disease.

Overall improvement rates after ventricular shunting in normal-pressure hydrocephalus are reported variably, but most series claim some improvement of dementia in approximately 50%. Figures for improvement are lower in idiopathic cases and about 60% of cases where a predisposing cause exists, e.g. head injury or meningitis.

Reduced levels of a number of enzymes have been demonstrated in brains of patients with Alzheimer's disease; a deficiency in choline acetyltransferase is the most marked of these.

Relative paucity of symptoms and signs of raised intracranial pressure is a feature of symptomatic chronic subdural haematoma in contrast to other space-occupying lesions.

References

1. Leading article. Chronic subdural haematoma. *Br Med J* 1979; 1: 433–434.
2. Editorial. Communicating hydrocephalus. *Lancet* 1977; 2: 1011–1012.
3. Terry RD. Editorial. Dementia: a brief and selective review. *Arch Neurol* 1976; 33: 1–4.
4. Hakim AM, Mathieson G. Dementia in Parkinson's disease: a neuropathologic study. *Neurology* 1979; 29: 1209–1214.
5. Jacobs L, Kinkel W. Computerized axial transverse tomography in normal pressure hydrocephalus. *Neurology* 1976; 26: 501–507.
6. Harrison MJG, et al. Multi-infarct dementia. *J Neurol Sci* 1979; 40: 97–103.
7. Boller F, et al. Parkinson's disease, dementia and Alzheimer's disease: clinicopathological correlations. *Ann Neurol* 1980; 7: 329–335.

180. Items D and E correct.

While the CT scan is a very useful tool in establishing the cause of coma, in most large series metabolic factors are more frequent than structural lesions; hence the CT scan is likely to be normal. Even in the presence of structural lesions, abnormalities are not always seen.

Cheyne-Stokes respiration (i.e. phases of hyperpnoea regularly alternating with apnoea) is a neurogenic alteration in respiratory control that usually results from intracranial causes; however, hypoxaemia, a prolonged circulation time and pulmonary congestion may amplify it. Sustained or prolonged, Cheyne-Stokes respiration usually implies bilateral dysfunction of neurologic structures lying deep in the cerebral hemispheres rather than in the brain stem; however, lesions in the upper pons occasionally can be associated with this breathing pattern. Most autopsy studies of patients with Cheyne-Stokes respiration have demonstrated mainly cortical or subcortical lesions with bilateral damage to corticospinal or corticobulbar pathways. It is frequently found in patients with hypertensive encephalopathy and metabolic disease. The onset of Cheyne-Stokes respiration may indicate the evolution of transtentorial herniation.

As a general rule the oculocephalic eye reflex movements remain intact when coma is the result of bilateral cerebral hemisphere dysfunction or due to metabolic cerebral dysfunction (intoxication with barbiturates, hypnotics and phenytoin being occasional exceptions). As a general rule the oculocephalic reflex (and caloric or oculovestibular responses) are absent in patients with coma due to brain stem lesions.

Apneustic breathing is a respiratory pattern with a prolonged pause at full inspiration. It is unusual but is of localising value, indicating damage to the respiratory control centres located at the mid or caudal pontine level in the region of the nucleus parabrachialis adjacent to the trigeminal motor nucleus. Apneustic breathing is usually seen in extensive pontine infarction but it may occur in patients with progressive brain stem function with transtentorial herniation or with severe anoxia or meningitis.

The pupillary pathways are relatively resistant to metabolic depression and therefore the presence of preserved pupillary light reflexes despite concomitant respiratory depression, caloric or oculovestibular unresponsiveness, rigidity or motor flaccidity, suggests metabolic coma. If asphyxia, anticholinergic or glutethimide ingestion or pre-existing pupillary disease can be ruled out, the absence of pupillary light reflexes strongly implies that the disease is structural rather than metabolic.

References

1. Plum F, Posner JB. The diagnosis of stupor and coma, 3rd Edn. Philadelphia: FA Davis, 1980.
2. North JB, Jennett S. Abnormal breathing patterns associated with acute brain damage. *Arch Neurol* 1974; 31: 338–344.

181. Item E correct.

Phenytoin is the drug of choice for generalised simple seizures (grand mal epilepsy). However, it is better to give it as a single dose treatment than in divided doses. It has a long biological half-life (24 hours) and therefore, once steady state is reached there is no advantage in more frequent dosage; patient compliance is generally better. The term 'generalised tonic-clonic seizures' is now preferred to 'grand mal epilepsy'.

It is desirable to use one agent and make sure that its plasma concentration is in the therapeutic range, rather than introducing second or even third drugs. In one study, 76–88% of patients were completely controlled on one drug when optimum serum drug concentrations were achieved and there was a 98% reduction in the rate of grand mal seizures. Polypharmacy increases the risk of chronic toxicity without necessarily controlling the seizure rate adequately, because the adverse effects are often additive. Furthermore, the addition of a second anticonvulsant drug to a patient's regimen may either increase or decrease the serum level of an existing drug (e.g. adding sulthiame to phenytoin can cause inhibition of phenytoin metabolism and raise the serum level with a risk of phenytoin toxicity). Conversely the addition of an inducer of hepatic enzymes such as phenobarbitone may lower phenytoin concentrations.

Phenytoin assays can be done using a variety of techniques, but they are reliable and widely available. They are essential in the management of epilepsy because of the well-defined but narrow therapeutic range for seizure control and the wide inter-subject variation in serum levels for any given dosage.

Phenytoin is hydroxylated by hepatic microsomal enzymes and this process is saturable (i.e. once a critical concentration has been reached, the rate of metabolism fails to increase in proportion to the serum concentration of the drug). This is important in the management of epilepsy, as it means that small changes in daily intake of the drug may disproportionately alter the serum level; therefore increments in dose need to be smaller as the therapeutic range is approached (i.e. 30–60 mg/day, with a serum level re-estimated 2–4 weeks later).

Phenytoin toxicity has been one of the problems confronting the physician attempting to control generalised seizures. The most characteristic side-effects are symptoms of cerebellar and vestibular dysfunction, with nystagmus, ataxia, diplopia and vertigo; behavioural changes of hyperactivity, confusion and hallucinations also occur. Increased seizure frequency may also occur at very high phenytoin concentrations; it is important to recognise this since treatment should not be by increasing drug dosage. Other side-effects (including blood dyscrasias, gastrointestinal disturbances, skin rashes and lymphadenopathy) are usually idiosyncratic effects, and gum hypertrophy and hirsutism are long-term side-effects.

References

1. Richens A, Dunlop A. Serum phenytoin levels in management of epilepsy. *Lancet* 1975; 2: 247–248.
2. Shorvon SD, et al. One drug for epilepsy. *Br Med J* 1978; 1: 474–476.

3. Richens A. Anticonvulsant interactions. *Curr Ther* 1977; May: 117–128.
4. From the NIH. Some side effects of phenytoin are studied. *JAMA* 1980; 243: 1038–1039.
5. Goodman LS, Gilman A, eds. The pharmacological basis of therapeutics, 6th Edn. New York: Macmillan, 1980: 454–455.

182. Items A, C, D and E correct.

Pregnancy has been clearly shown to be associated with a progressive fall in plasma levels of anticonvulsant drugs whilst the patient continues on a steady dose. This may be one reason for the increase in seizures which occurs during pregnancy in epileptic patients.

The increased drug requirement falls rapidly after delivery but may take 1–6 months to return to the normal state.

There is increased risk of haemorrhage in babies when the mother is taking anticonvulsants, especially barbiturates. The bleeding seems to be due to lack of the vitamin K-dependent clotting factors. Bleeding occurs earlier than in classical haemorrhagic disease of the newborn. It may occur within 24 hours of birth or even before delivery. Vitamin K can be given to the mother before delivery. Fresh frozen plasma would be the emergency therapy.

Cleft lip or palate occurs in about 2 per 1000 births and if the mother is on treatment for epilepsy the rate rises, according to different studies, to 3–25 per 1000. There is an increase also in relation to congenital heart disease. Total fetal malformations in control groups ranged from 20–50 per 1000 live births and in treated epilepsy groups from 70 to almost 200 per 1000 live births.

This increased risk of fetal malformation is not necessarily due to teratogenic effect of the drugs and only part of the relatively small increase in risk could be due to the drugs.

There is increased risk of abnormality when the mother with epilepsy is not taking any anticonvulsant and similarly the risk is increased when the father has epilepsy.

References

1. Lander CM, et al. Plasma anticonvulsant concentrations during pregnancy. *Neurology* 1977; 27: 128–131.
2. Mountain KR, et al. Neonatal coagulation defect due to anticonvulsant drug treatment in pregnancy. *Lancet* 1970; 1: 265–268.
3. Stumpf DA, Frost M. Seizures, anticonvulsants and pregnancy. *Am J Dis Child* 1978; 132: 746–748.
4. Shapiro S, et al. Anticonvulsants and parental epilepsy in the development of birth defects. *Lancet* 1976; 1: 272–275.

183. Items C, D and E correct.

A delay in the visual-evoked potential is commonly found in patients with multiple sclerosis but not necessarily only those with objective evidence of demyelination involving the visual pathways.

Raised antibodies to measles and the presence of specific

histocompatability antigens have been described but are not useful in establishing the diagnosis in individuals.

Paroxysmal phenomena consist of brief, often frequent, stereotyped neurologic symptoms referable particularly to brain stem function. These can sometimes be precipitated by movement and might consist of dysarthria or painful tonic seizures. The suggested mechanism is that transversely spreading activation of axons occurs within a partially demyelinated lesion. Such symptoms invariably respond dramatically to carbamazepine and frequently after a period of weeks or months it is possible to withdraw therapy.

It has been known for many years that changes in body temperature as well as electrolyte balance might interfere with nerve conduction. This does happen in multiple sclerosis; for example, after a hot bath the patient can have transient dysfunction, or after exercise, lose vision in one eye. Increasing the temperature does slightly increase the conduction velocity at all levels of demyelination until a temperature is reached at which conduction suddenly fails. The temperature at which blocking occurs gets progressively lower as the degree of demyelination increases. If the myelin sheath is reduced to a quarter of its normal thickness then the fibres become very thermosensitive.

While there is no diagnostic laboratory test for multiple sclerosis, the most widely accepted general finding is that of localised synthesis of immunoglobulin within the CNS. It is generally agreed that at least 80% of patients with multiple sclerosis will have an oligoclonal pattern of the gammaglobulin subfractions in the CSF.

References

1. McDonald WI, Halliday AM. Diagnosis and classification of multiple sclerosis. *Br Med Bull* 1977; 33: 4–8.
2. Thompson EJ. Laboratory diagnosis of multiple sclerosis: immunological and biochemical aspects. *Br Med Bull* 1977; 33: 28–33.

184. Item B correct.

Clinical and simple laboratory tests can distinguish complete visual loss of ocular, optic nerve, cerebral or non-organic origin. Consensual and direct pupillary responses to light require intact afferent visual pathway to the level of the lateral geniculate body as well as intact efferent pathways via the oculomotor nerves.

Optokinetic nystagmus is induced by passage of pattern contours before the eyes. It represents a complex oculomotor reflex which involves parietal lobe centres and occipital optomotor fibres which descend in the internal sagittal layer and which are medial to the optic radiations in their posterior course through the parietal lobe. Optokinetic nystagmus is triggered by visual impulses at a cerebral level and requires an intact visual pathway. It is more closely related to movement or contour recognition than to visual acuity. However, it is an excellent test of gross visual function and provides positive evidence of sight in infants, malingerers and hysterical patients as well as in profoundly retarded or aphasic subjects.

Pupillary accommodation and convergence depends on the co-operation of the patient. It involves the oculomotor nerve, ciliary ganglion and short posterior ciliary nerves. The mid-brain anteromedian nucleus of Edinger-Westphal has a rostral portion concerned with accommodation and a caudal portion which elicits pupillary constriction. Vision is not a prerequisite for the accommodation response, which can be tested in blind subjects by proprioceptive fixation of the fingertips.

Posterior electroencephalogram abnormalities are not necessarily specific for lesions of the visual cortex and conversely patients with cortical blindness due to ischaemia may have relatively normal electroencephalograms.

An absent visual evoked potential would indicate a significant organic lesion involving central vision mechanisms; however, it does not necessarily indicate that visual acuity is singificantly reduced. Patients with mulptile sclerosis may have grossly abnormal or absent visual evoked potentials due to previous demyelinating lesions in the optic nerves but visual acuity may be relatively unimpaired. Similarly if a major refractive error is present then an abnormal visual evoked potential may be recorded in the presence of an intact visual pathway.

Reference

1. Glaser JS. Neuro-ophthalmology. Hagerstown: Harper and Row, 1978.

185. Items B, C, D and E correct.

Tetracyclines have little direct nephrotoxicity but they have a potent anti-anabolic effect on metabolism leading to the excessive formation of urea and presumably other toxic breakdown products of protein. Thus they can induce a uraemic syndrome without anuria or obvious oliguria when given to patients with pre-existing renal disease. Most are contraindicated in patients with impaired renal function — either acute or chronic.

Amongst the tetracyclines, doxycycline is the one not contraindicated in patients with renal impairment. It is largely eliminated by a non-hepatic gastrointestinal pathway.

The aminoglycosides and cephalosporins are variably nephrotoxic and accumulate in the proximal renal tubule cells, which may be damaged by them.

An increasing number of drugs, including antibiotics and anti-inflammatory drugs, are being reported as inducing renal failure due to interstitial nephritis. Patients are often polyuric, have normal or large kidneys and eosinophilia is common. The serum creatinine and urea rise in spite of these findings.

If nephrotoxicity due to gentamicin or kanamycin is present, the use of potent loop diuretics may well exacerbate the problem. In a shocked or very ill oliguric patient it is particularly dangerous to combine frusemide and aminoglycoside antibiotics.

References

1. Editorial. Cephalosporin nephrotoxicity. *Lancet* 1979; 1: 962.
2. Editorial. Antibiotic damage to damaged kidneys. *Lancet* 1978; 2: 558–559.

186. Items A, D and E correct.

It has been known for a long time that alkalosis shifts potassium (K) into cells. It has now been established that bicarbonate administration will have this effect without necessarily altering pH.

Dialysis commonly removes much less than 15–20 mmol of K per litre exchange and this is very small relative to total body K of 3000–4000 mmol. The manoeuvre is effective in treating hyperkalaemia because it induces metabolic shifts due to glucose, buffer-base, etc.

Significant loss of total body K in non-oedematous patients is not common. However, careful monitoring of K levels in patients on digitalis may indicate a need for K supplements, or adjuvant K-sparing diuretics, to avoid toxicity problems.

Except in 'acute on chronic' situations (including infection, acidosis, administration of K etc.), hyperkalaemia is not often a major problem in stable chronic renal failure prior to dialysis therapy. This is because an increase in the fractional excretion of potassium is one of the homeostatic mechanisms occurring in chronic renal failure (in an attempt to maintain normal plasma levels).

References

1. Tannen RI, ed. Potassium homeostasis. *Kidney Internat* 1977; 11: 389–515.
2. Stockigt JR. Potassium metabolism. *Anaesth Intens Care* 1977; 5: 317–325.

187. Items A, B, C and E correct.

In most situations hyperkalaemia reflects either a failure of renal excretion of potassium or a redistribution of potassium between cells and extracellular fluid, often due to changes in acid-base balance. Adaptive increases in renal potassium excretion can usually maintain external potassium balance provided renal function is normal. Hyperkalaemia is rare in patients with chronic renal tubular failure until the glomerular filtration rate is less than 10% of normal. However, under certain circumstances, life-threatening hyperkalaemia may occur in patients with only modest degrees of renal impairment.

Hypoaldosteronism may be due to generalised adrenal insufficiency or an isolated defect in the zona glomerulosa. The latter is becoming increasingly recognised in older patients as well as in patients with diabetes or interstitial renal disease. It is characterised by a reduced aldosterone secretion, low plasma renin levels, mild hyperkalaemia and in some cases, reduced sensitivity to the kaluretic effect of aldosterone. Hyperkalaemia tends to occur when potassium supplements or potassium-sparing diuretics are administered.

Both insulin and renal potassium excretion play a part in the body's defence against hyperkalaemia. In diabetic patients requiring insulin who also have selective hypoaldosteronism and in diabetic patients treated with potassium-sparing diuretics, a paradoxical hyperkalaemia may occur following the administration of hypertonic glucose. Hypertonicity produces a redistribution of potassium from intracellular to extracellular fluid. The effect of diabetic ketoacidosis on potassium levels is affected by several factors including impairment of renal function and, perhaps, a degree of insulin resistance due to acidosis.

A decreased ability to excrete potassium may occur in a number of renal tubular disorders including systemic lupus erythematosus, sickle cell disease, amyloidosis and following renal transplantation. Whether this is due to refractoriness of the renal tubules or unresponsiveness of the renin-aldosterone system, is not known for certain. The clinical implication is that, in these conditions, the use of potassium supplements or potassium-sparing diuretics is potentially hazardous.

Like most other diuretics, frusemide and ethacrynic acid which act on the loop of Henle cause hypokalaemia. The mechanisms for this include increased availability of sodium in the distal tubule, secondary hyperaldosteronism induced by increased renin production and a tendency to hypovolaemia, and a metabolic alkalosis relating to hyperaldosteronism and hypovolaemia.

References

1. Cox M, et al. The defense against hyperkalaemia: the roles of insulin and aldosterone. *N Engl J Med* 1978; 299: 525–532.
2. Better OS. Editorial. Nonazotemic hyperkalaemia following kidney transplantation. *Miner Electrolyte Metab* 1980; 3(4): 167–171.

188. Items B, C and D correct.

Serum sodium levels reflect osomolality, and hyponatraemia is more commonly due to excess water retention than to sodium depletion, i.e. it represents dilution of body osmolality; thus treatment is usually by restriction of water intake. Persistent secretion of 'excess' anti-diuretic hormone (ADH) will lead to hyponatraemia in patients who continue to drink because, in the presence of ADH, the kidney cannot generate appropriate solute-free (dilute) urine. Chlorpropamide, amitriptyline and carbamazepine are three of the drugs (others include cyclophosphamide, tolbutamide, vincristine and thioridazine) which stimulate the secretion or potentiate the action of ADH. Hypothyroidism, adrenal insufficiency and hypopituitarism may also be associated with hyponatraemia.

Oedematous patients given potent diuretics may also develop hyponatraemia. There are several physiological mechanisms for this but it is important to recognise patients with hypokalaemia and potassium depletion in whom replacement of potassium may restore sodium concentrations towards normal levels. Hypokalaemia leads to inappropriate ADH secretion which becomes more appropriate with potassium replenishment.

Hyperlipidaemia and hyperproteinaemia cause 'pseudo-hyponatraemia' because the mass of lipid or protein occupies a significant volume of plasma. In these patients the true sodium osmotic activity and concentration in plasma water is normal.

Lithium carbonate, demeclocycline, methoxyfluorane and amphotericin all have the opposite effect, causing a diabetes insipidus-like situation and hypernatraemia by interference either with ADH secretion or its action on the renal tubule.

References

1. Fichman MP, et al. Diuretic-induced hyponatremia. *Ann Intern Med* 1971; 75: 853–863.
2. Brenner BM, Stein JH (eds). Sodium and water homeostatis. New York: Churchill Livingstone, 1978.
3. Flear CTG, et al. Hyponatraemia: mechanisms and management. *Lancet* 1981; 2: 26–31.
4. Kennedy PGE, et al. Severe hyponatraemia in hospital inpatients. *Br Med J* 1978; 2: 1251–1253.
5. Thomas TH, et al. Severe hyponatraemia: a study of 17 patients. *Lancet* 1978; 1: 621–624.
6. Fuisz RE. Hyponatremia. *Medicine* (Baltimore) 1963; 42: 149–170.
7. Friedler RM, et al. Hyponatremia and hypernatremia. *Clin Nephrol* 1977; 7: 163–172.

189. Items D and E correct.

The fluorescent bacterial antibody test, which was claimed to distinguish upper from lower urinary tract infection, has an appreciable rate of false-positive results (approximately 30%).

Single high-dose antibiotic therapy has been demonstrated to be effective in the treatment of uncomplicated lower urinary tract infection. However, single dose therapy would be inappropriate in this patient where the presence of loin pain and fever makes upper urinary tract infection likely.

If intravenous pyelography is performed subsequently and found to be normal, there is no indication for a micturating cystourethrogram. Even if reflux were demonstrated, in the absence of renal scarring it is likely to be mild. Ureteric reimplantation is probably only of benefit in young children with severe vesico-ureteric reflux accompanied by renal scarring or intrarenal reflux with infection.

In a survey of 55 women with proven urinary tract infection on catheter specimens, involvement of the upper urinary tract was demonstrated in 9 out of 10 with *Proteus* infections, compared with 11 out of 30 with *E. coli* infections.

References

1. Editorial. Single-dose treatment of urinary tract infections. *Lancet* 1981; 1: 26.
2. Andriole VT. Urinary tract infections in pregnancy. *Urol Clin North Am* 1975; 2: 485–498.
3. Montgomerie JZ. Urinary tract infection. In: Gopnick HC (ed). Current nephrology. Boston: Houghton Mifflin, 1978; 2: 285–304, and 1979; 3: 295–308.

190. Items A, D and E correct.

Urinary tract infections can recur because of bacterial persistence after chemotherapy or because of re-infection. The former usually occurs within 6 weeks of stopping therapy, while re-infection involves a different organism from that producing the original infection.

Bacterial persistence is commonly caused by infection stones and in men by chronic bacterial prostatitis. Infection stones consist of urea-splitting bacteria, frequently *Proteus mirabilis*, embedded within struvite (magnesium ammonium phosphate) or apatite (calcium phosphate) calculi. Pyelolithotomy often does not achieve the intended cure because bacteria-laden concentrations are left behind. A combination of antibiotics, pyelolithotomy and chemical dissolution of residual fragments with an organic acid solution has been successful.

Chronic bacterial prostatitis is the most common cause of recurrent urinary tract infections in men. The diagnosis is established by quantitative microbiological studies performed on divided urinary specimens and prostatic fluid. Co-trimoxazole has been found to be the most effective drug of choice and a treatment period of 12 weeks has been recommended.

Other possible causes of bacterial persistence include atrophic unilateral pyelonephritis, thought to be related to reduced complement activity and leukocyte function, and the persistence of aberrant bacterial forms which have defective cell walls.

In women most recurrences are re-infections rather than bacterial persistence. There is no evidence that a prolonged course of therapy will decrease the subsequent number of re-infections after cessation of treatment, but chemoprophylaxis (e.g. nocturnal co-trimoxazole or nitrofurantoin) has been shown to reduce the incidence of re-infection.

References

1. Gleckman RA. Recurrent urinary tract infections: therapeutic considerations. *Postgrad Med* 1979; 65(2): 156–159.
2. Whitworth JA. Management of asymptomatic bacteriuria. *Aust NZ J Med* 1981; 11; 321–328.

191. Items A and E correct.

The small, scarred, contracted kidney of reflux nephropathy is thought to result from the effects of gross vesicoureteric reflux on the kidney in the first few years of life, usually in association with infection. New scars rarely form in affected kidneys after the age of 4–5 years.

The correction, by re-implantation, of continuing gross vesicoureteric reflux in adults will not improve renal function or reduce the incidence of urinary tract infection, nor cure associated hypertension.

Hypertension is a frequent late complication of reflux nephropathy. It is usually benign and relatively easy to control but occasionally it may follow an accelerated and malignant course. 15% of patients with reflux nephropathy present in adulthood with hypertension or its complications. Frequently there is no symptom of urinary tract disease and no history of infection. In situations where there is unilateral parenchymal renal disease and hypertension, the high-blood pressure may be cured by the removal of the afftected kidney, but this does not occur invariably.

There is no evidence at the present time that the renin-angiotensin system has a causative role in the maintenance of non-malignant hypertension associated with unilateral reflux nephropathy.

References

1. Savage JM, et al. Renin and blood-pressure in children with renal scarring and vesicoureteric reflux. *Lancet* 1978; 2: 441–444.
2. Bailey RR, et al. Renal vein renin concentration in the hypertension of unilateral reflux nephropathy. *J Urol* 1978; 120:21–23.
3. Hodson J. Reflux nephropathy. *Med Clin North Am* 1978; 62(6); 1201–1221.
4. Kincaid-Smith P, Becker G. Reflux nephropathy and chronic atrophic pyelonephritis: a review. *J Infect Dis* 1978; 138: 774–780.
5. Bailey RR. The relationship of vesico-ureteric reflux to urinary tract infection and chronic pyelonephritis — reflux nephropathy. *Clin Nephrol* 1973; 1: 132–141.

192. Items A, B and E correct.

Adults polycystic kidney disease is inherited as an autosomal dominant character. The manner in which the abnormal gene initiates the pathological process in the kidney, which results in multiple cyst formation, remains obscure. Animal experiments suggest that the condition in man may be due to the chronic effects of some toxic metabolite produced in the body as a result of an inherited metabolic disorder. About one-third of patients with polycystic kidney disease have multiple liver cysts but it is extremely uncommon for these cysts to cause liver dysfunction.

Renal function deteriorates very gradually and most patients who develop end-stage renal failure do so in the fourth or fifth decade. End-stage renal failure occurs in 70% of patients who live to the age of 65 years. In Australasia, 9% of patients entering dialysis/ transplantation programmes have a diagnosis of polycystic renal disease.

The most important complication of the disease, apart from renal failure, is hypertension. Control of high blood pressure is important in conservative management.

In general, patients with polycystic kidney disease are good candidates for haemodialysis or renal transplantation. Those who have had recurrent urinary tract infections or who have very large kidneys may require nephrectomy before renal transplantation surgery.

References

1. Mitcheson HD, et al. Clinical aspects of polycystic disease of the kidneys. *Br Med J* 1977; 1: 1196–1199.
2. Salvatierra D, et al. End stage polycystic kidney disease: management by renal transplantation and selective use of preliminary nephrectomy. *J Urol* 1976; 115: 5–7.

193. Items C and E correct.

In this case an intravenous pyelogram would help to exclude obstruction and would confirm the renal size. It is not contraindicated by the degree of renal failure but should be performed by giving a high dose of dye without dehydration. A radionuclide study may give similar information with less discomfort and risk.

Occasionally analgesic nephropathy can produce haematuria and acutely swollen kidneys with necrotic papillae in situ, but this is unlikely in this case. Usually there are more leukocytes in the urine. Resolving urinary infection may present with smooth enlarged kidneys but red cell casts and haematuria of glomerular type are not usual.

A renal biopsy is strongly indicated to identify glomerulonephritis or interstitial nephritis perhaps induced by co-trimoxazole. The smooth enlarged kidneys, red cell casts, mild hypertension, previous normal creatinine and normal size heart all support a diagnosis of acute nephritis or interstitial nephritis.

Renal biopsy may well reveal (as it did in this case) crescentic glomerulonephritis with perhaps linear IgG staining of glomerular basement membrane. Early diagnosis before severe oliguria allows early institution of therapy (steroids, cyclophosphamide or chlorambucil, perhaps with plasma exchange). Once oliguria is established recovery is less likely. Haematuria and mild proteinuria together with renal pain are not uncommon in acute crescentic or rapidly progressive nephritis.

Aortography is not an appropriate immediate investigation unless the intravenous pyelogram or radionuclide study shows one non-functioning kidney, which is unlikely.

A peripheral blood eosinophilia is not uncommon in drug-induced interstitial nephritis, which can also complicate acute glomerulonephritis. Renal gallium-67 scanning is often strongly positive in acute interstitial nephritis.

References

1. Beirne GJ, et al. Idiopathic crescentic glomerulonephritis. *Medicine* (Baltimore) 1977; 56: 349–381.
2. Leading Article. Plasmapheresis and severe glomerulonephritis. *Br Med J* 1979; 1: 434–435.
3. Boulton WK, Couser WG. Intravenous pulse methylprednisolone therapy of acute crescentic rapidly progressive glomerulonephritis. *Am J Med* 1979; 66: 495–502.
4. Becker GJ, et al. Plasmapheresis in the treatment of glomerulonephritis. *Med J Aust* 1977; 2: 693–696.
5. Cameron JS. Diseases of the urinary system. Treatment of glomerulonephritis by drugs. *B Med J* 1977; 1: 1457–1459.
6. Glassock RJ. A clinical and immunopathologic dissection of rapidly progressive glomerulonephritis. *Nephron* 1978; 22: 253–264.
7. Harmer D, et al. (Correspondence). Plasmapheresis in fulminating crescentic nephritis. *Lancet* 1979; 1: 679.

8. Sieberth HG, Maurin N. The therapy of rapidly progressive glomerulonephritis. *Klin Wochenschr* 1983; 61: 1001–1010.
9. Bolton WK. Pulse methylprednisolone therapy of polyarteritis nodosa (PAN) acute crescentic rapidly progressive glomerulonephritis (AC-RPGN). *Kidney Int* 1982; 21: 145.
10. Pusey CD, Lockwood CM. Plasma exchange and immunosuppressive drugs in the management of severe glomerulonephritis. *Prog Clin Biol Res* 1982; 106: 91–104.

194. Items C, D and E correct.

Understanding of the pathogenesis of bone disease in chronic renal failure has been greatly assisted by the discovery that vitamin D is hydroxylated and activated in the kidney. After absorption from the gut or synthesis in skin, vitamin D_3 is hydroxylated in the liver to the main circulating form, 25-hydroxyvitamin D_3. This is further activated by 1-hydroxylation in the renal tubules to produce the most active vitamin D derivative — 1,25-dihydroxy D_3 Hydroxylation may occur at other positions, particularly the 24 and 26 positions. It is not yet clear whether these metabolites are inactive and represent a way of suppressing vitamin D_3 function or whether they have different actions to the major metabolite. Most vitamin D preparations, whether natural or synthetic, act largely on the gut to increase calcium absorption. There are also actions on the kidney to decrease calcium excretion and on the bone to increase calcium release, all of these actions tending to raise the extracellular calcium concentration. It has been proposed that some derivatives, particularly 24,25-dihydroxy D_3, may promote bone mineralisation, but this action is in doubt.

There are major interactions between vitamin D_3 and its metabolites and parathyroid hormone. For instance, the level of parathyroid hormone appears to determine which vitamin D_3 metabolite is produced in the kidney. In renal failure there is a complex disturbance of vitamin D_3 and parathyroid hormone function, the major components of which appear to be: failure to hydroxylate vitamin D_3 in the kidney, producing low levels of 1,25-dihydroxy D_3; low intestinal absorption of calcium leading to hypocalcaemia; raised levels of parathyroid hormone and of its breakdown products and resistance to the action of parathyroid hormone. Failure to hydroxylate vitamin D_3 may be due to direct damage to kidney tubules or to suppression of the 1-hydroxylase enzyme by hyperphosphataemia, uraemia or other stimuli. Raised levels of parathyroid hormone are probably due to hypocalcaemia brought about by failure to absorb calcium from the gut (due to deficiency of 1,25-dihydroxyvitamin D_3), to hyperphosphataemia or other factors.

These complex inter-reactions result in a very high incidence of histological bone disease in people with chronic renal failure of more than 12 months duration, although symptomatic or clinical bone disease is uncommon. The usual histological picture is one of secondary hyperparathyroidism or 'mixed bone disease', i.e. a combination of hyperparathyroidism with resorption and failure of mineralisation. In some instances a pure form of osteomalacia may be found and such patients usually have low levels of 25-hydroxyvitamin D_3, evidence of bone toxicity from trace elements (particularly aluminium), or some other factors such as hypophosphataemia.

Vitamin D is the treatment of choice in patients with bone disease who are undergoing haemodialysis. Newer forms of vitamin D, notably 1,25-dihydroxyvitamin D_3 or a synthetic analogue 1-alphahydroxyvitamin D_3, are available and have the advantage of a shorter duration of action and a lower incidence of vitamin D_3 toxicity. Dihydrotachysterol (AT 10) has similar advantages, but vitamin D_3 itself is very long-acting, being stored in fat, increases the level of 25-hydroxyvitamin D_3 and is much more prone to cause prolonged toxicity.

It is likely that all forms of vitamin D act through enhancing gastrointestinal absorption of calcium, although it is possible that there are other subtle differences between the action of the various metabolites. Patients who already have a high or normal calcium are usually less suitable for treatment with vitamin D preparations. If they have evidence of osteomalacia they are less likely to respond to vitamin D, and other contributing causes, particularly aluminium toxicity, should be considered. Patients wih hyperparathyroidism and normal or high serum calcium levels are difficult to treat with vitamin D because of the risk of hypercalcaemia and should preferably be treated with subtotal parathyroidectomy.

Reference

1. Haussler MR, McCain TA. Basic and clinical concepts related to vitamin D metabolism and action. *N Engl J Med* 1977; 297: 974–983, 1041–1050.

195. Item C correct.

The patient is likely to have idiopathic hypercalciuria due to either an enhanced calcium absorption from the gut or a renal calcium leak. In a middle-aged man in the absence of symptoms and with a normal plasma calcium level it is unnecessary to investigate for an underlying neoplasm or metabolic bone disorder.

The presence of hypercalciuria should be determined in relation to the dietary calcium. In normal subjects an increase in calcium intake from 10 to 25 mmol/day has a minimal effect on urinary calcium excretion, but in patients with idiopathic hypercalciuria it causes a marked increase. Hypercalciuria is considered to be present when daily calcium excretion exceeds 0.1 mmol/kg of body weight on a 25 mmol calcium diet.

In patients with idiopathic hypercalciuria there is a tendency to hypophosphataemia, increase in 1,25-dihydroxyvitamin D_3 synthesis and increase in intestinal calcium absorption. Three separate mechanisms have been proposed to explain the pathogenesis of idiopathic hypercalciuria: a primary intestinal hyperabsorption of calcium; a primary renal tubular loss of calcium; and subtle primary hyperparathyroidism. Differential diagnosis is based on the calcaemic responses to oral calcium and the appropriateness of the coincident parathyroid response as assessed by the levels of cyclic AMP in the urine.

	Absorptive hypercalciuria	Renal hypercalciuria	Subtle primary hyperparathyroidism
Serum calcium	Significant increase	Minimal increase	Significant increase
Nephrogenous cyclic AMP	Reduced further from subnormal	Reduced from normal	Reduced from normal

Allopurinol may decrease the rate of calcium oxalate stone formation in subjects with marginal hyperuricosuria but would not be recommended after only a single episode in a patient with normal plasma urate level.

There is sound experimental and clinical therapeutic evidence that thiazide diuretics will reduce hypercalciuria and hence reduce the tendency to form calcium stones in patients with recurrent urolithiasis.

Restriction of calcium intake is not indicated because it may lead to enhanced oxalate obsorption from the gut and increased urinary oxalate. Restriction of dietary oxalate may be marginally beneficial though most urinary oxalate is derived from metabolic sources rather than from the gut.

A high fluid intake in stone-formers is advisable both day and night. In the absence of hypercalcaemia, polyuria is unlikely to be clinically significant and would not prevent stone formation during low nocturnal urinary flow.

References

1. Broadus AE, Thier SO. Metabolic basis of renal-stone disease. *N Engl J Med* 1979; 300: 839–845.
2. Melick R. Nephrolithiasis. *Aust NZ J Med* 1979; 9: 718–721.
3. Coe FL. Hyperuricosuric calcium oxalate nephrolithiasis. *Kidney Int* 1978; 13: 418–426.
4. Yendt ER, Cohanim M. Prevention of calcium stones with thiazides. *Kidney Int* 1978; 13: 397–409.
5. Williams HE. Oxalic acid and the hyperoxaluric syndromes. *Kidney Int* 1978; 13: 410–417.
6. Coe FL, Favus MJ. Nephrolithiasis. In: Isselbacher KJ, et al (eds). Harrison's Principles of internal medicine, 9th Edn. New York: McGraw-Hill, 1980: 1349–1353.

196. Items B, D and E correct.

Idiopathic oedema is a common disorder occurring exclusively in women. It may be significant that is was described only some years after the introduction of oral diuretics. It is characterised by complaints of recurrent abdominal swelling and swelling of the face, hands, and feet.

Obesity is sometimes an associated problem and certainly, there is usually a preoccupation with weight. The diagnosis is essentially one of exclusion, and conditions such as heart failure, cirrhosis, nephrotic syndrome, allergy and local venous obstruction need to be considered. During periods of weight gain (as much as 5 kg in 24–48 hours) oliguria and sodium retention are usually noted. Mild forms of the condition may be quite common. Those which are severe enough to require investigation are usually associated with a history of taking diuretics, and sometimes other drugs, particularly laxatives. In these cases it is likely that the diuretic aggravates and perpetuates the condition by activating mechanisms for sodium retention.

Persistent use of diuretics may also lead to hypokalaemia and hyperuricaemia. In a number of cases cessation of the diuretics has been accompanied by a considerable rise in weight followed by a spontaneous diuresis and natriuresis after about a week. The retention of sodium and water in these cases was directly related to the intensity of the stimulation of the renin-angiotensin-aldosterone system by the diuretics. However, it should be noted that a number of patients stated that they had oedema prior to taking diuretics and in not all cases did weight return to normal after diuretics were stopped. In these cases an additional mechanism potentiating sodium retention appears to be present.

Patients with idiopathic oedema have been described as obsessional about their weight and appearance but it is difficult to know whether this is an important causative factor or whether it develops as a result of the tendency to oedema. Patients often attempt to control their food intake to lose weight but usually state that this is unsuccessful. It is possible that periods of sodium retention are stimulated by periods of severe voluntary restriction of carbohydrate intake.

Various explanations for idiopathic oedema have been advanced, particularly alterations in the interplay between oestrogen and progesterone and the renin-angiotensin-aldosterone system. Changes in the secretion or sensitivity to prolactin or antidiuretic hormone have also been postulated. Hypokalaemia due to diuretics may also contribute to sodium retention either directly or through stimulation of prostaglandin secretion. Correction of potassium deficiency is important, particularly when attempts are made to cease diuretic therapy.

Idiopathic oedema is difficult to treat, but a few points can be made. It it generally agreed that diuretic therapy perpetuates and may aggravate the situation by creating mild volume depletion and stimulating sodium resorption. While stopping diuretics is desirable, it is not always possible or practical. Changing to a potassium-sparing diuretic, particularly spironolactone, may improve the situation. Restriction of sodium and calorie intake should not be forgotten but is usually inadequate and not received well by the patient. Other approaches to the treatment of idiopathic oedema include the administration of bromocriptine, which reduces prolactin secretion, or captopril.

References

1. MacGregor GA, et al. Is 'idiopathic' oedema idiopathic? *Lancet* 1979; 1: 397–400.
2. Ferris TF, Bay WH. Idiopathic oedema. In: Brenner BM, Stein JH (eds). Sodium and water homeostasis. Vol 1, Contemporary issues in nephrology. New York: Churchill Livingstone, 1977; 131–153.

197. Items A and C correct.

Hypertension in renal disease is common, and often severe, causing further vascular damage to an already compromised organ. Good control of blood pressure may improve renal function in some patients and at least slow the rate of deterioration in others. Polycystic kidney disease often presents with hypertension.

In the majority of patients with renal failure hypertension is salt- or volume-dependent, although there is a disturbed relationship between ECF volume and the renin-angiotensin system. Most patients on dialysis have their blood pressure controlled by weight removal and only a few (usually those with previous accelerated hypertension) show gross elevations of plasma renin activity or angiotensin II.

Hypertension in most renal transplant recipients is due to a combination of steroids, sodium retention and chronic rejection. Stenosis of the donor renal artery or excessive renin production from the recipients own remnant kidneys are much less common causes.

References

1. Moczek WJ, et al. The value of aggressive therapy in the hypertensive patient with azotemia. *Circulation* 1969; 40: 893–904.
2. Davies DL, et al. Abnormal relation between exchangeable sodium and the renin-antiotensin system in malignant hypertension and hypertension with chronic renal failure. *Lancet* 1973; 1: 683–686.

198. Items A, D, and E correct.

Hodgkin's disease may occasionally be complicated by minimal change nephrotic syndrome. These two conditions may be linked immunologically by a disorder of cell-mediated lymphocyte function. When nephrosis complicates carcinoma or non-Hodgkin's lymphoma, the glomerular pathology is usually membranous glomerulonephritis, probably indicative of immune complex deposition, as it is in nephrosis complicating captopril treatment.

Bee-stings, lithium and non-steroidal anti-inflammatory agents such as naproxen, fenoprofen, phenylbutazone and sulindac have also been incriminated as causes of minimal change disease.

References

1. Moorthy AV, et al. Nephrotic syndrome in Hodgkin's disease; evidence for pathogenesis alternative to immune complex deposition. *Am J Med* 1976; 61: 471–477.
2. Greenstone M, et al. Acute nephrotic syndrome with reversible renal failure after phenylbutazone, *Br Med J* 1981; 282: 950–951.
3. Clive DM, Stoff JS. Renal syndromes associated with non steroidal anti-inflammatory drugs. *N Engl J Med* 1984; 210: 563–572.

199. Items B and D correct.

Idiopathic membranous glomerulonephritis accounts for about 20% of adult cases of glomerulonephritis. The place of oral steroid treatment is debatable but it is certainly not curative. An early UK trial using high doses of prednisone for 6 months or more showed no benefit and the mortality was higher in the treated group compared to controls. A recent US collaborative study using a shorter, alternate-day regimen suggested earlier remission of symptoms in the treated group, but there were insufficient data to clearly demonstrate a long-term beneficial effect on renal function. An unpublished Australian trial showed some apparent benefits in the group treated with steroids, cyclophosphamide and anticoagulants.

An underlying malignancy may be found in 10% of patients, so this is well worth looking for in a man of this age: the renal disease may be the presenting symptom. Although a membranous nephropathy is one of the pathological presentations of SLE, this diagnosis would be unlikely in an elderly man.

Microscopic haematuria is common in membranous glomerulonephritis but macroscopic haematuria would suggest either a bladder tumour or renal vein thrombosis, a particular complication of this condition.

The natural history of this condition is generally benign. 20–30% of cases may show complete or partial remission over many years and only a minority will require a dialysis/transplant programme.

References

1. Collaborative Study of the Adult Idiopathic Nephrotic Syndrome. A controlled study of short term prednisone treatment in adults with membranous nephropathy. *N Engl J Med* 1979; 301: 1301–1306.
2. Gluck MC, et al. Membranous glomerulonephritis. Evolution of clinical and pathological features. *Ann Intern Med* 1973; 78: 1–18.
3. Row PG, et al. Membranous nephropathy. Long-term follow-up and association with neoplasia. *Q J Med* 1975; 44: 207–239.

200. Items A, C and D correct.

It has been convincingly shown in many studies that blood transfusions increase the survival of subsequently performed renal allografts. This has now been demonstrated prospectively and there appears to be a graded response, i.e. the greater the number of transfusions, the better the graft survival. It would appear that all varieties of red cell preparation with the exception of frozen cells are capable of this effect; there is still some debate as to whether perioperative transfusion during transplant surgery imparts any beneficial effect or whether all the blood must be administered preoperatively. However, no study has yet shown an effect of blood transfusion on patient survival after transplantation, as opposed to graft survival.

Iron overload will accompany repeated transfusions in dialysed patients as it does in those with thalassaemia. Aluminium intoxication in dialysis patients, however, is usually the result of excessive aluminium in the water used for dialysate preparation.

Reference

1. Opelz G, et al. Induction of high kidney graft survival rate by multiple transfusion. *Lancet* 1981; 1: 1223–1225.

CW01003420

FORD

ESCORT & ORION

Sept 1980 to Sept 1990

All Ford Escort and Orion models except Van, Combi, Diesel and RS1600i models. Does **not** cover 'revised' Escort and Orion range introduced in September 1990.

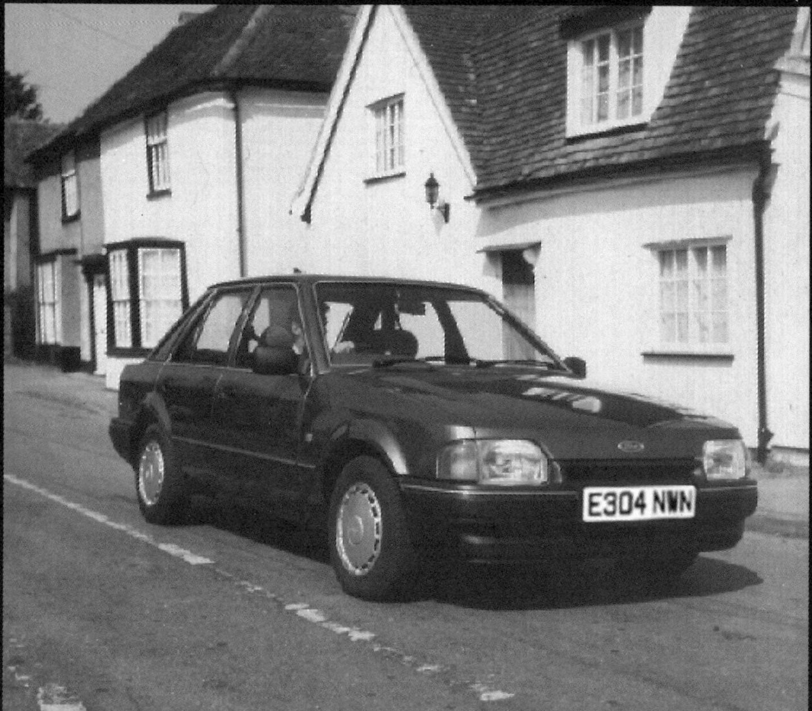

HANDBOOK & DRIVERS GUIDE

by Steve Rendle

Full details of all servicing and repair tasks for the models covered by this Handbook can be found in the relevant Owners Workshop Manual - OWM **686** for the Ford Escort and OWM **1009** for the Ford Orion.

(1812 – 1W1)

Haynes THE BOOK ®

A Haynes Handbook
and Drivers Guide
© Haynes Publishing 1994

Printed and published by
J H Haynes & Co Ltd Sparkford
Nr Yeovil Somerset BA22 7JJ
England

ISBN 1 85010 812 9

British Library Cataloguing in Publication Data. A catalogue record of this book is available from the British Library

All rights reserved. No part of this book may be reproduced or transmitted in any form or by any means, electronic or mechanical, including photocopying, recording or by any information storage or retrieval system, without permission in writing from the copyright holder

ABCDEFGHIJKLMN

ACKNOWLEDGEMENTS

We gratefully acknowledge the assistance of RoSPA in compiling the information used in this Handbook. Thanks are also due to Duckhams Oils who provided lubrication data and to Britax who supplied information on child safety. Certain illustrations, including the cover photography, are the copyright of the Ford Motor Company Limited and are used with their permission. Additional photographs were supplied by Quadrant Picture Library/Auto Express. Thanks are also due to all those people at Sparkford who helped in the production of this Handbook.

We take great pride in the accuracy of information given in this Handbook, but vehicle manufacturers make alterations and design changes during the production run of a particular vehicle of which they do not inform us. No liability can be accepted by the authors or publishers for loss, damage or injury caused by any errors in, or omissions from, the information given.

CONTENTS

ABOUT THIS HANDBOOK

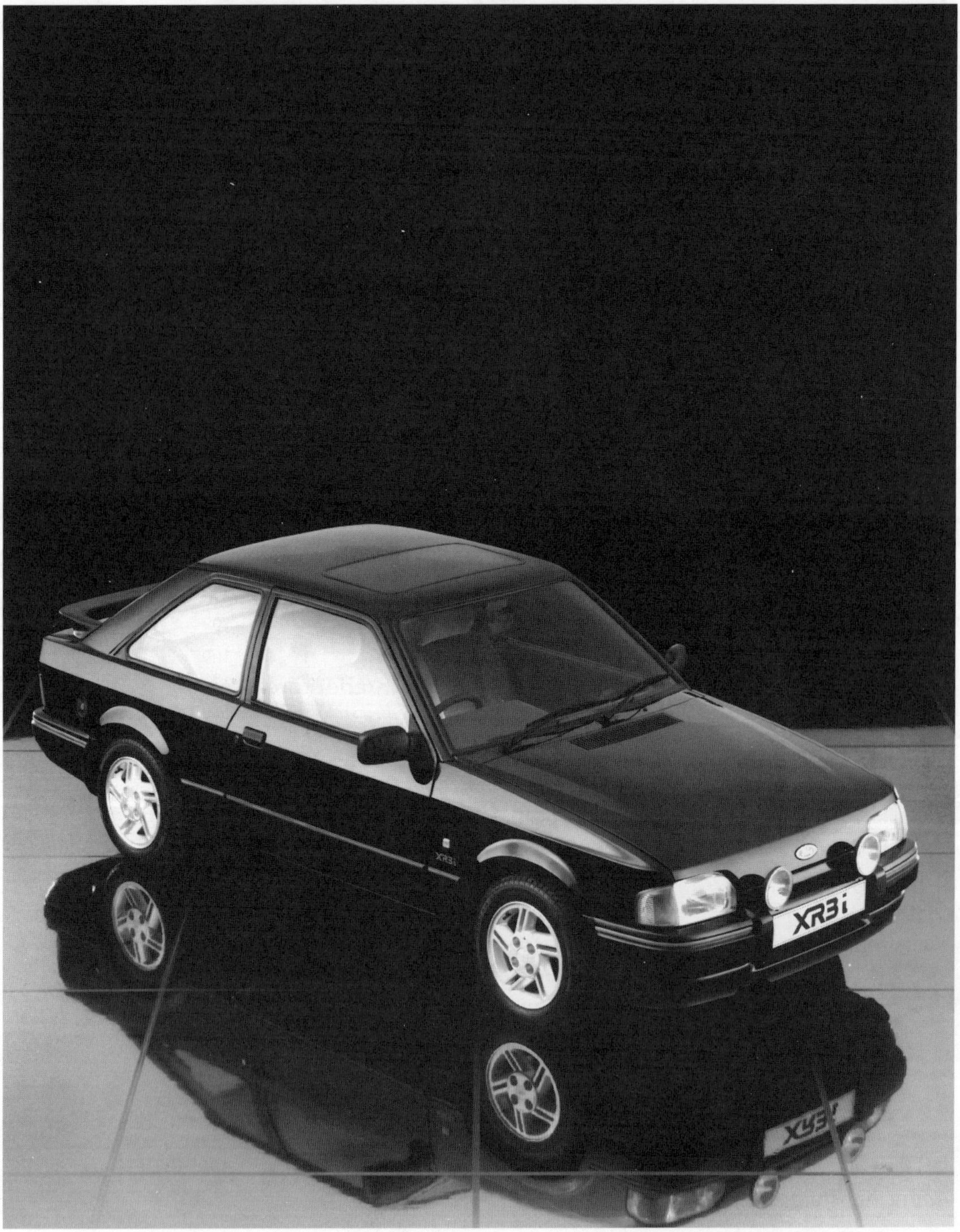

The idea behind this Handbook is to help you to get the most out of your motoring.

Apart from the things that every owner needs to know, to deal with unexpected mishaps like a puncture or a blown light bulb, you'll find clearly presented information on road safety, hints on driving abroad, and tips on how to prepare your car for the MOT test. We've also included details of local radio frequencies to help you avoid those inevitable 'jams', and there's a Section on what to do in the unfortunate event of an accident.

For those not familiar with their car, there's a Section to explain the location and the operation of the various controls and instruments. Additionally, there's a Section on fault finding, and a useful glossary of car jargon.

Garage labour charges usually form the major part of any car servicing bill, and we hope to help you to reduce those bills by carrying out the more straightforward routine servicing jobs yourself. If you're about to start carrying out your own servicing for the first time, we aim to provide you with easy-to-follow instructions, enabling you to carry out the simpler tasks which perhaps you've left to a garage or a 'car-minded' friend in the past. Even if you prefer to leave regular servicing to a suitably qualified expert, by using this book you'll be able to carry out regular checks on your car to make sure that your motoring is safe and hopefully trouble-free. You'll also find advice on buying suitable tools, and safety in the home workshop.

Some readers of this Handbook may not yet have bought an Escort or Orion, so we've included a brief history of the range, and some useful tips on buying and selling.

All in all, we hope that this book will prove a handy companion for your motoring adventures, and hopefully we'll help to reduce the problems which inevitably crop up in everyday driving. If you're bitten by the DIY bug, and you're keen to tackle some of the more advanced repair jobs on your car, then you'll need our **Owners Workshop Manual** for your particular model (OWM 686 for Escort models, or OWM 1009 for Orion models). These manuals give a step-by-step guide to all the repair and overhaul tasks, with plenty of illustrations to make things even clearer.

Happy motoring!

6 THE ESCORT/ORION FAMILY

From top to bottom:
Escort Ghia (1980)
Escort 5-door Estate (1980)
Escort Cabriolet (1984)

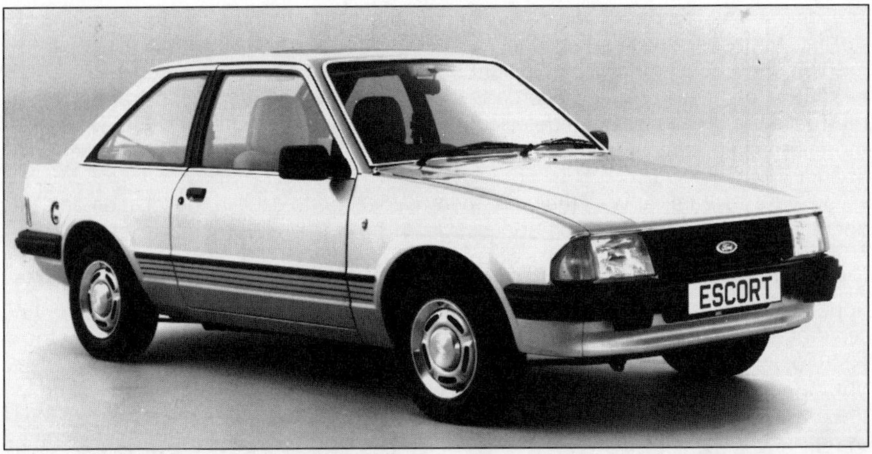

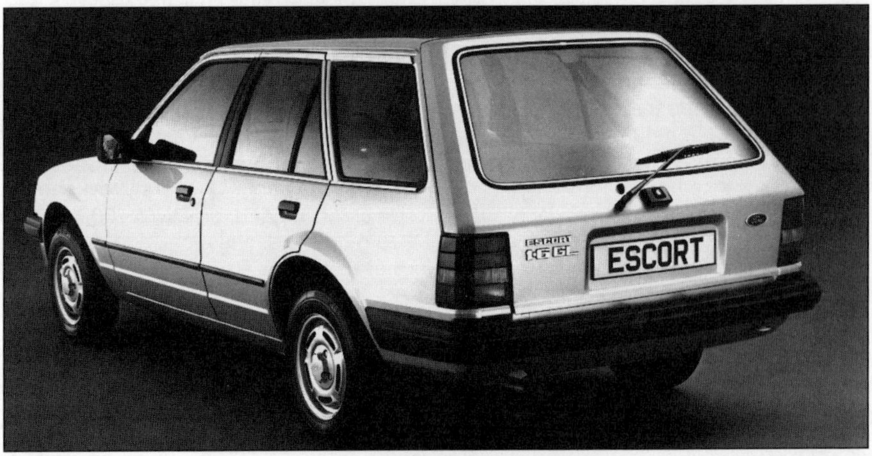

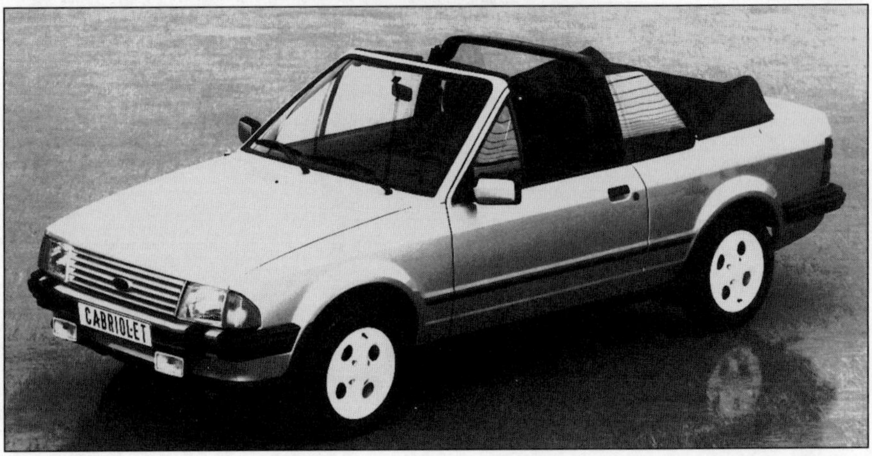

The 'MK 3' Escort was first introduced into the UK in the Autumn of 1980. The most important change made from previous Escort models, apart from the obvious difference in shape, was the change to front-wheel-drive.

To begin with, only a 3 or 5-door Hatchback bodystyle was available, but 3- & 5-door Estate versions soon followed. In 1983 the Orion 4-door Saloon and the 2-door Escort Cabriolet models were launched. In 1986, the whole range was facelifted and heavily revised to incorporate many improvements over the original design, and these later Escort models are often referred to as 'MK 4's. Models were produced with 1.1, 1.3, 1.4 & 1.6 litre engines, 4- & 5-speed manual gearboxes and 3-speed & CTX automatic transmissions, and with a number of different trim levels, from the Base Hatchback, Saloon and Estate, to the racing-inspired RS Turbo Hatchback model.

All members of the Escort/Orion family share a similar mechanical layout, and they all use the same family of engines and gearboxes, although many detailed modifications and improvements were made during the ten years of production.

Most of the mechanical components of the vehicles are fairly conventional, and the main systems are designed to keep servicing time and costs as low as possible. The electronic ignition system (not applicable to certain 1.1 litre models), clutch, brakes, wheel bearings, etc, are all routine-maintenance-free, and should only require attention when certain items need to be renewed.

All the engines are of 4-cylinder in-line layout, and are mounted transversely at the front of the car, with the gearbox positioned on the left-hand end of the engine (when viewed from the driver's seat).

A wide range of standard and optional equipment is available across the model ranges, including items such as sunroofs, electric windows, central door locking and, on certain models, anti-lock brakes.

With the wide availability of spare parts, these cars are ideal for the enthusiastic amateur mechanic, who wants to keep running costs to a minimum.

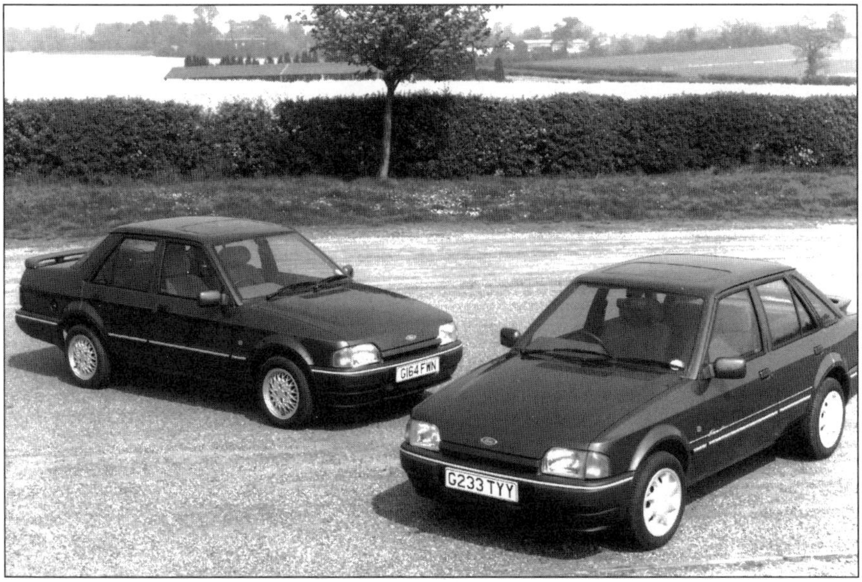

▲ *Escort Eclipse and Orion Equipe (1989)*

THE ESCORT/ORION FAMILY

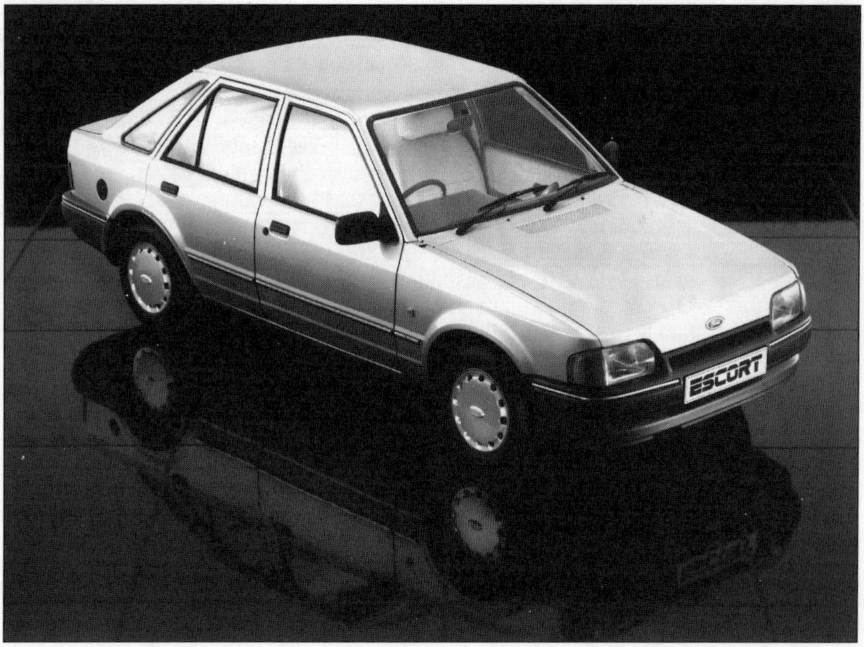

▲ *Escort L (1986)*

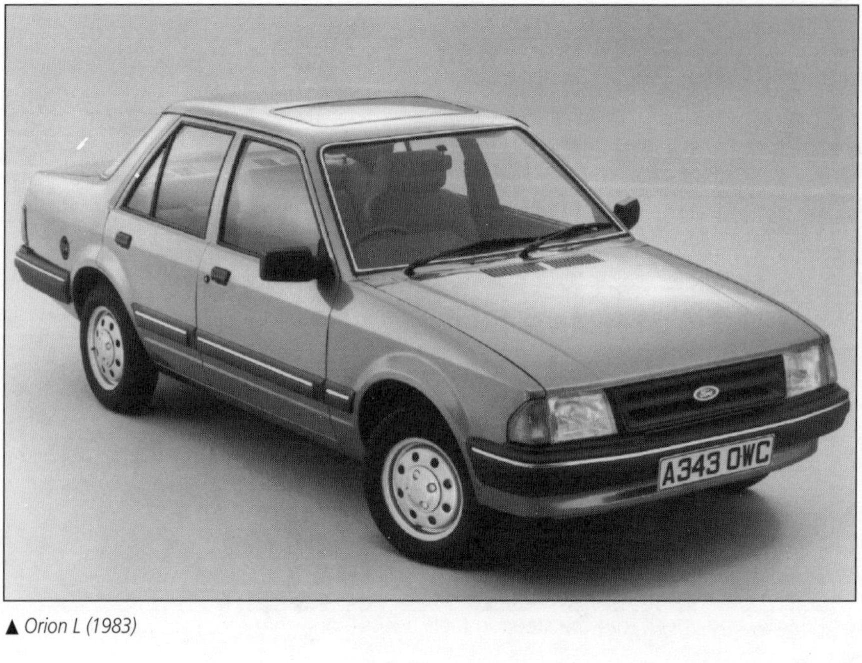

▲ *Orion L (1983)*

GENERAL TIPS ON BUYING

- **Don't rush out and buy the first car to catch your attention**
- **Always buy from a recognised dealer in preference to buying privately**
- **Have the car checked over by someone knowledgeable before you buy it**
- **In general, you get what you pay for!**

Before buying a second-hand car, it's worthwhile doing some homework to try and avoid some of the pitfalls waiting for the unwary. First of all, don't rush out and buy the first car to catch your attention (all that glitters is not gold!), and remember that much of the responsibility is yours when it comes to the soundness of the deal, especially when buying a car privately.

Wherever possible, buy from a recognised dealer, and check that the dealer is a member of the Retail Motor Industry Federation, as this will provide you with certain legal safeguards if you have any problems. If you buy from a dealer, you are covered by the Sale Of Goods Act, which in summary states that the goods must be fit for their intended purpose, the goods must be of proper quality, and the goods must be as described by the seller. If you're buying a car privately, ask to see the service receipts and the MOT certificates going back as long as the car has been in the possession of the current owner (this will help to establish that the car hasn't been stolen, and that the recorded mileage is genuine), and always ask to view the car at the seller's private address (to make sure that the car isn't being sold by an unscrupulous dealer posing as a private seller). Check the vehicle documents for obvious signs of forgery and, if in doubt, contact the DVLA and give them details of the Registration Document, as they will be able to run a check on its authenticity.

As far as the soundness of the car itself is concerned, a genuine service history is helpful. This is provided by the service book supplied with the car when new, which should be completed and officially stamped by an authorised garage after each service. Cars with a full service history (fsh) usually command a higher price than those without.

To check the condition of a car, a professional examination is well worthwhile, if you can afford it, and organisations such as the AA and RAC will be able to provide such a service. Otherwise, you must trust your own judgement, and/or that of a knowledgeable friend. Although it's tempting, try not to overlook the mechanical soundness of the car in favour of the overall appearance. It's relatively easy to clean and polish a car every week, but when were the brakes and tyres last checked? Above all, safety must always take priority. Don't view a car in the wet, as water on the bodywork can give a misleading impression of the condition of the paintwork. First of all, check around the outside of the car for rust, and for obvious signs of new or mis-matched paintwork which might show that the car has been involved in an accident. Check the tyres for signs of unusual wear or damage, and check that the car 'sits' evenly on its suspension, with all four corners at a similar height. Open the bonnet and check for any obvious signs of fluid leakage (oil, water, brake fluid), then start the engine and listen for any unusual noises – some background noise is to be expected on older cars, but there should be no sinister rattles or bangs! Also listen to the exhaust to make sure that it isn't 'blowing' indicating the need for renewal, and check for signs of excessive exhaust smoke. Black smoke may be caused by poorly adjusted fuel mixture, which can usually be rectified fairly easily, but blue smoke usually indicates worn engine components, which may prove expensive to repair. Finally, drive the car, and test the brakes, steering and gearbox. Make sure that the car doesn't pull to one side, and check that the steering feels positive and that the gears can be selected satisfactorily without undue harshness or noise. Listen for any unusual noises or vibration, and keep an eye on the instruments and warning lights to make sure that they are working and indicating correctly.

If all proves satisfactory, try to negotiate a suitable deal, but remember that a dealer has to work to a profit margin, and it's unlikely that you'll find a good car for a silly price. Always obtain a receipt for your money.

On the whole, it's true to say that you get what you pay for. Above all, don't be rushed into making a hasty decision.

POINTS TO LOOK FOR WHEN BUYING AN ESCORT/ORION

In addition to the points outlined previously, there are a few special points to look for when buying an Escort or Orion.

In general, the later models built from 1986 onwards, are an all-round improvement on the earlier models, and will prove a better buy if your budget allows.

Corrosion is not usually a problem on Escorts and Orions, but there are a few areas which are prone to trouble. Firstly, check for stone chips on the bonnet, on the front valance (beneath the front bumper), and on the sill panels (under the doors) which can cause unsightly surface rust. Open the bonnet and check the inside surfaces of the front wings either side of the engine compartment. If rust is evident, it's best to reject the car, as in the worst cases welding will be required to cure the problem. Another source of trouble is the area around the battery tray (particularly underneath) which is prone to corrosion due to battery acid being washed over the metal by rain water.

On models with plastic bumpers, check for any signs of damage or cracks, as these components are expensive to renew.

CVH type engines (1.3 litre up to 1986, and all 1.4 & 1.6 litre models), are prone to problems with a build-up of black sludge inside the engine if regular oil changes are not carried out. To check for this, remove the oil filler cap from the top of the engine and run a finger around the inside of the hole. If sludge is present, reject the car. Another point to note for CVH engines is that the camshaft drivebelt should be renewed after 36 000 miles. If you're not sure whether this has been done, it's sensible to have the necessary work carried out as soon as you buy the car, as if the drivebelt breaks in service, very serious and expensive engine damage can occur.

On early models, an automatic choke may be fitted, which can prove troublesome, causing poor starting and excessive fuel consumption. Later models have manual chokes.

Other possible problem areas are the contact breaker type distributor on early models which is prone to failure, and the self-adjusting clutch mechanism (fitted to all models) which can cause problems when the components wear.

Escorts and Orions are plentiful on the secondhand market, and it shouldn't be difficult to find a good car which will give trouble-free service.

GENERAL TIPS ON SELLING

- **Make sure that the car is clean and tidy**
- **Make sure that all of the service documents, registration document etc, are available for inspection**
- **Ask yourself ... 'Would I buy this car?'**

Obviously when selling a car, bear in mind the points which the prospective buyer should be looking for, as described in the above sections. It goes without saying that the car should be clean and tidy, as first impressions are important. Any fluid leaks should be cured, and there's no point in trying to disguise any major bodywork or mechanical problems.

If you're trading the car in with a dealer, you will always get a lower price than if you sell privately, but you can be fairly sure that there will be less comeback to you should any unexpected problems develop. If selling privately, don't allow the buyer to take the car away until you have his/her money, and it's a good idea to ask him/her to sign a piece of paper to say that he/she is happy to buy the car as viewed, just in case any problems develop later on. Give a receipt for the money paid.

Note: *All figures are approximate, and will vary depending on model*

DIMENSIONS [mm (in)]

Overall length

Escort Hatchback and Cabriolet models	**4040** to **4070** (159.2 to 160.4)
Escort Estate models	**4100** to **4140** (161.5 to 163.1)
Orion models	**4220** to **4240** (166.3 to 167.1)

Overall width

All models	**1640** to **1750** (64.6 to 69.0)

Overall height

All models	**1380** to **1410** (54.4 to 55.6)

WEIGHTS [kg (lb)]

Nominal kerb weight

Escort Hatchback models	**855** to **980** (1885 to 2161)
Escort Cabriolet models	**930** to **995** (2051 to 2194)
Escort Estate models	**885** to **965** (1951 to 2129)
Orion models	**895** to **945** (1973 to 2084)

Maximum roof rack load

All models	**75** (165)

Maximum towing weight (for trailer or caravan)

All except 1.1 litre models	**900** (1980)
1.1 litre models	**540** (1188)

Maximum trailer/caravan noseweight

All models	**50** (110)

12 CONTROLS AND EQUIPMENT

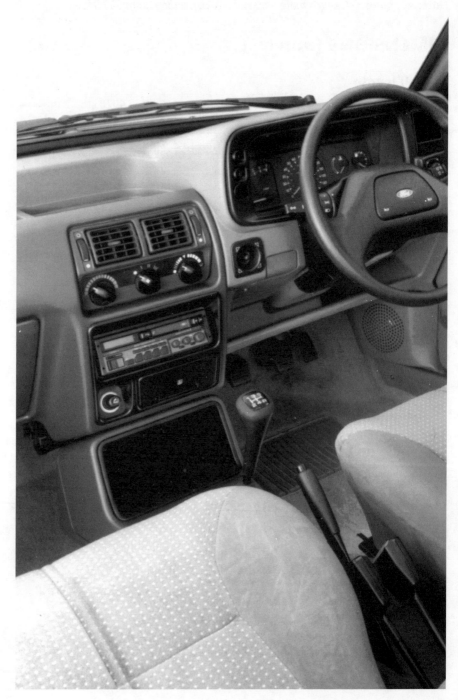

For those not familiar with the Escort/Orion models, this Section will help to identify the instruments and controls. Typical instrument panel layouts are shown in the accompanying illustrations. The operation of most equipment is self-explanatory, but some items require further explanation to ensure that their use is fully understood.

Note that not all items are fitted to all models.

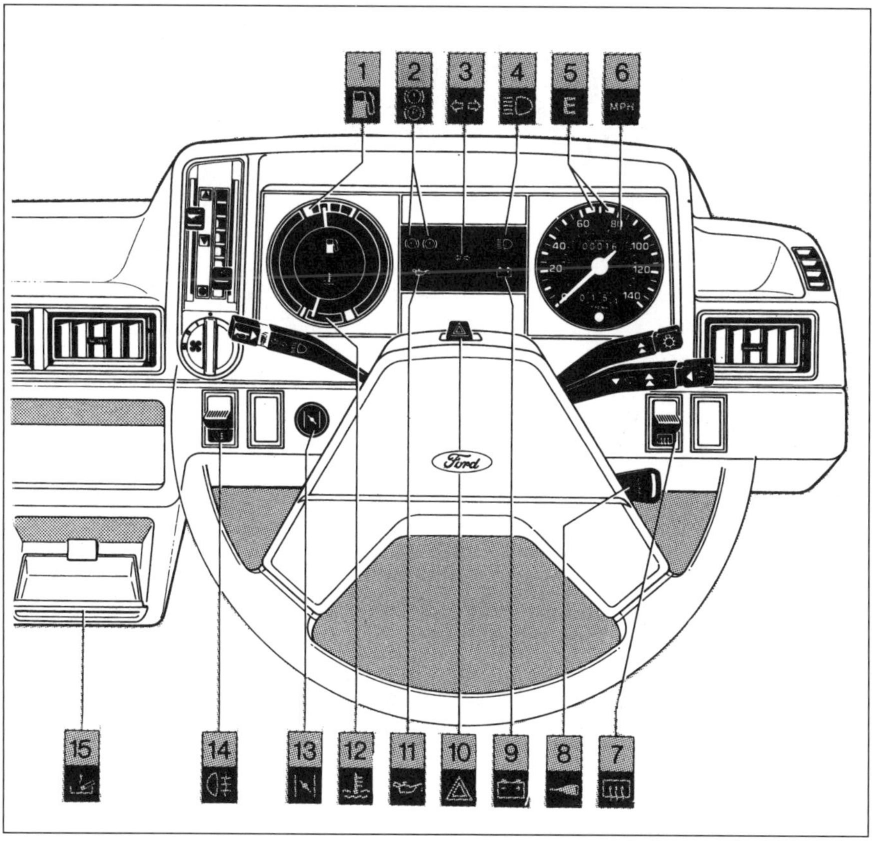

▲ *Typical instrument panel layout for 'low series' Escort models up to 1986*

1. *Fuel gauge*
2. *Handbrake on/low brake fluid level warning light*
3. *Direction indicator warning light*
4. *Headlight main beam warning light*
5. *Econolights*
6. *Speedometer*
7. *Heated rear window switch*
8. *Ignition switch/steering lock*
9. *Ignition warning light*
10. *Hazard flasher switch*
11. *Low oil pressure warning light*
12. *Temperature gauge*
13. *Choke control*
14. *Rear foglight switch*
15. *Ashtray*

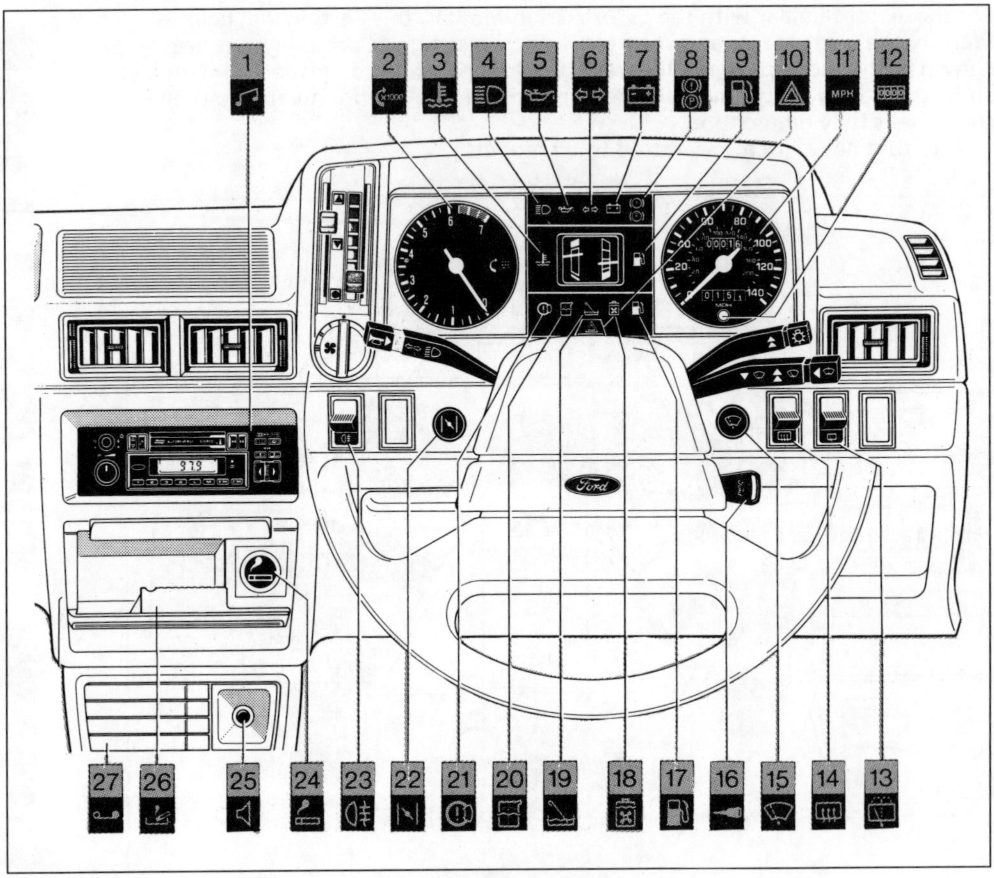

▲ *Typical instrument panel layout for 'high series' Escort models up to 1986*

1 *Radio*
2 *Tachometer*
3 *Temperature gauge*
4 *Headlight main beam warning light*
5 *Low oil pressure warning light*
6 *Direction indicator warning light*
7 *Ignition warning light*
8 *Handbrake on/low brake fluid level warning light*
9 *Fuel gauge*
10 *Hazard flasher switch*
11 *Speedometer*
12 *Trip meter reset button*
13 *Tailgate wash/wipe switch*
14 *Heated rear window switch*
15 *Variable intermittent wipe control*
16 *Ignition switch/steering lock*
17 *Low fuel level warning light*
18 *Low coolant level warning light*
19 *Low oil level warning light*
20 *Low washer fluid level warning light*
21 *Brake pad wear warning light*
22 *Choke control*
23 *Rear foglight switch*
24 *Cigarette lighter*
25 *Loudspeaker balance control*
26 *Ashtray*
27 *Cassette stowage compartment*

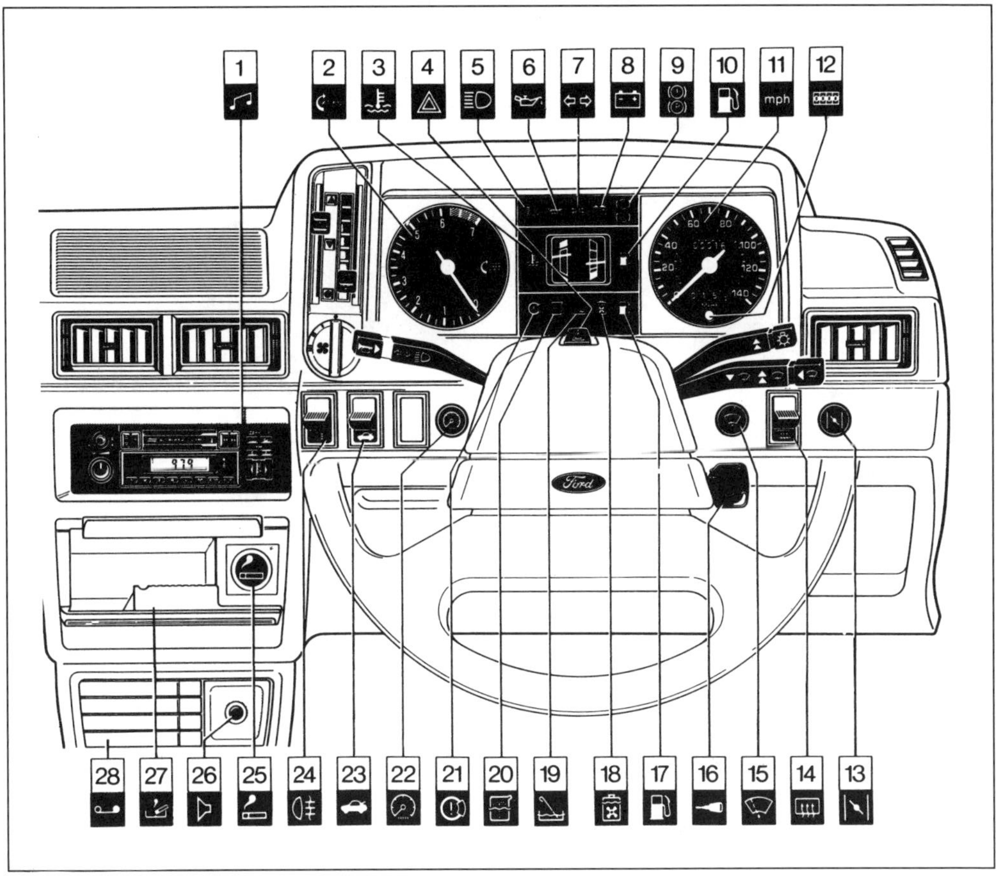

▲ *Typical instrument panel layout for 'high series' Orion models up to 1986*

1 *Radio*
2 *Tachometer*
3 *Temperature gauge*
4 *Hazard flasher switch*
5 *Headlight main beam warning light*
6 *Low oil pressure warning light*
7 *Direction indicator warning light*
8 *Ignition warning light*
9 *Handbrake on/low brake fluid level warning light*
10 *Fuel gauge*
11 *Speedometer*
12 *Trip meter reset button*
13 *Choke control*
14 *Heated rear window switch*
15 *Variable intermittent wipe control*
16 *Ignition switch/steering lock*
17 *Low fuel level warning light*
18 *Low coolant level warning light*
19 *Low oil level warning light*
20 *Low washer fluid level warning light*
21 *Brake pad wear warning light*
22 *Instrument illumination control*
23 *Remote boot release*
24 *Rear foglight switch*
25 *Cigarette lighter*
26 *Loudspeaker balance control*
27 *Ashtray*
28 *Cassette stowage compartment*

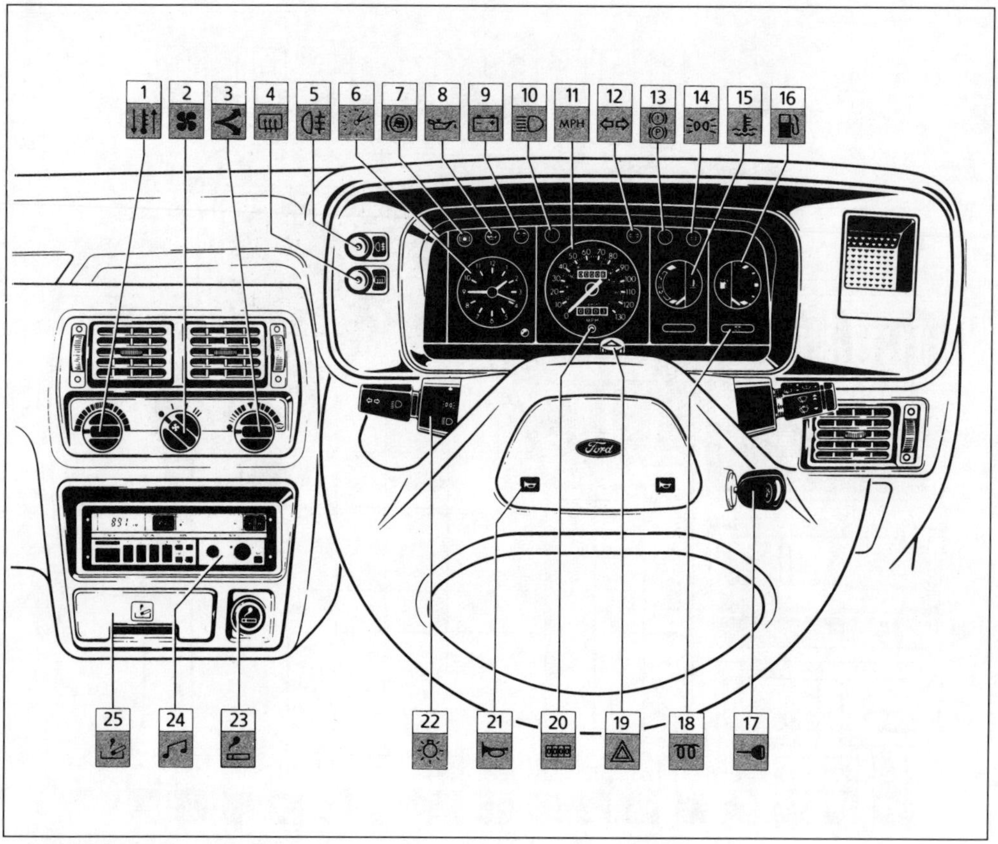

▲ *Typical instrument panel for 'low series' Escort/Orion models from 1986*

1 *Air temperature control*
2 *Booster fan switch*
3 *Air distribution control*
4 *Heated rear window switch*
5 *Rear foglight switch*
6 *Clock*
7 *ABS warning light*
8 *Low oil pressure warning light*
9 *Ignition warning light*
10 *Headlight main beam warning light*
11 *Speedometer*
12 *Direction indicator warning light*
13 *Handbrake on/low brake fluid level warning light*
14 *Sidelight/tail light warning light*
15 *Temperature gauge*
16 *Fuel gauge*
17 *Ignition switch/steering lock*
18 *Glow plug warning light (Diesel models only)*
19 *Hazard flasher switch*
20 *Trip meter reset button*
21 *Horn pad*
22 *Multi-function switch*
23 *Cigarette lighter*
24 *Radio*
25 *Ashtray*

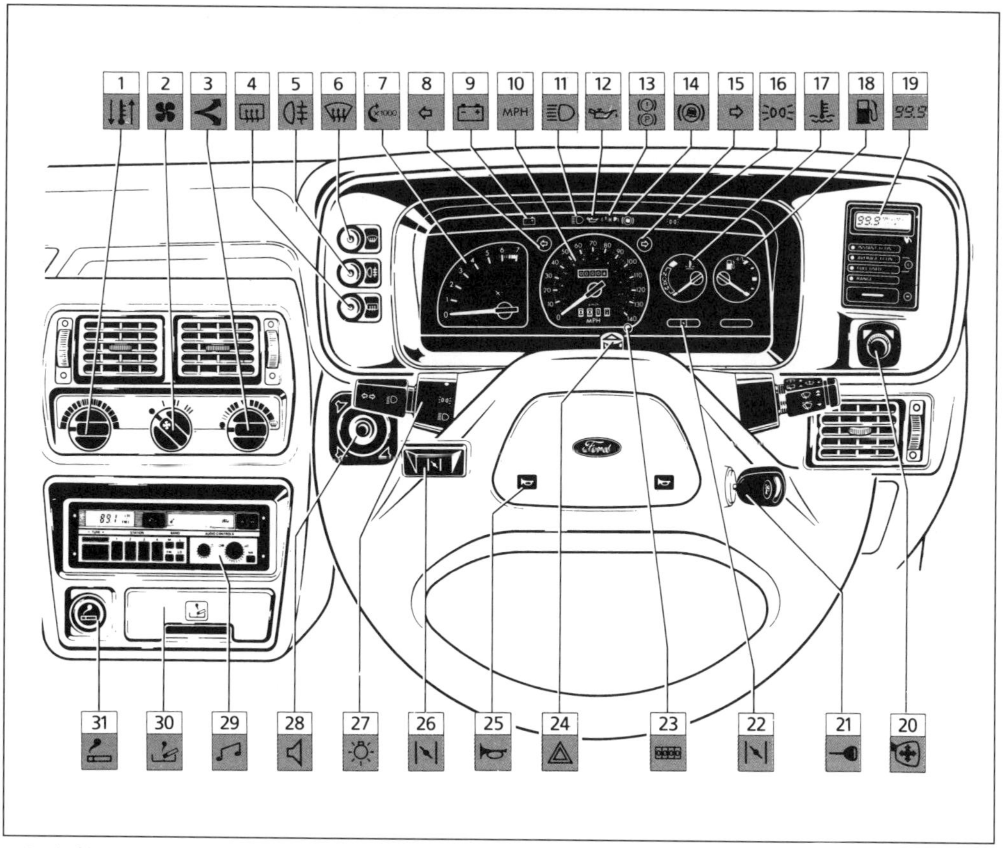

▲ *Typical instrument panel layout for 'high series' Escort/Orion models from 1986*

1 *Air temperature control*
2 *Booster fan switch*
3 *Air distribution control*
4 *Heated rear window switch*
5 *Rear foglight switch*
6 *Heated windscreen switch*
7 *Tachometer*
8 *Direction indicator warning light (left)*
9 *Ignition warning light*
10 *Speedometer*
11 *Headlight main beam warning light*
12 *Low oil pressure warning light*
13 *Handbrake on/low brake fluid level warning light*
14 *ABS warning light*
15 *Direction indicator warning light (right)*
16 *Sidelight/tail light warning light*
17 *Temperature gauge*
18 *Fuel gauge*
19 *Fuel computer*
20 *Electric door mirror switch*
21 *Ignition switch/steering lock*
22 *Manual choke warning light*
23 *Trip meter reset button*
24 *Hazard flasher switch*
25 *Horn push*
26 *Choke control*
27 *Multi-function switch*
28 *Loudspeaker balance control*
29 *Radio*
30 *Ashtray*
31 *Cigarette lighter*

DRIVER'S INSTRUMENTS AND CONTROLS

Speedometer

Indicates the car's road speed, and incorporates a mileage recorder. Some models have a trip meter, which can be reset by pressing the button protruding from the instrument.

Tachometer ('Rev Counter')

Indicates engine speed in revolutions per minute (rpm or rev/min). For normal driving and the best fuel economy the engine speed should be kept in the 2000 to 4000 rpm range. The red band indicates the maximum permissible engine speed.

Fuel gauge

Indicates the quantity of fuel remaining in the tank. When the needle enters the red band, there are approximately 8 litres (1.8 gallons) of fuel remaining.

Temperature gauge

Indicates the engine coolant temperature. As the engine warms up, the needle should move from the blue (cold) end of the scale into the middle region. If the needle remains in the blue section, or enters the red (hot) section, a fault is indicated and advice should be sought (refer to *'Fault finding'* on page 124).

Do not continue to run an engine which shows signs of overheating.

Clock

Apart from the analogue type, three digital types have been used:

ANALOGUE TYPE

To adjust the time, push in the button and turn it.

DIGITAL TYPE

To adjust the time, switch on the ignition. Press the button on the left to change the hour setting, and press the button on the right to change the minutes setting. To synchronise the clock with an exact time signal, press and hold both buttons, then release the buttons at the time signal, and set the time as described previously.

MULTI-FUNCTION DIGITAL TYPE (EARLY MODELS)

The clock can display the date, and has a timer feature. To operate the clock, the ignition must be switched on.

Adjusting time

To change the hours setting, press the upper recessed button **(F)** once, using a pointed instrument such as a ballpoint pen. The display will show the hour number on the left, and either 'A' for am or 'P' for pm on the right. The hour number will increase by one each time the button is pressed again. Four seconds after the button is last pressed, the display will show normal time, but with the newly selected hour number.

To change the minutes setting, press the lower recessed button **(G)** once. The display will still show normal time, but the clock will have stopped, and the minute number will increase by one each time the button is pressed again. To restart the clock after setting the time, press the **stop/start** button **(C)**. If the clock is set slightly ahead of actual time, it can be synchronised with a time signal by pressing the **stop/start** button on the signal.

Date display

To display the date, press the **select** button **(A)** once. The date will be displayed for four seconds, after which the time will reappear.

Adjusting date

To set the date, obtain the date display as described previously. To set the day, immediately press the top recessed button **(F)** once. The date will increase by one each time the button **(F)** is pressed. To set the month, press the bottom recessed button **(G)** immediately after obtaining the date display. The month number will increase by one each time button **(G)** is pressed. Four seconds after either recessed button is released, the display will show normal time.

Timer

To operate the timer, with the display showing the time, press the **select** button **(A)** twice. The timer can now be started by pressing the **stop/start** button **(C)**. Pressing the **stop/start**

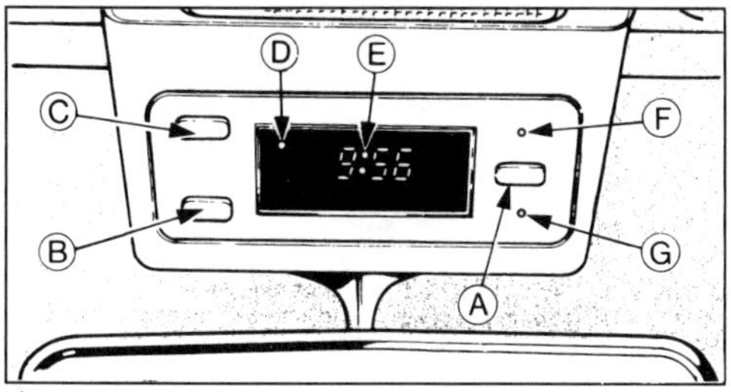

▲ *Multi-function digital clock*
A *Select button*
B *Reset button*
C *Stop/start button*
D *Timer symbol*
E *Colon*
F & G *Recessed adjustment button (early models only)*

button again will stop the timer and freeze the display. A third press will restart the timer from where it stopped. The timer will count to 59 minutes 59 seconds, and then roll over to 1 hour 00 minutes and continue to count at one minute intervals. When the timer reaches 59 hours 59 minutes, it automatically resets to 0 and continues counting.

Either of the two other displays can be selected when the timer is working. To display the time, press the **select** button once, and to display the date, press the **select** button again. To reset the timer to zero with the clock showing time, press the **select** button twice to display the timer, then to zero the timer press the **reset** button **(B)**. The display can now be set to show the normal time by pressing the **select** button, or the timer can be restarted by pressing the **stop/start** button. The recorded time, when the timer was stopped, will be stored in the memory until the timer is restarted again, even if the ignition is switched off. If the ignition is switched off when the timer is still running, it will continue to count until the ignition is switched on again and the timer is stopped or reset; the timer can therefore be used to record actual journey time.

MULTI-FUNCTION DIGITAL TYPE (LATER MODELS)

The clock can display the date, and has a timer feature. No display is shown with the ignition switched off, but the display can be recalled for 4 seconds by pressing the **select** button **(A)**. One press will display time, and further presses will display the date and timer. The ignition must be switched on to carry out all setting and adjustments.

Adjusting time and date

The time and date must be set using the following sequence. With the display showing the time, press the **reset** button **(B)** once. The display should flash showing '12H' or '24H' depending on whether the display has been set to the 12 or 24 hour format. Press the **stop/start** button **(C)** to change the format. Press the **reset** button again. The hour number on the left will flash. If the 24 hour format was selected, the minute number on the right will remain stationary, but if the 12 hour format was selected, an 'A' for am or 'P' for pm will appear in place of the minutes. Press the **stop/start** button to increase the hour number as required. Press the **reset** button again. The minute number on the right of the display will now flash. Press the **stop/start** button to increase the minute number. Press the **reset** button again. The date will now be displayed, with the day number flashing on the left, and the month number stationary on the right. Press the **stop/start** button to increase the day number. Press the **reset** button again. The display now shows the date with the day stationary on the left, and the month number flashing on the right. Press the **stop/start** button to increase the month number. When the adjustments are complete, press the **reset** button to return to the time display. To return to the time display at any point during the procedure, press the **select** button.

Date display

To display the date, press the **select** button **(A)** once. The date will be displayed for four seconds, after which the time will reappear.

Timer

The operation of the timer is the same as described for the earlier type of multi-function clock.

Fuel computer

Provides information on fuel level, distance and economy. There is also an audible warning to indicate low fuel level. The computer is controlled by three pushbuttons, and a tone will sound to indicate that a button has been pressed. The **function** button **(E)** is used to switch between the four functions of the computer, and indicator lights show which function has been selected.

INSTANT ECONOMY

Shows the instantaneous fuel consumption, and this figure will change rapidly as driving conditions change during acceleration, braking, etc.

AVERAGE ECONOMY

Shows the average fuel consumption since the function was last reset.

FUEL USED

Shows the quantity of fuel used since the function was last reset.

RANGE

Gives an estimate of the distance the car will travel on the fuel remaining in the tank. To remind the driver that the fuel level is low, an audible warning will sound when the range decreases to 50, 25 and 10 miles (80, 40 and 20 km) respectively. To stop the warning, any of the three buttons can be pressed, but in any case, the warning will stop automatically after sounding five times. Approximately 5 litres (1 gallon) of fuel are left in the tank when the range indicates 0. The computer will automatically calculate a new range when more than 9 litres (2 gallons) of fuel are added to the tank.

When the ignition is switched on, the computer shows the last selected display as long as the range is not less than 50 miles (80 km), in which case the audible warning will sound and the range will be displayed to remind the driver that the fuel level is low. Pressing the **clear** button **(G)** while in the 'Fuel Used' function sets the value to 0. Pressing the **clear** button while in the 'Average Economy' function sets the value to the current 'Instant Economy' value. Pressing the **mode** button **(F)** changes the units displayed from metric to imperial, and vice versa.

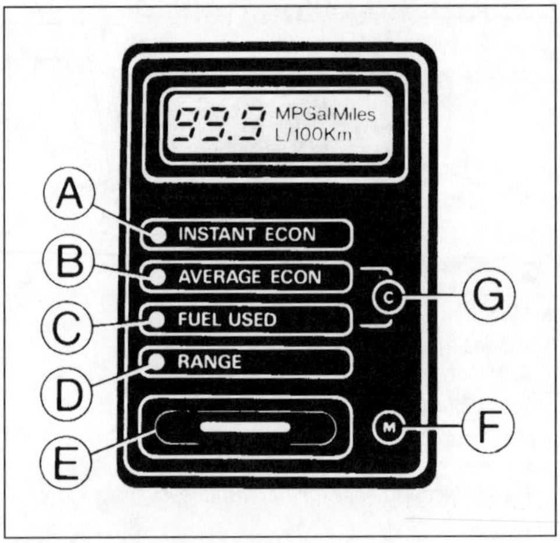

▲ *Fuel computer*
A *Instant Economy indicator*
B *Average Economy indicator*
C *Fuel Used indicator*
D *Range indicator*
E *Function button*
F *Mode button*
G *Clear button*

Warning lights

These lights warn the driver of a fault, or inform the driver that a particular device is in operation.

HANDBRAKE ON/LOW BRAKE FLUID LEVEL WARNING LIGHT

Warns that the handbrake is applied, or the brake fluid level is low. If the light comes on whilst driving, and the handbrake is fully released, stop immediately and check the brake fluid level (refer to *'Regular checks'* on page 72).

Do not continue to drive the car if a brake fluid leak is suspected.

LOW OIL PRESSURE WARNING LIGHT

Warns that the engine oil pressure is low. If the light stays on for more than a few seconds after start-up, it's likely that the engine is worn and advice should be sought. If the light comes on whilst driving, switch off the engine immediately and seek advice.

IGNITION WARNING LIGHT

Acts as a reminder that the ignition circuit is switched on if the engine isn't running, and acts as a no-charge warning light. If the light stays on after starting, or comes on whilst driving, the battery is not charging properly. The battery may therefore become fully discharged (resulting in a 'flat' battery), and the best course of action is to stop and seek advice.

MANUAL CHOKE WARNING LIGHT

Acts as a reminder that the choke is in operation. The light will go out when the choke control is pushed in.

HEADLIGHT MAIN BEAM WARNING LIGHT

Acts as a reminder that the headlight main beam is switched on.

SIDELIGHT/TAIL LIGHT WARNING LIGHT

Acts as a reminder that the side lights and tail lights are switched on.

DIRECTION INDICATOR WARNING LIGHT(S)

Show(s) that the direction indicators are switched on.

ABS (ANTI-LOCK BRAKING SYSTEM) WARNING LIGHT

This light should come on when the ignition is switched on and the handbrake is applied. If the light stays on when the handbrake is released, or comes on whilst driving, there is a fault in one of the ABS circuits. Normal braking will still be available, but the braking system should be checked by a Ford dealer as soon as possible.

ECONOLIGHTS

These lights provide a rough indication as to how economically the car is being driven. As a guide, aim to drive so that the lights come on only momentarily, or not at all. The amber light will come on when the car is being driven less economically, and the red light will come on when the car is being driven uneconomically. In practice, it will be very difficult to drive without causing the lights to come on at some stage, especially when accelerating.

Auxiliary warning system

Consists of five lights which are connected to sensors to monitor various fluid levels and front brake pad wear. When the ignition is first switched on, the auxiliary warning lights will all come on for approximately 5 seconds. Check that the lights all go out before starting the engine. The function of each individual light is as follows.

BRAKE PAD WEAR WARNING LIGHT

Indicates that the front brake pads are worn to the stage where they require renewal. If the light comes on, the pads should be renewed as soon as possible.

LOW OIL LEVEL WARNING LIGHT

Indicates that the oil level has reached the 'MIN' mark on the dipstick. If the light comes on, the oil level should be topped up as soon as possible (refer to *'Regular checks'* on page 70). Note that the oil level check only works during initial start-up, and does not work with the engine running.

LOW COOLANT LEVEL WARNING LIGHT

Indicates that the coolant level has reached the 'MIN' mark on the reservoir. If the light comes on, the coolant level should be topped up as soon as possible (refer to *'Regular checks'* on page 71).

LOW FUEL LEVEL WARNING LIGHT

Comes on when there are approximately 8 litres (1.8 gallons) of fuel left in the tank.

LOW WASHER FLUID LEVEL WARNING LIGHT

Indicates that the windscreen washer fluid reservoir is below quarter full.

Ignition switch/steering lock

The switch has four positions as follows:

- **O** Ignition off, steering locked
- **I** Ignition off, accessory circuits on, steering unlocked
- **II** Ignition on, and all electrical circuits on
- **III** Starter motor operates (release the key immediately the engine starts)

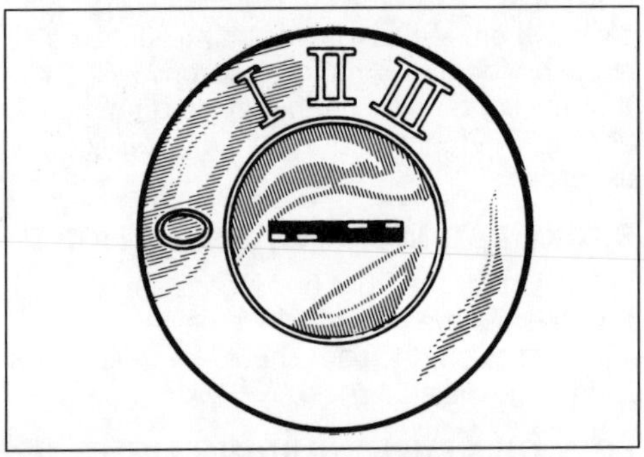

▲ *Ignition switch/steering lock key positions*

Choke

The choke control should be pulled out as necessary to start a cold engine, and should be gradually pushed in as the engine warms up, until the car can be driven smoothly with no choke. Note that some models have an automatic choke.

Gearbox

MANUAL GEARBOX

Either a 4- or 5-speed gearbox may be fitted. The gear positions follow the usual 'H' pattern, but the method of selecting reverse gear varies depending on model:

4-speed gearbox

On earlier gearboxes, reverse gear is positioned to the left of 1st gear. Reverse is selected by moving the lever fully left from the neutral position, then pressing down against spring pressure and pushing forwards.

On later gearboxes, reverse gear is positioned to the left of 1st gear. Reverse is selected by moving the lever fully left from the neutral position, then pressing down against spring pressure, and then pushing further left and forwards.

5-speed gearbox

On earlier gearboxes, reverse gear is positioned opposite 5th gear. Reverse is selected by moving the lever fully right from the neutral position, then pushing down against spring pressure and pulling rearwards.

On later gearboxes, reverse gear is positioned opposite 5th gear. Reverse is selected by moving the lever fully right from the neutral position against spring pressure before pulling rearwards.

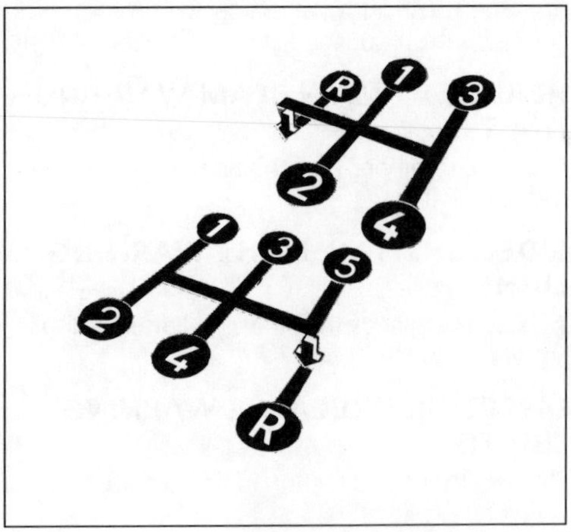

▲ *Gear lever positions (early manual gearboxes)*

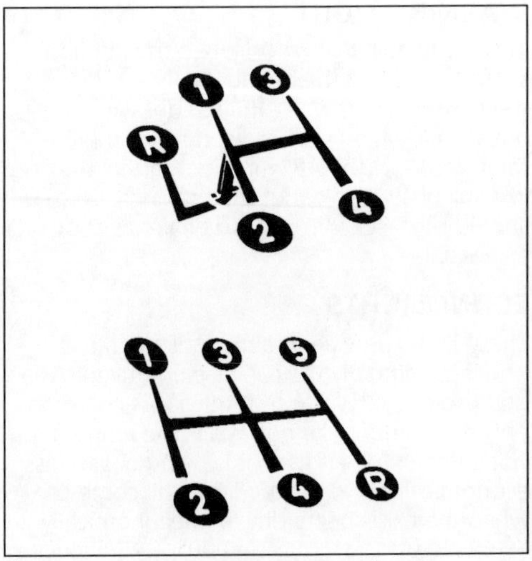

▲ *Gear lever positions (later manual gearboxes)*

CONVENTIONAL AUTOMATIC TRANSMISSION

There are 6 selector positions:

P – locks the transmission and should be used when parking. The engine can be started. Only select **P** after parking when the car is stationary, and always apply the handbrake.

R – selects **Reverse** gear.

N – selects **Neutral**. The engine can be started. No power is transmitted to the wheels.

D – selects **Drive**. The transmission will change gear automatically using 1st, 2nd and 3rd gears.

2 – allows the transmission to change automatically between 1st and 2nd gears only. Useful when driving up or down hills, or when driving through a series of bends. It will also reduce wheelspin when moving away in slippery conditions.

1 – locks the transmission in 1st gear. It should only be used when driving up or down extremely steep slopes.

The handbrake or footbrake must be applied before selecting **R**, **D**, **2** or **1**, when the car is stationary. Don't select positions **1** or **2** at speeds of more than 60 mph (97 km/h). To select positions **R** and **P**, the selector lever must first be pushed down in the **N** position. The lever must also be pushed down to move it out of the **P** position. To move out of the other positions, the selector lever must be moved sideways first.

CTX AUTOMATIC TRANSMISSION

There are 5 selector positions:

P, R and **N** – have the same functions as described for the conventional automatic transmission.

D – selects **Drive**. The transmission will infinitely vary the gear ratio between the lowest and highest available.

L – gives increased engine braking. Should be used when driving up or down steep slopes.

The handbrake or footbrake must be applied before selecting **R**, **D**, or **L** when the car is stationary. To select positions **R** and **P**, the selector lever must first be pushed down in the **N** position. The lever must also be pushed down to move it out of the **P** position. To move out of the other positions, the selector lever must be moved sideways first.

Multi-function switch (models up to 1986)

Controls the direction indicators, headlight flash & main beam, and horn. On models fitted with driving lights, these operate with the headlight main beam and headlight flash.

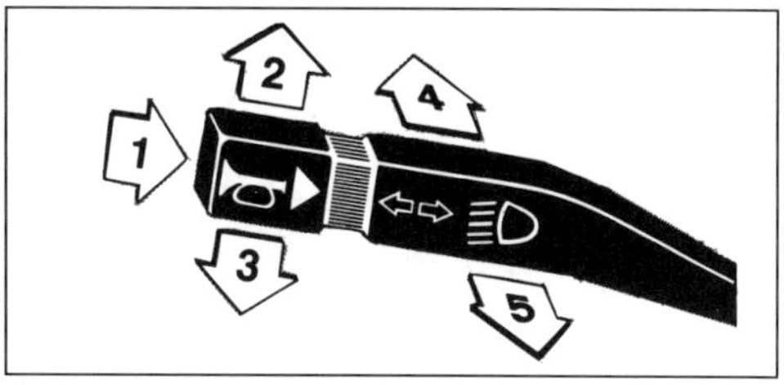

▲ *Multi-function switch (models up to 1986)*
1 Horn
2 Right direction indicator
3 Left direction indicator
4 Headlight main beam
5 Headlight flash

Multi-function switch (models from 1986)

Controls the direction indicators, sidelights/tail lights and headlights, and headlight flash and main beam. On models fitted with driving lights, these operate with the headlight main beam and headlight flash.

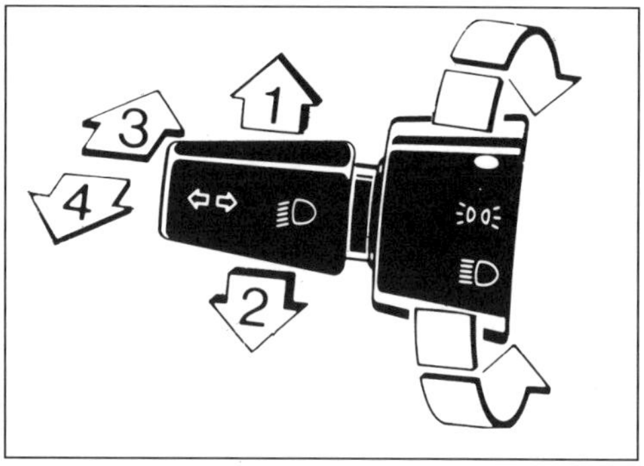

▲ *Multi-function switch (models from 1986)*
1 Right direction indicator
2 Left direction indicator
3 Headlight main beam
4 Headlight flash
Turn collar at base of switch to switch on sidelights/tail lights or headlights

Exterior lights switch (models up to 1986)

Controls the sidelights/tail lights and headlights.

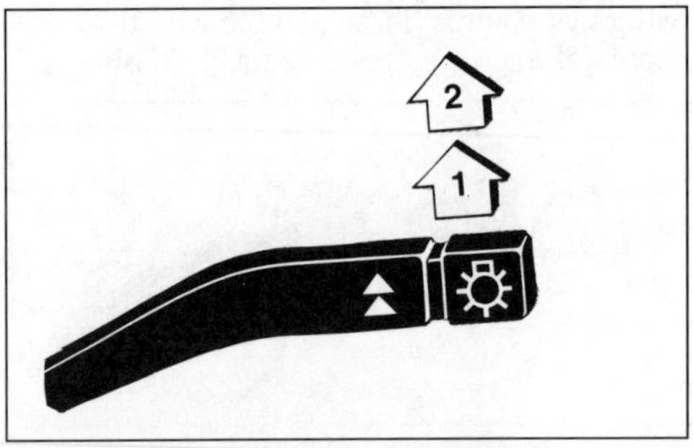

▲ *Exterior lights switch (models up to 1986)*
- ***1*** *Sidelights/tail lights*
- ***2*** *Headlights*

Windscreen wash/wipe switch (models up to 1986)

Controls the windscreen wipers and washers. Where fitted, the headlight washers will operate at the same time as the windscreen washers when the headlights are switched on. On certain models with intermittent wipe, the interval between wipes can be varied using the knob provided on the facia. Turn the knob clockwise to increase the interval, or anti-clockwise to decrease the interval.

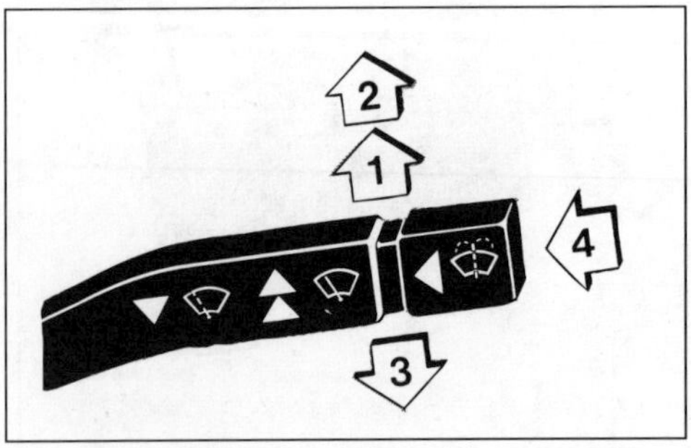

▲ *Windscreen wash/wipe switch (models up to 1986)*
- ***1*** *Normal wiper speed*
- ***2*** *Fast wipe*
- ***3*** *Single wipe or intermittent wipe (depending on model)*
- ***4*** *Windscreen washers*

Tailgate wash/wipe switch (models up to 1986)

Depress the switch to the first position to operate the wiper. Depress the switch further and hold it depressed to operate the washer.

Windscreen and tailgate (where applicable) wash/wipe switch (models from 1986)

Controls all the wash/wipe functions. On certain models with intermittent wipe, the interval between wipes can be varied using a collar at the base of the switch. Turn the collar clockwise to increase the interval, or anti-clockwise to decrease the interval.

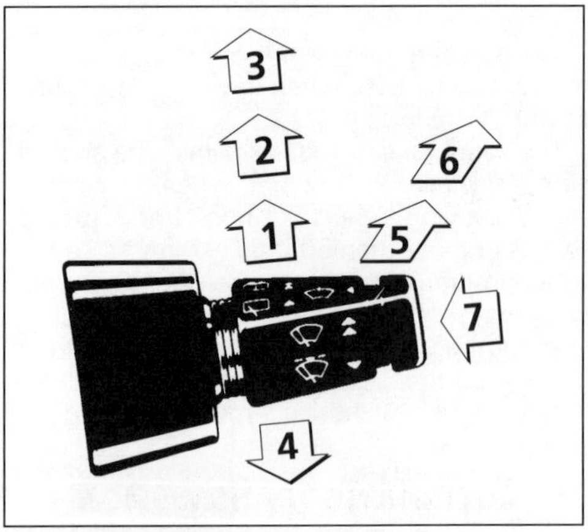

▲ *Windscreen and tailgate (where applicable) wash/wipe switch (models from 1986)*
- ***1*** *Single 'flick' wipe*
- ***2*** *Normal wiper speed*
- ***3*** *Fast wipe*
- ***4*** *Intermittent wipe*
- ***5*** *Tailgate wipe*
- ***6*** *Tailgate wash*
- ***7*** *Windscreen washers*

Heating and ventilation controls (models up to 1986)

Lever **A** – controls the temperature: up for hot, and down for cold, with variable settings in between.

Lever **B** – controls the distribution of the air between the windscreen (up) and the car floor area (down) with variable settings in between. When the lever is fully down, the airflow is shut off.

Switch **C** – controls the booster fan. The fan may have two or three speeds, and the switch may be of rotary or rocker type depending on model.

The airflow through the louvred vents in the facia is controlled independently using the knurled wheel at the side of each vent to increase or decrease the amount of air, and by moving the position of the slats to control the direction.

Side vents at each end of the facia operate with the windscreen demister vents to de-mist the side windows.

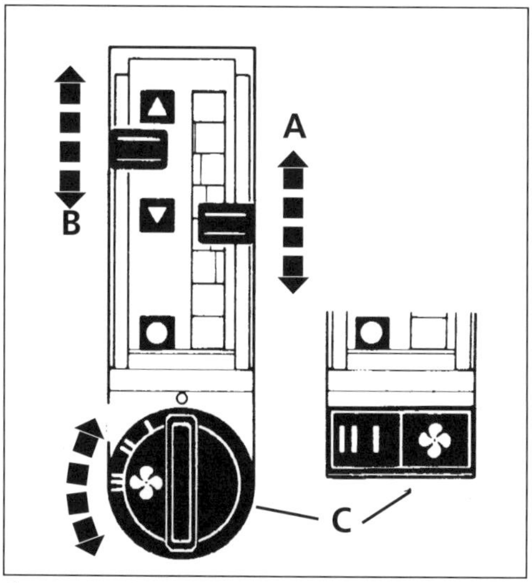

▲ *Heating and ventilation controls (models up to 1986)*
A *Air temperature control*
B *Air distribution control*
C *Booster fan switch (alternative types)*

Heating and ventilation controls (models from 1986)

Knob **A** – controls the temperature: right for hot, and left for cold, with variable settings in between.

Knob **B** – controls the booster fan which has three speeds.

Knob **C** – controls the distribution of the air between the windscreen (right) and the car floor area (left), with variable settings in between. If the knob is moved fully to the left, the airflow is shut off.

The airflow through the louvred vents in the facia is controlled independently using the knurled wheel at the side of each vent to increase or decrease the amount of air, and by moving the position of the slats to control the direction.

Side vents at each end of the facia operate with the windscreen demister vents to de-mist the side windows.

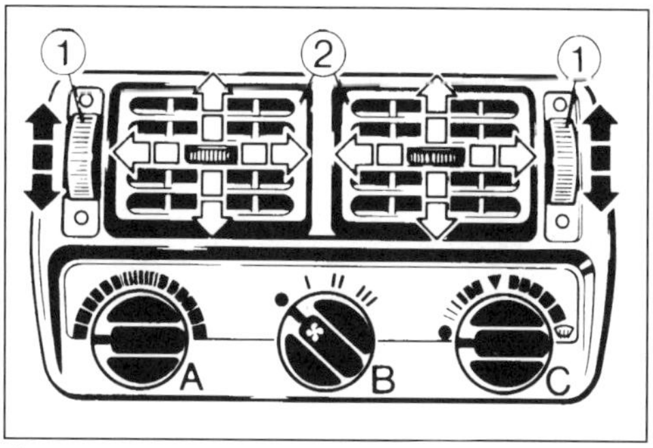

▲ *Heating and ventilation controls (models from 1986)*
1 *Knurled wheel*
2 *Slats*
A *Air temperature control*
B *Booster fan switch*
C *Air distribution control*

Hazard flasher switch

Operates the flashers regardless of the position of the ignition switch.

Rear foglight switch

Operates the rear foglights provided that the headlights are switched on at dipped beam.

Heated rear window switch

Operates the heated rear window provided that the ignition is switched on. It's recommended that the device is switched off as soon as demisting is complete, as drain on the battery is very high (some models are fitted with a timer which switches the element off automatically after 10 minutes).

Electric door mirror switch (models up to 1986)

The switch assembly is located in the centre console. To adjust the driver's mirror, move switch **(2)** to the right, then move switch **(1)** in the required direction. To adjust the passenger's mirror, move switch **(2)** to the left.

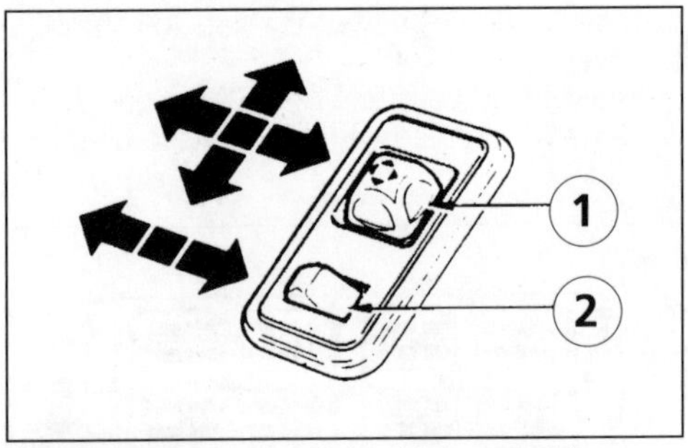

▲ *Electric door mirror switch (models up to 1986)*
*For **1** and **2** see text*

Electric door mirror switch (models from 1986)

The switch has three positions to adjust the driver's and passenger door mirrors:

A – the passenger's door mirror can be adjusted by moving the knob in the required direction

B – off

C – the driver's door mirror can be adjusted by moving the knob in the required direction

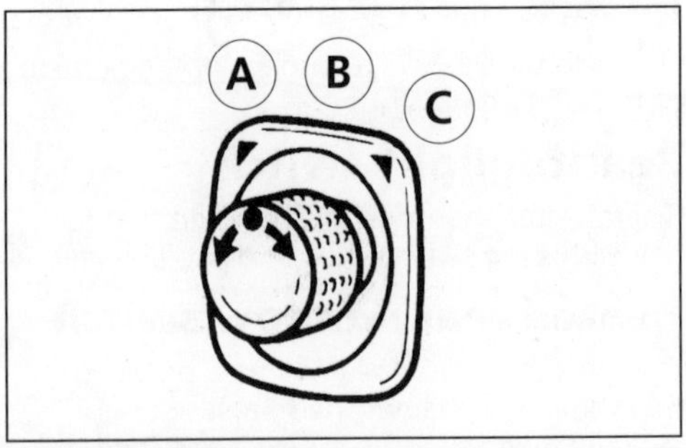

▲ *Electric door mirror switch (models from 1986)*
*For **A**, **B** and **C** see text*

Heated windscreen switch

Operates the windscreen heating element provided that the engine is running.

Heated front seats switch

Mounted either in the facia or the centre console, operates the heating elements with the ignition key in position **I** or **II**. To avoid battery drain it should only be used with the engine running.

Loudspeaker balance control

Adjusts the sound balance between the front, rear, left, and right of the car by moving the joystick in the required direction.

Instrument illumination control

Adjusts the brightness of the instrument illumination when the exterior lights are switched on.

Remote boot/tailgate release

Operates provided that the engine is not running.

Bonnet release lever

Mounted under the steering column. Pull the lever to release the bonnet, then lift the bonnet safety catch (slightly above and right of Ford badge) to open the bonnet.

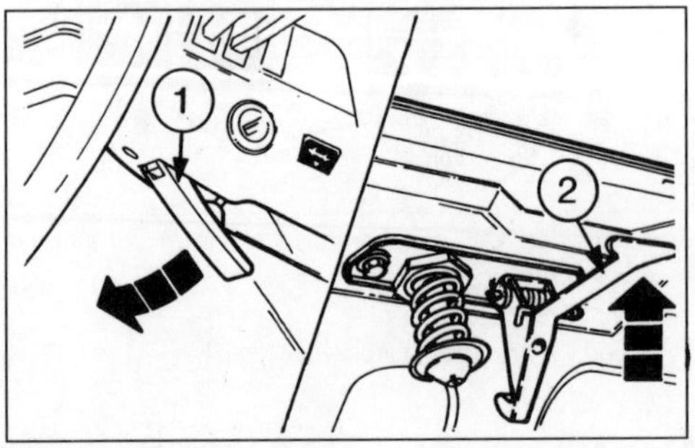

▲ *Bonnet release mechanism*
***1** Bonnet release lever*
***2** Safety catch*

INTERIOR EQUIPMENT

Cigarette lighter

Operates regardless of the position of the ignition switch. Press the lighter in, then release it, and wait until it pops out ready for use.

Electric windows

Switches mounted in the front door armrests raise and lower the front windows with the ignition switched on. Two switches are provided on the driver's side so that the driver can control the passenger's side window. Press the top of the switch to lower the window,

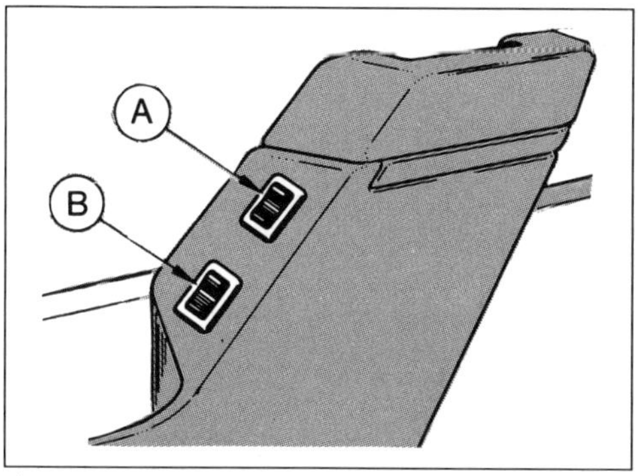

▲ *Electric windows switches – driver's side (models up to 1986)*
A *Passenger's side window switch*
B *Driver's side window switch*

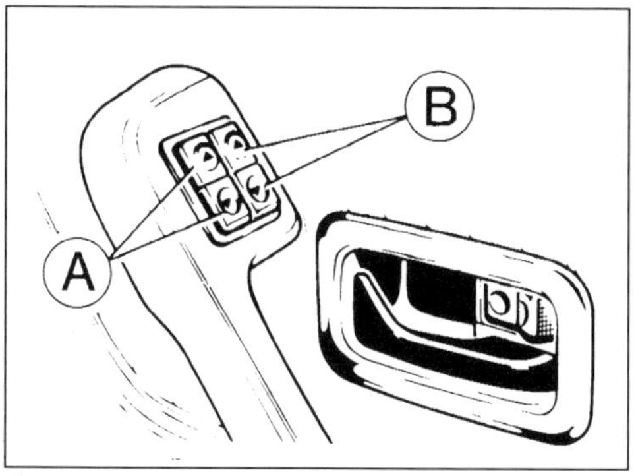

▲ *Electric windows switches – driver's door (models from 1986)*
A *Driver's side window switch*
B *Passenger's side window switch*

and the bottom of the switch to raise the window. Keep the switch pressed until the window reaches the desired position.

Sunroof

The sunroof is of the tilt/sliding type. To open the sunroof, ease the winder handle out of its recess, and turn it anti-clockwise. Turn the handle clockwise to close the sunroof. To tilt the rear edge of the sunroof, ease the winder handle out of its recess, and turn it clockwise, overcoming the resistance (open the facia side air vents to prevent a partial vacuum inside the car with the roof in this position). The sun-blind can be moved to any position when the sunroof is closed or tilted, and moves back when the sunroof is opened.

Dipping rear view mirror

Pull back the lever under the mirror to reduce the glare from the lights of following vehicles.

Seat belts

The operation of the seat belts is self-explanatory for most models, but certain points require additional explanation.

FRONT SEAT BELTS (THREE-DOOR AND CABRIOLET MODELS)

On some models, the outer lower end of the belt is free to slide along a steel bar. When putting the belt on, it's essential to ensure that the belt has moved to the front of the bar, and has not been prevented from sliding forward by a rear seat passenger, or luggage by behind the seat. Similarly, when the belt is released, ensure that it returns to the rear of the bar and does not lie in the door aperture.

REAR SEAT BELTS (ALL MODELS)

The centre rear seat belt is of the lap type, and must be manually adjusted for fit by the wearer. The tongue and the buckle of the lap strap are identified by a white spot, and the lap strap tongue should never be locked into a buckle without this identifying spot. To tighten the belt, pull the webbing through the adjuster and move the plastic clip to hold the end of the belt. To lengthen the belt, turn the adjuster at right-angles to the belt, then press the tongue into the adjuster housing and pull the webbing through the adjuster.

REAR SEAT BELTS (CABRIOLET)

The two side belts are of the lap type, with retractors which lock when the user stops extracting the webbing. To put on one of these belts, make sure that the webbing is fully retracted; then pull the webbing out in a continuous steady movement without stopping, until it's fully extracted, and push the tongue on the end of the belt into the buckle until a click is heard. Allow the webbing to retract, when it should automatically lock. A release button is provided on the back of the retractor housing, so that the webbing can be pulled out further from any partly extended position.

Front seat adjustment

SEAT SLIDING CONTROL

To move a seat backwards or forwards, pull the lever located under the front of the seat away from the door on models up to 1986, or to the right on models from 1986; then slide the seat to the required position. Release the lever, and ensure that the seat has locked in position by gently rocking it backwards and forwards.

SEAT BACK RELEASE (THREE-DOOR MODELS)

Pull up the lever on the side of the seat, and tilt the seat back to allow access to the rear seats.

SEAT RECLINING CONTROL

Turn the wheel on the inside bottom edge of the seat to alter the angle of the seat back. If the seat is moved fully forwards, it is possible to recline the seat back further.

SEAT LUMBAR ADJUSTMENT

Certain models have a wheel on the inside edge of the seat back which can be used to adjust the lumbar support.

Adjustable head restraints

The head restraints can be adjusted for height by pulling up or down (do not force the head restraint beyond the upper stop position), and the angle can be adjusted by tilting backwards or forwards.

Folding rear seats

Either a full width or a split rear seat back may be fitted, depending on model.

ESCORT HATCHBACK AND ESTATE MODELS

Maximum load capacity is obtained by folding the rear seat cushion forwards against the front seats before folding down the rear seat back(s). On five-door models, the rear doors must first be opened to allow enough space for the seat cushion to fold. Pull the cushion forward using the looped tab provided.
To fold the rear seat back(s) down, pull the relevant release catch(es) at the top of the seat back(s), then fold the seat back(s) forwards. When returning the seat back(s) to the normal position, hold the top(s) of the rear seat belt(s) forwards to avoid trapping, and make sure that the seat back locking catch(es) engage properly. Where applicable, also make sure that the seat cushion locks into position, and that the seat belts are not trapped.

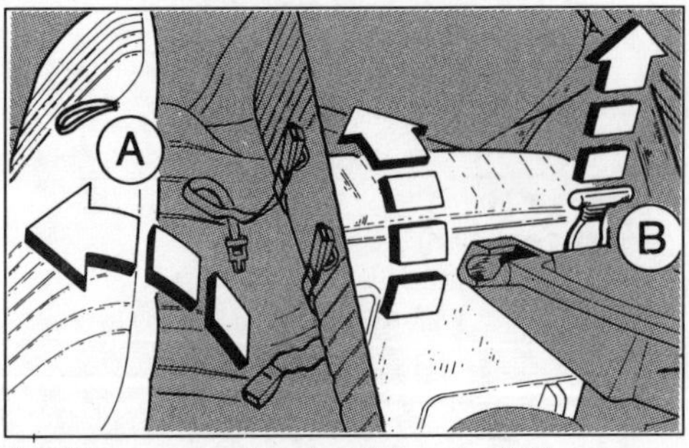

▲ *Folding rear seats (Escort models up to 1986)*
A *Seat cushion looped tab*
B *Seat back release catch*

ESCORT CABRIOLET MODELS

The seat is folded in exactly the same way as described for other Escort models, except that the seat back catch is located in the boot. If the car is to be driven with the folding roof open, and the seat back folded down, the roof protective cover must be secured with both rubber straps which are fixed to the front edge of the roof stowage tray. The straps should be clipped to the press studs located in the centre of the protective cover.

When the seat back is returned to its normal position, make sure that the catch is fully engaged.

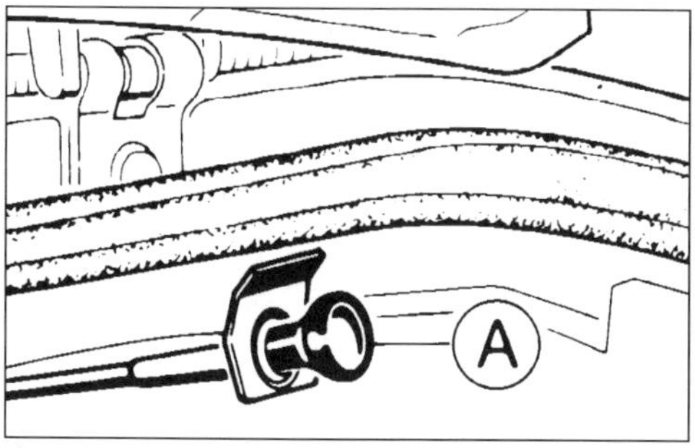

▲ *Folding rear seat back release catch **(A)** – Escort Cabriolet models*

ORION MODELS

The procedure is exactly the same as described for Escort models, except that the seat cushion cannot be folded forwards.

Rear parcel shelf

On Escort models with a rear parcel shelf, the shelf can be removed by unhooking the cords from the tailgate, and pulling the shelf rearwards and upwards.

EXTERIOR EQUIPMENT

Door locks (models up to 1986)

To lock a front door, either close it and turn the key in the lock or, with the door open, press the lock interior plunger (located at the top of the door below the window), then close the door, making sure that the exterior handle is held up.

To lock a rear door, hold the door open, press the lock interior plunger, then close the door. The rear door locks incorporate childproof catches, operated by pushing the small lever on the back edge of the door downwards.

Door locks (models from 1986)

The locks are similar to those already described for earlier models, with the following differences:

Instead of plungers on the tops of the doors, rocker switches are provided to lock the doors from inside the car. The switches are located in the recesses above the door interior handles, and red indicators on the switches are visible when the doors are unlocked.

The driver's door can only be locked by using the key after closing the door.

Central door locking system

The system can be operated from the driver's door on models up to 1986, or from the driver's door and passenger's door on models from 1986. On the earlier models, the front passenger's door and the tailgate/boot lid locks can be operated independently of the driver's door. On the later models, only the tailgate/boot lid lock can be operated independently. It's only possible to operate the system with the doors closed, either by locking from outside using the key, or from inside using the lock interior plunger or rocker switch (as applicable).

Manually-operated folding roof (Escort Cabriolet models)

The roof must only be opened when the car is stationary. To open the roof, working on each side of the car, press the locking catch **(B)**

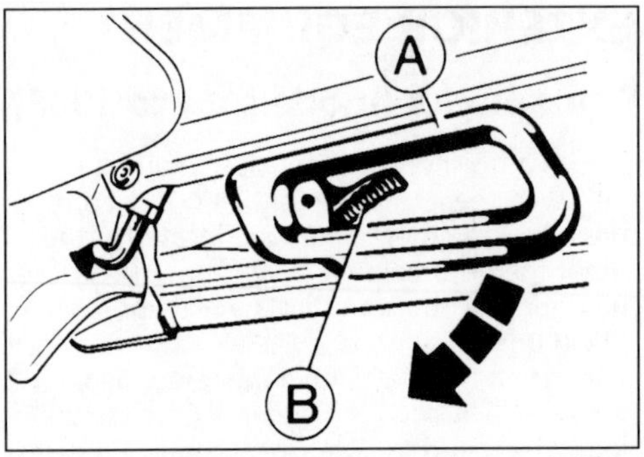

▲ *Folding roof locking handle **(A)** and locking catch **(B)***

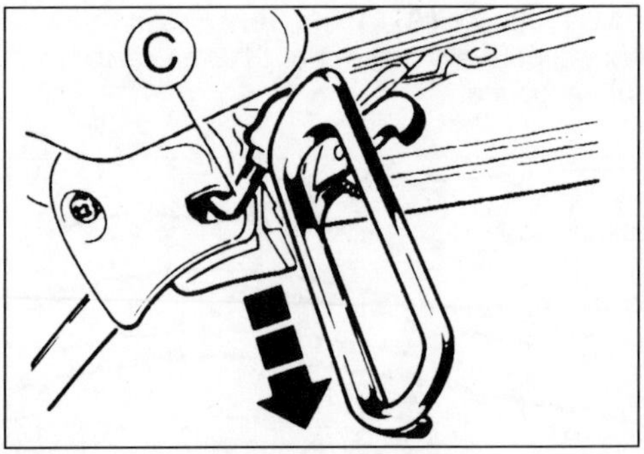

▲ *Folding roof latching hook **(C)***

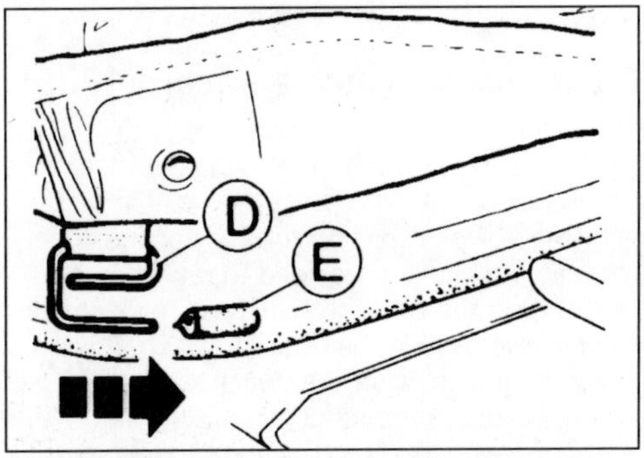

▲ *Folding roof protective cover clips **(D)** and looped tabs **(E)***

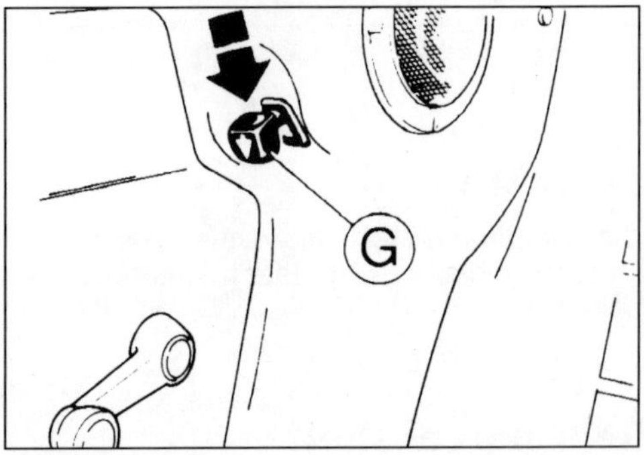

▲ *Folding roof release knob **(G)***

upwards, and hold in this position while pulling the locking handle **(A)** downwards. Pull both the locking handles **(A)** down firmly until the latching hooks **(C)** are in the released position, then push both handles up again. From outside the car, grasp the roof under the front edge, then lift it upwards and push it to the rear. Working at each side, press the middle of the hinged frame down until the locking mechanism engages with an audible click. From behind the car, slide the protective cover from the rear over the folding roof, then hook both the clips **(D)** on the protective cover into the looped tabs **(E)** which are located on the rear edge of the folding roof. Pull the protective cover forwards and fasten all the press studs.

To close the roof, first remove the protective cover, unclipping the press-studs individually to avoid straining the fabric. Press down each release knob **(G)** to release the folding roof. With the roof released, pull it as far forward as possible. Working at each side, hold the latching hook **(C)** up, and pull the locking handle **(A)** down and forwards as far as possible until the latching hook **(C)** engages with the latching plate. When both latching hooks are in position, push each locking handle upwards to its locked position.

Power-operated folding roof (Escort Cabriolet models)

Before opening the roof, make sure that all items are removed from the rear parcel shelf, and make sure that the boot lid is securely closed. Also make sure that all passengers are clear of the roof hinged framework. Don't try to operate the roof with the roof latches engaged.

To open the roof, working on each side of the car, press the locking catch **(B)** upwards, and hold in this position while pulling the locking handle **(A)** downwards. Pull both the locking handles **(A)** down firmly until the latching hooks **(C)** are in the released position, then push both handles up again. Turn the ignition switch to position **I**, then press the lower part of the roof operating switch (on the centre console) until the roof is fully open. From behind the car, slide the protective cover from the rear over the folding roof, then hook both the clips **(D)** on the protective cover into the looped tabs **(E)** which are located on the rear edge of the folding roof. Pull the protective cover forwards and fasten all the press studs.

To close the roof, first remove the protective cover, unclipping the press-studs individually to avoid straining the fabric. Turn the ignition key to position **I**, then press the upper part of the roof operating switch until the roof is fully closed. Working at each side, hold the latching hook **(C)** up, and pull the locking handle **(A)** down and forwards as far as possible until the latching hook **(C)** engages with the latching plate. When both latching hooks are in position, push each locking handle upwards to its locked position.

If the power roof mechanism fails, the roof can be closed manually as follows:

Remove the protective cover as described previously, and open the boot lid. Open the hydraulic pump cover which is on the left-hand side of the boot, and fully open the 'T'-shaped tap on the pump by turning it fully anti-clockwise to the stop. Close the boot lid. It's recommended that two people close the roof by grasping each latch, and pulling the roof closed evenly on both sides at roughly the same speed as when it closes under power. Secure the front of the roof as described previously, then open the boot lid again, and close the tap on the hydraulic pump by turning it fully clockwise. Refit the pump cover and close the boot lid. If it's necessary to open the roof manually, reverse the procedure just described.

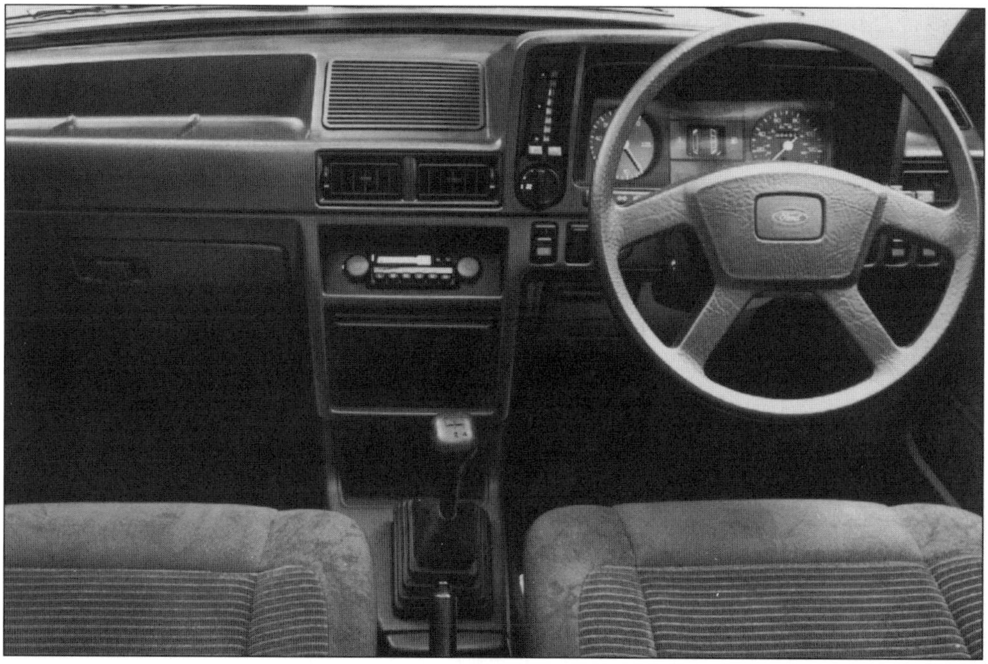

ACCIDENTS AND EMERGENCIES

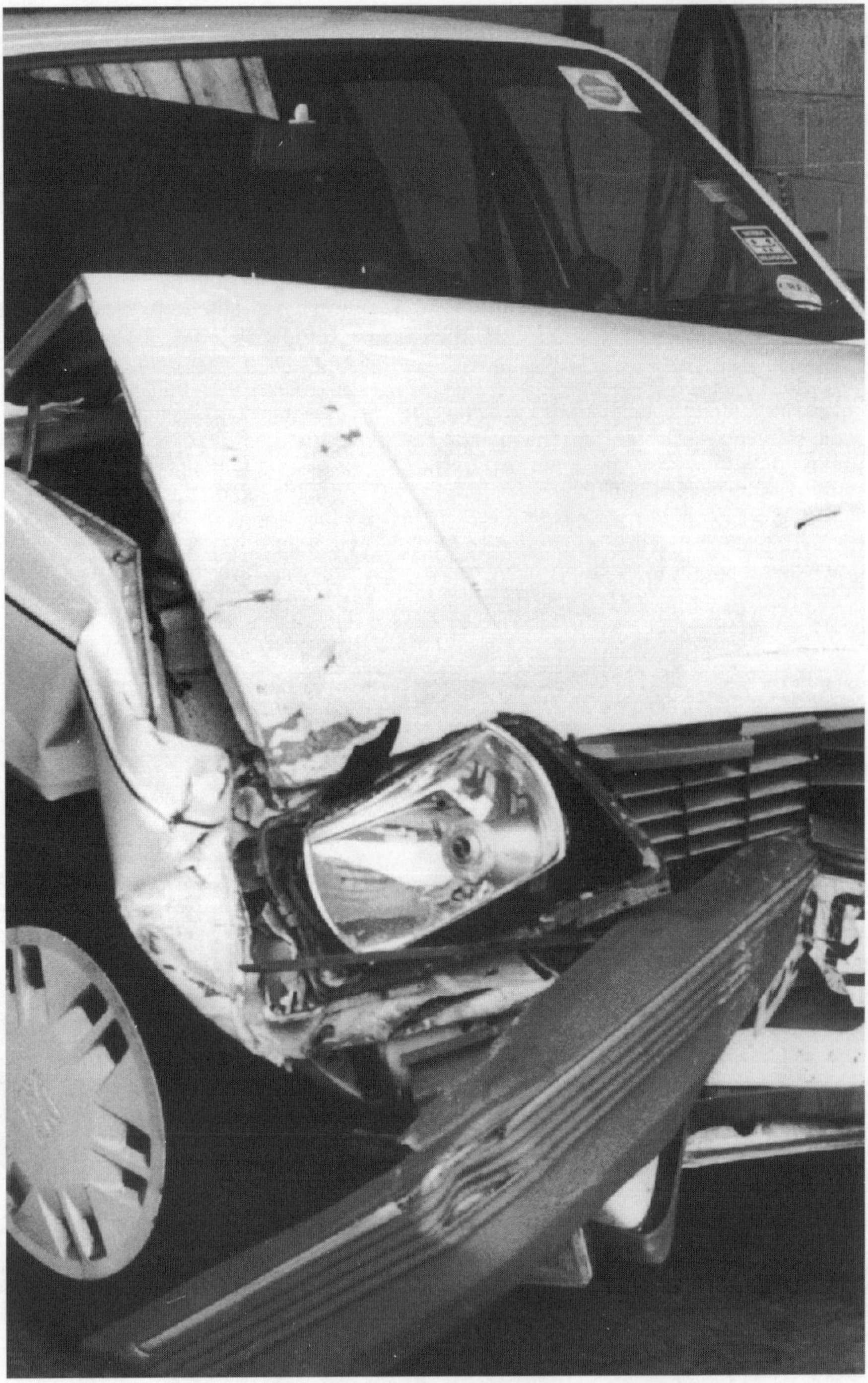

In the event of an accident, the first priority is safety. This may seem obvious, but in the heat of the moment, it's very easy to overlook certain points which may worsen the situation, or even cause another accident. The course of action to be taken will vary depending on how serious the accident is, and whether anyone is injured, but always try to think clearly, and don't panic.

We don't suggest that you consult this Section at the scene of an accident, but hopefully the following advice will help you to be better prepared to deal with the situation should you be unfortunate enough to appear on the scene of an accident or become involved in one yourself.

HOW TO COPE WITH AN ACCIDENT

Deal with any possible further danger

Further collisions and fire are the dangers in a road accident.

- **If possible warn other traffic**

  Where possible, switch on the car's hazard warning flashers.
  If a warning triangle is carried, position it a reasonable distance away from the scene of the accident, to give approaching drivers sufficient warning to enable them to slow down. Decide from which direction the approaching traffic will have least warning, and position the triangle accordingly.
  If possible, send someone to warn approaching traffic of the danger which exists, and to encourage the traffic to slow down.

- **Switch off the ignition and impose a 'No Smoking' ban**

  This will reduce the possibility of fire, should there be a petrol leak.

Call for assistance

Send someone to call the emergency services (dial 999), and make sure that all the necessary information is provided to the operator. Give the exact location of the accident, and the number of vehicles and if applicable the number of casualties involved. Refer to the *'Motorway breakdowns'* Section on page 42 for details of how to call for assistance on a motorway.

- **Call an ambulance**
  If anyone is seriously injured or trapped in a vehicle.

- **Call the fire brigade**
  If anyone is trapped in a vehicle, or if you think that there is a risk of fire.

- **Call the police**
  If any of the above conditions apply, or if the accident is a hazard to other traffic. In most cases, the accident must be reported to the police within 24 hours even if none of the above conditions apply (refer to *'Requirements of the law in the event of an accident'* on page 36).

Administer first aid

Refer to *'First aid'* on page 34.

Provide your details

If you are involved in the accident as a driver or car owner, provide your personal and vehicle details to anyone having reasonable grounds to ask for them. Also inform the police of the details of the accident as soon as possible, if not already done.

FIRST AID

Always carry a first aid kit

If possible, learn first aid by attending a suitable course – contact the St John Ambulance Association or Brigade, St Andrew's Ambulance Association or the British Red Cross Society in your local area for details. These organisations will also be able to provide further training in heart massage and mouth-to-mouth resuscitation which could enable you to save someone's life in an emergency.

Before proceeding with any kind of first aid treatment, deal with any possible further danger, and call for assistance, as described previously in this Chapter.

To help remember the sequence of action which should be followed when dealing with a seriously injured casualty, use the **ABC** of emergency first aid.

Casualties remaining in vehicles

Any injured people remaining in vehicles should not be moved unless there is a risk of further danger (such as from fire, further collisions etc).

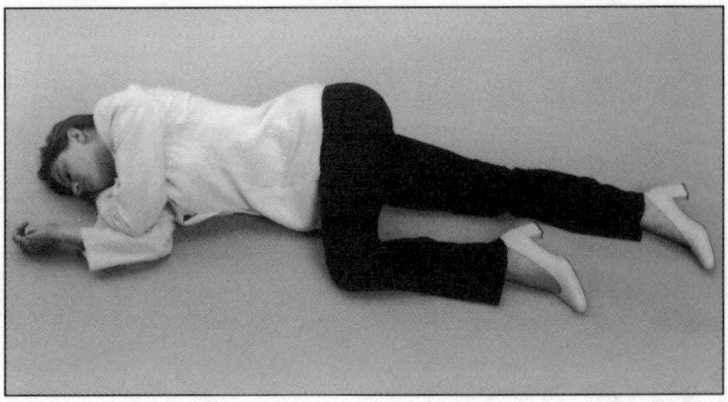

▲ *The recovery position*

Casualties outside the vehicles

Recovery position

To prevent the possibility of an unconscious but breathing casualty choking or suffocating, he/she must be placed in the recovery position.

Lie the casualty on his/her side. Bend the leg and position the arms as shown to support the head.

First aid for other injuries

Always treat injuries in the following order of priority:

- Ensure that the casualty has a clear airway. If not treat as described opposite.
- Put any breathing, unconscious casualty into the recovery position as described previously.
- Treat any severe bleeding by applying direct pressure to the wound. Maintain the pressure for at least 10 minutes and apply a suitable clean dressing. If the wound continues to bleed, apply further pressure and dressings **over** that already in place. If bleeding from a limb, and as long as the limb is not broken, lift the affected limb to reduce the bleeding.
- Broken limbs should not be moved, unless the casualty has to be moved in order to avoid further injury. Support the affected limb(s) by placing blankets, bags, etc, alongside.
- Burns should be treated with plenty of cold water as soon as possible. Don't attempt to remove any clothing, but cover with a clean dressing.

Reassurance

The casualty may be in shock, but prompt treatment will minimise this. Reassure the casualty confidently, avoid unnecessary movement, and keep him/her comfortable and warm. Make sure that the casualty is not left alone.

Give the casualty NOTHING to eat, drink or smoke.

A

Airway

- **Check for breathing**

Check that the airway is clear. If the casualty is breathing noisily or appears not to be breathing at all, remove any obvious obstruction in the mouth and tilt the head back as far as possible. Breathing may then start.

B

Breathing

- **If breathing has stopped**

If after clearing the airway the casualty still appears not to be breathing, look to see if the chest or abdomen is moving. Place your ear close to the casualty's mouth to listen and feel for breathing, and look to see if there's any movement of the chest. If you can't detect anything, you must start breathing for the casualty (mouth-to-mouth resuscitation).

To do this, pinch the casualty's nostrils firmly, keep his/her chin raised, and seal your lips around the casualty's mouth. Breathe out through your mouth into the casualty until the chest rises, then remove your mouth and allow the casualty's chest to fall. Give one further breath.

If giving mouth-to-mouth resuscitation to a child, remember that an adult's lungs are significantly larger than those of a child. Care must be taken not to overinflate a child's lungs, as this may cause injury.

- **Check for a pulse at the base of the neck**

If the heart is beating, continue to breathe into the casualty at a rate of one breath every 5 seconds, until he/she is able to breathe unaided, then place the casualty in the recovery position (refer to *'Recovery position'* opposite).

C

Circulation

- **If the heart has stopped**

If there is no pulse at the neck, then external chest compression (heart massage) must be started.

To do this, if the casualty is still in the vehicle, he/she must be removed and laid on his/her back on the ground. Kneel down on one side of the casualty. Feel for the lower half of the casualty's breastbone and place the heel of one of your hands on this part of the bone, keeping your fingers off the casualty's chest. Cover this hand with your other hand, interlocking your fingers. Keeping your arms straight and vertical, press the breastbone down about 4 to 5 centimetres (1½ to 2 inches). The pressure should be smooth but not jerky. Do this 15 times, at the rate of just over once a second. It may help you to count aloud as you press.

Follow this by 2 breaths as described under *'Breathing'*.

Repeat the cycle of 2 breaths followed by 15 compressions, twice more, ending with 2 breaths, then re-check the pulse.

- **If there is still no pulse**

Repeat the cycle 9 times and then check the pulse. Continue this procedure until there is a pulse or until professional help arrives.

REQUIREMENTS OF THE LAW IN THE EVENT OF AN ACCIDENT

The following is taken from the Road Traffic Act of 1988.

If you are involved in an accident – which causes damage or injury to any other person, or another vehicle, or any animal (horse, cattle, ass, mule, sheep, pig, goat or dog) not in your vehicle, or roadside property:

You must

- stop;
- give your own and the vehicle owner's name and address and the registration mark of the vehicle to anyone having reasonable grounds for requiring them;
- if you do not give your name and address to any such person at the time, report the accident to the police as soon as reasonably practicable, and in any case within 24 hours;
- if anyone is injured and you do not produce your certificate of insurance at the time to the police or to anyone who has with reasonable grounds required its production, report the accident to the police as soon as possible, and in any case within 24 hours, and either produce your certificate of insurance to the police when reporting the accident or ensure that it is produced within seven days thereafter at any police station you select.

ESSENTIAL DETAILS TO RECORD AFTER AN ACCIDENT

If you're involved in an accident, note down the following details which will help you to complete the accident report form for your insurance company, and will help you if the police become involved.

- The name and address of the other driver and those of the vehicle owner, if different.
- The name(s) and address(es) of any witness(es) (independent witnesses are particularly important).
- A description of any injury to yourself or others.
- Details of any damage caused to the vehicles involved or other property.
- The name and address of the other driver's insurance company and, if possible, the number of his/her certificate of insurance.
- The registration number of the other vehicle (check this against the tax disc if possible).
- The number of any police officer attending the scene.
- The location, time and date of the accident.
- The speed of the vehicles involved.
- The width of the road, details of road markings and signs, the state of the road surface, and the weather conditions.
- Any marks or debris on the road relevant to the accident.
- A rough sketch showing the vehicle positions before and after the accident. It's helpful to make a note of the vehicle positions in terms of distance from fixed landmarks, such as lamp posts, buildings, etc.
- Whether any of the other vehicle occupants were wearing seat belts.
- If the accident occurred at night or in poor visibility, whether vehicle lights or street lights were switched on.
- If you have a camera, take a picture of the vehicles and the scene.

If the other driver refuses to give you his/her name and address, or if you consider that he/she has committed a criminal offence, inform the police immediately.

Use this page to record all the relevant details in the event of an accident.
You should transfer all the information recorded on this page onto the Motor Vehicle Accident Report form which you can obtain from your insurance company.

OTHER DRIVER DETAILS

FULL NAME OF DRIVER:

ADDRESS:

POST CODE:

HOME TELEPHONE: WORK TELEPHONE:

DRIVING LICENCE NUMBER: ISSUED:

DATE OF BIRTH: DATE DRIVING TEST PASSED:

TYPE OF LICENCE: (tick box) Full ☐ Provisional ☐ Heavy Goods ☐

PERMITTED GROUPS:

FULL NAME OF OWNER:

ADDRESS:

POST CODE:

TELEPHONE:

INSURANCE COMPANY:

POLICY NUMBER:

AGENT OR BROKER:

TELEPHONE:

OTHER VEHICLE DETAILS

MAKE: MODEL:

YEAR: CC:

REGISTRATION NUMBER:

ACCIDENT REPORT DETAILS

CIRCUMSTANCES OF ACCIDENT

DATE: TIME: am/pm

PLACE: (Street or Road)

TOWN: COUNTY:

SPEED: WERE THE POLICE CALLED? Yes ☐ No ☐

If 'Yes' give details of Police Constabulary concerned:

DETAILS OF WHAT HAPPENED (Please use the page opposite to make a rough sketch map)

WHAT WAS THE WEATHER LIKE?

INDEPENDENT WITNESS 1

TELEPHONE:

INDEPENDENT WITNESS 2

TELEPHONE:

DETAILS OF ANY INJURIES SUSTAINED BY EITHER PARTY:

ACCIDENT REPORT SKETCH MAP

Essential items to include in your sketch map:

- The layout of the road and its approaches.
- The directions and identities of both vehicles.
- Their relative positions at the time of impact.
- The road signs and road markings.
- Names of the Streets and Roads.

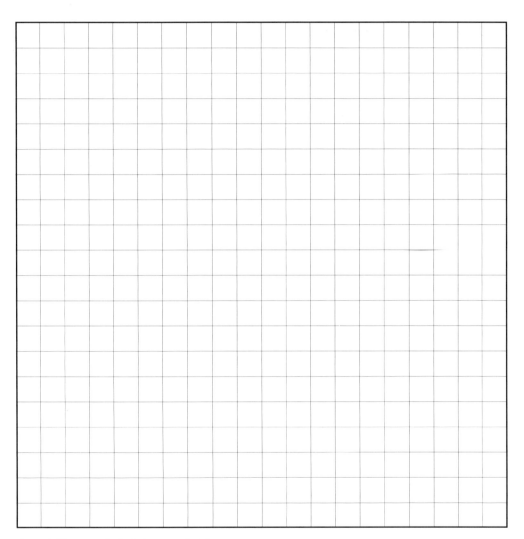

HOW TO COPE WITH A FIRE

Fire is unpredictable, and particularly dangerous when cars are involved because of the presence of petrol, which is highly inflammable.

It's sensible to carry a fire extinguisher on board your car, but bear in mind that the average car fire extinguisher is suitable for use only on the smallest of fires.

In the event of your car catching fire:

- **Switch off the ignition.**
- **Get any passengers and yourself out of the car and well away from danger.**
- **Impose an immediate 'No Smoking' ban.**
- **DO NOT expose yourself, or anyone else, to unnecessary risk in an attempt to control the fire.** Minor fires can be controlled using a suitable extinguisher, but always use an extinguisher at arms-length, and bear in mind that a small vehicle fire can develop into a serious situation without warning.
- **Call for assistance, if necessary** - refer to *'How to cope with an accident'* on page 33.

HOW TO COPE WITH A BROKEN WINDSCREEN

There are a number of national specialist companies who offer roadside assistance to drivers who suffer broken windscreens, and it's a good idea to carry the 'phone number of a suitable specialist in your car for use in such situations. Some car insurance policies enable the use of such companies at preferential rates, and it's worth enquiring about this when obtaining insurance quotes.

- **Most of the windscreens fitted to modern cars are of the laminated type.** Laminated windscreens are made from layers of glass and plastic (usually two layers of glass sandwiching a layer of plastic) which prevents the windscreen from shattering, and preserves the driver's vision in the event of the screen suffering an impact.

  A sharp impact may crack the outer glass layer, but clear vision is usually maintained.

  Obviously, if the windscreen is damaged, it should be replaced at the earliest opportunity, but there is no need to curtail your journey unless the damage is particularly serious.
- **Some older cars may be fitted with toughened windscreens.** If a toughened windscreen suffers an impact, the glass will normally stay intact, but severe 'crazing' will usually occur which is likely to seriously affect the driver's vision.

  If a toughened windscreen breaks, stop immediately, and seek assistance. **DO NOT** attempt to knock the broken glass out of the windscreen frame, as this is likely to result in injury to yourself, and damage to the car. Driving without a windscreen is extremely dangerous and should not be attempted.

WHAT TO DO IF YOUR CAR IS BROKEN INTO OR VANDALISED

If you are unfortunate enough to have your car broken into or vandalised, do not attempt to drive your car away from the scene unless you are satisfied that no damage has been caused which could affect the car's safety.

Where possible notify the police before moving your car, and inform your insurance company at the earliest opportunity.

In the unfortunate event of a breakdown, the first priority must always be safety – never risk causing an accident by attempting to move the car or trying to work on it if it's in a dangerous position.

Joining one of the national motoring organisations such as the AA or the RAC can provide you with a recovery and assistance service should you break down. It may also save you money, as local garages often charge high rates to provide a recovery service.

This Section provides advice on the course of action to follow should you break down. There are also Sections covering the procedure to follow for towing, and on how to cope with two of the more common causes of breakdowns – a puncture, and a flat battery.

Breakdowns on an ordinary road (not a motorway)

Most importantly of all, common sense must be used, but the following advice should prove helpful.

- **Warn approaching traffic,** to minimise the risk of a collision. Where possible, switch on the car's hazard warning flashers, and at night leave the sidelights switched on.
  If a warning triangle is carried, position it a reasonable distance away from the scene of the breakdown, to give approaching drivers sufficient warning to enable them to slow down. Decide from which direction the approaching traffic will have least warning, and position the triangle accordingly.
  If possible, send someone to warn approaching traffic of the danger which exists, and to encourage the traffic to slow down.
- **Get the passengers out of the car** as a precaution should the car be hit by another vehicle. The passengers should move well away from the car and approaching traffic, up (or down) an embankment, or into a nearby field for example.
- **If possible, move the car to a safe place.** If the car cannot be safely driven or pushed to a place of safety, call a recovery service to provide assistance. *Don't expose yourself or anyone else to unnecessary danger in order to move the car.*
- **If the car can't be safely moved, turn the steering wheel towards the side of the road.** If the car is hit it will then be pushed into the side of the road, not into the path of traffic.
- **Try to find the cause of the problem.** Only attempt this if the car is in a safe position away from traffic. Refer to the *'Fault finding'* on page 123 for details.
- **If necessary call for assistance** from one of the national motoring organisations if you're a member, or from a local garage who can provide a recovery service.

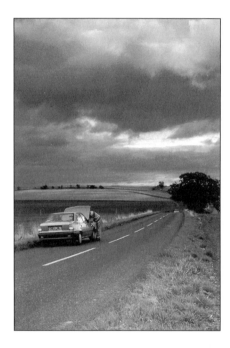

Motorway breakdowns

In the event of a motorway breakdown, due to the speed and amount of traffic there are a few special points to consider, and the following advice should be followed.

- **If possible, switch on the car's hazard warning flashers, and at night leave the sidelights switched on.**
- **DO NOT open the doors nearest to the carriageway, and DO NOT stand at the rear of the car, or between it and the passing traffic.**
- **Get the car off the carriageway and onto the hard shoulder as quickly as possible, and as far to the left as possible** – never forget the danger from passing traffic. Turn the steering wheel to the left so that the car will be pushed away from the carriageway if hit from behind.
- **If you can't move the car off the carriageway** – get everyone out of the car and well away from the carriageways (up/down an embankment, or into a nearby field for example) as quickly as possible. Never forget the danger from passing traffic. Call for assistance as described below. Attempt to warn approaching traffic of your car's presence by signalling from well to the back of the hard shoulder, NOT the carriageway. DO NOT put yourself at risk. Face the approaching traffic, and be prepared to move quickly clear of the hard shoulder onto the verge if any vehicles pull onto the hard shoulder.
- **Get the passengers out of the car** – as a precaution should the car be hit by another vehicle. The passengers should move well away from the car and approaching traffic, up (or down) an embankment, or into a nearby field for example. If animals are being carried, it may be advisable to leave them in the vehicle. In any case, animals and children **must** be kept under tight control.
- **Call for assistance** – using the nearest emergency telephone on your side of the carriageway. NEVER cross the carriageways to use the emergency telephones.
  The direction of the nearest telephone is indicated by an arrow on the marker post behind the hard shoulder (the marker posts are positioned 100 metres/300 feet apart). Each telephone is coded with details of its location, and the operator will automatically be informed of your position on the motorway when you make the call.
  Give the operator details of your car type and registration number and, if you're a member of one of the motoring organisations, ask the operator to arrange assistance.
- **Don't leave your car unattended for a long period.**

Changing a wheel

- **First of all, make sure that the car is in a safe position.** It may be safer to drive the car slowly forwards and risk damaging the wheel, than to risk causing an accident.
- **If you're in any doubt** as to whether you can safely change the wheel without putting yourself or other people at risk, call for assistance.
- **All the tools required to change a wheel are kept in the boot**
  However, if you're carrying any luggage in the boot, you'll need to move it for access to the spare wheel.
  On Saloon and Hatchback models, lift the floor mat up to expose the spare wheel.
  On Estate models, a cover panel must be lifted up.
  The spare wheel is secured in place with a bolt which must be unscrewed before the wheel can be lifted out.
  The jack and the wheel brace (a spanner for unscrewing the wheel bolts) are secured to the underside of the spare wheel.

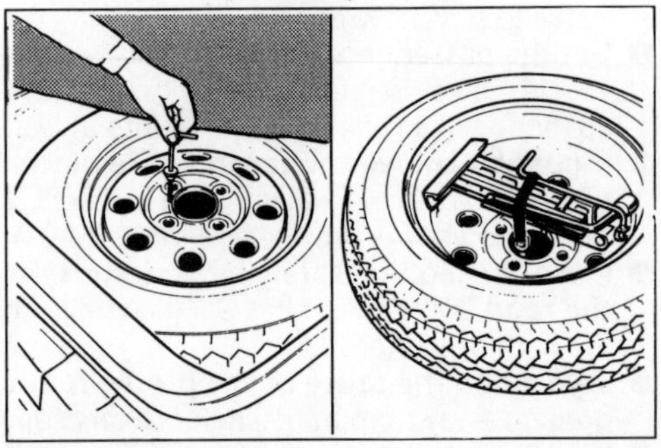

▲ *Spare wheel, jack and wheel brace location in boot (Hatchback model)*

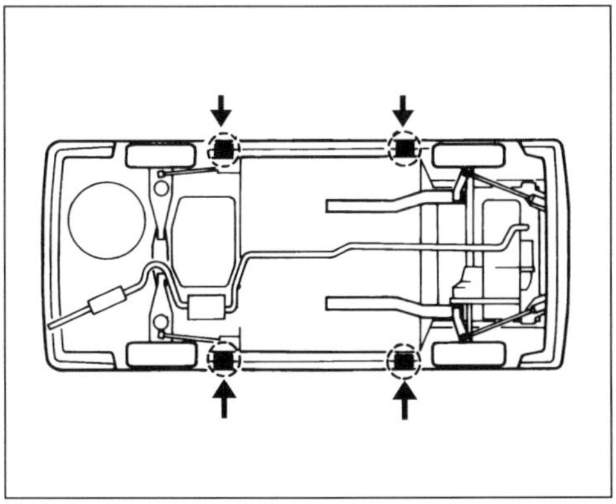

▲ *Jacking points for use with the car jack when changing a wheel*

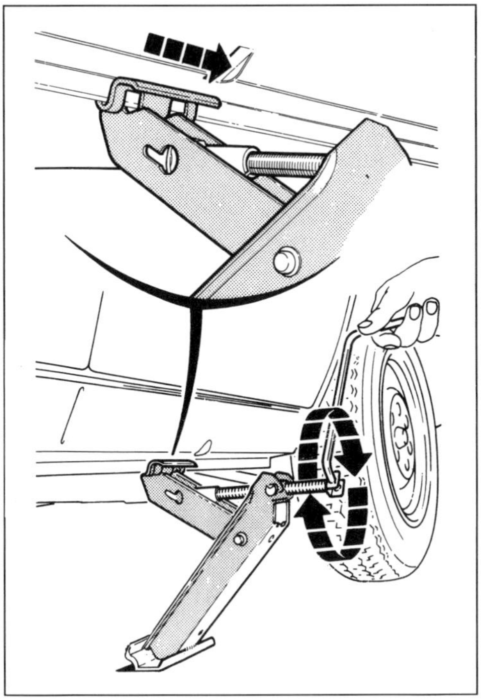

▲ *Using the car jack*

- **Lift the spare wheel and the tools out of the boot.** Place them on the ground. Don't put any luggage back in the boot yet, as the wheel with the punctured tyre will have to be fitted in the spare wheel well.
- **Make sure that the handbrake is applied**, and select reverse gear on models with a manual gearbox, or position **P** on models with automatic transmission.
- **Prise off the wheel trim** (where applicable), which covers the wheel bolts on the wheel with the puncture, using the blade-shaped end of the wheel brace.
- **Slacken the four wheel bolts** by at least half a turn, with the wheel on the ground, using the wheel brace. If you carry a length of piping for just such emergencies, slide it over the end of the wheel brace to make it easier to unscrew the bolts.
- **Before jacking the car**, make sure that the ground is solid enough to safely take the jack, and try to find something to chock the wheel diagonally opposite the one to be changed (two large stones or pieces of wood).
- **The jacking points** are shown in the accompanying illustration, and small cut-outs in the flange under the car show their locations.
- **Choose the jacking point nearest the wheel to be changed**, and engage the channel in the head of the jack with the flange under the car.
  Unfold the jack handle, then turn the handle until the large plate on the bottom of the jack is resting evenly on the ground. Carry on turning the jack handle slowly to raise the car until the wheel is clear of the ground, making sure that the car doesn't move on the jack.
  As a safety precaution, the spare wheel can be positioned under the side of the car which has been jacked up, to reduce the possibility of injury or damage if the jack slips.
- **Unscrew all the wheel bolts**, then remove the wheel. Sometimes it may be necessary to tap the wheel in order to remove it, but if this is done, make sure that the car doesn't move on the jack.
- **Fit the spare wheel to the car**, and tighten the wheel bolts in a crosswise order, then slowly lower the car to the ground.
- **Remove the jack, and fully tighten the wheel bolts**. There is no need to strain yourself doing this, just make sure that the bolts are tight.
- **Refit the wheel trim,** where applicable.

- **Stow the wheel** which has been removed in the boot, together with the jack and wheel brace.
- **Remove the wheel chocks**, and make a final check to ensure that all tools and debris have been cleared from the roadside
- **Select neutral,** where applicable, before starting up and driving away.

Towing

If your car needs to be towed, or you need to tow another car, special towing eyes are provided at the front and rear of the car. On RS Turbo models, a plastic cover must be unclipped from the front spoiler for access to the front towing eye.

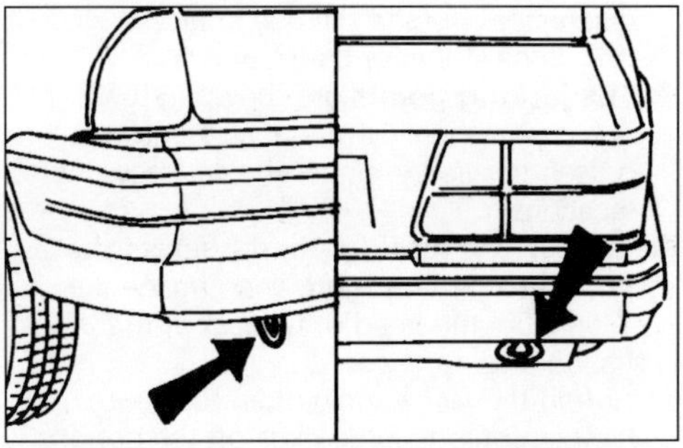

▲ *Towing eye locations (arrowed) – Hatchback model*

When being towed, the ignition key should be turned to position **II** (steering lock released, and ignition warning light on). This is necessary for the direction indicators, horn and brake lights to work.

Note that when being towed, the brake servo does not work (because the engine is not running). This means that the brake pedal will have to be pressed harder than usual to operate the brakes, so allowance should be made for greater stopping distances. If the breakdown doesn't prevent the engine from running, the engine could be started and allowed to idle so that the servo operates while towing.

When a car with an automatic transmission is being towed, the gear selector lever should be moved to the **N** position. To avoid damage to the transmission, do not tow the car any faster than 30 mph (50 km/h) or any further than 30 miles (50 km).

An 'On tow' notice should be displayed prominently at the rear of the car on tow to warn other drivers.

Make sure that both drivers know details of the route to be taken before moving off, as it is difficult, and dangerous, to try to communicate once underway.

Before moving away, the tow car should be driven slowly forwards to take up any slack in the tow rope.

The driver of the car on tow should make every effort to keep the tow rope tight at all times, by gently using the brakes if necessary, particularly when driving downhill.

Drive smoothly at all times, particularly when moving away from a standstill. Allow plenty of time to slow down and stop when approaching junctions and traffic queues.

Starting a car with a flat battery

Apart from old age (most batteries should last for at least three years), a battery will normally only go flat if there is a fault in the charging circuit (indicated by a continuously glowing ignition warning light), or when a particular circuit (eg headlights) is left on for a long time with the engine switched off.

To start a car with a flat battery, you can either use a push or tow start (models with manual gearbox only), or a set of jump leads.

TOW/PUSH STARTING

The method used to start the engine is the same whether the car is being towed or being pushed but, if the car is to be towed, first read the previous Section on towing for details of where to connect the tow rope.

Proceed as follows:

1 Turn the ignition key to position **II** to switch on the ignition.
2 If the engine is cold, on models with a manual choke, pull out the choke control.
3 Depress the accelerator pedal.
4 Depress the clutch pedal and select third gear. Hold the clutch pedal down.
5 Tow or push the car, and slowly release the clutch pedal. The engine will turn over, and should start (don't worry about the car 'juddering' as the engine turns). If the car is being towed, as soon as the engine starts,

depress the clutch pedal and *gently* brake the car so that you don't run into the tow vehicle.

STARTING USING JUMP LEADS

Note: *Starting using jump leads can be dangerous if done incorrectly. If you're uncertain about the following procedure, it's recommended that you ask someone suitably qualified to do the jump starting for you.*

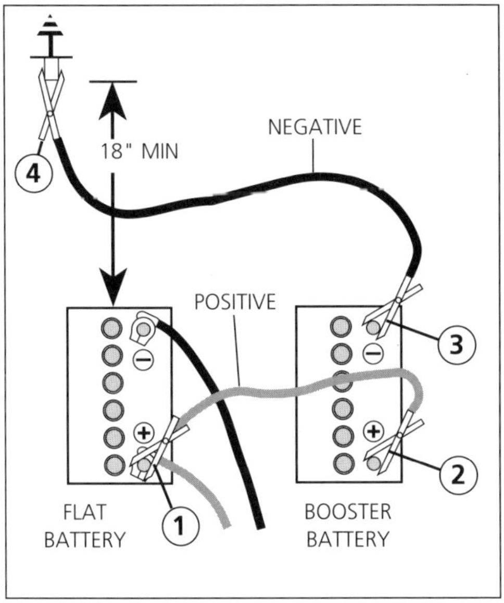

▲ *Jump start lead connections for negative earth vehicles – connect leads in order shown*

Before attempting to use jump leads, there are a few important points to note.

First of all, use only proper jump leads which have been specifically designed for the job.

Make sure that the booster battery (the fully charged battery) is a 12-volt type.

Position the two vehicles close enough together to connect the leads, but **do not** allow the vehicles to touch.

Turn off all electrical circuits.

DO NOT allow the ends of the two jump leads to touch at any time during the following procedure. Proceed as follows.

1 Open the vehicle bonnets, and connect one end of one of the jump leads (usually the red one) to the positive (+) terminal of the flat battery, and the other end to the positive terminal of the booster battery.

2 Connect one end of the other jump lead to the negative (–) terminal of the booster battery, and connect the other end to a suitable earth point on the car with the flat battery at least 50 cm (18 in) away from the battery (eg a clean, bare metal area on the engine block or body). Make sure that all the lead clips are secure.

3 Start the engine of the vehicle with the booster battery and let it run for a few minutes, then start the engine of the car with the flat battery in the normal way.

4 When the engine is running smoothly, disconnect the jump leads in exactly the reverse order to that in which they were connected.

What to carry in case of a breakdown

Carrying the following items may help to reduce the inconvenience and annoyance caused if you're unlucky enough to break down during a journey:

- Alternator drivebelt (refer to *'Servicing'* on page 94 for details of renewal)
- Spare fuses (refer to *'Bulb, fuse and relay renewal'* on page 118 for details of renewal)
- Set of principal light bulbs (refer to *'Bulb, fuse and relay renewal'* on page 113 for details of renewal)
- Battery jump leads (refer to *'Starting a car with a flat battery'* on page 44 for details of starting using jump leads)
- Tow-rope (refer to *'Towing'* on page 44 for details of towing procedure)
- Litre of engine oil (refer to *'Regular checks'* on page 70 for details of checking oil level)
- Torch

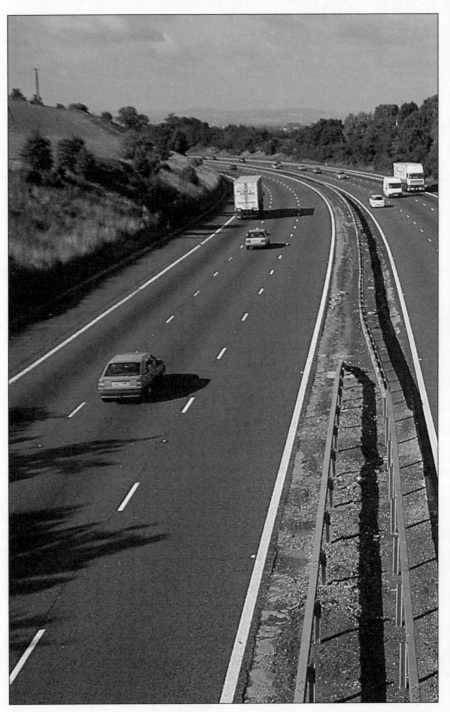

In the UK, more people are injured or killed every year due to road accidents than through any other single cause.

Car manufacturers are paying more attention to passive safety when designing new cars, but drivers must ultimately take active responsibility for ensuring the safety of themselves, their passengers, and just as importantly, other road users.

There will always be accidents on the roads, but taking the time to read the following advice may help you to avoid such a mishap.

The following Sections aim to give advice which will help you to reduce the risk of becoming involved in an incident when driving, not necessarily by changing the way that you drive, but simply by making you aware of some of the potential risks which can easily be avoided. For more information and practical advice on road safety, it is well worth considering taking part in one of the various courses provided by organisations such as RoSPA and the Institute of Advanced Motorists.

BEFORE STARTING A JOURNEY

As a driver, before beginning a journey it's important to make sure that you're comfortable so that you can concentrate on driving without any unnecessary distractions. Spending a few moments carrying out a few simple checks and adjustments will help to make your journey more relaxing, safer and hopefully trouble-free.

Driver comfort

Before driving, make sure that you're comfortable, and that you can operate all the controls easily, particularly if someone else has recently driven the car.

- **Seat**
  Make sure that the seat is positioned a comfortable distance from the steering wheel and the pedals, so that you can operate all the controls comfortably
- **Seat back**
  Make sure that the seat back is adjusted to give your back plenty of support. Your back should rest against the seat, and there should be no need to lean forwards from the seat back. You should be able to reach the steering wheel comfortably, and you should be able to turn the wheel easily without stretching.
- **Head restraint**
  If a head restraint is fitted, it should be adjusted to support your head in the event of an accident. Your head should not rest against the restraint during normal driving and, as a rough guide, the restraint is correctly positioned when its top is in line with your eyes. Similarly, make sure that any passenger head restraints are adjusted correctly if passengers are being carried.
- **Mirrors**
  All the mirrors should be adjusted so that they give a clear view behind the car without the need to move your head unnecessarily.
- **Steering column**
  If the car is fitted with an adjustable steering column, adjust the column so that the steering wheel can be reached comfortably, and the wheel can be turned easily without stretching.

Checks

If you're planning a long journey, refer to *'Regular checks'* on page 69, and make sure that you carry out all the checks mentioned before setting off. Also make sure that you know where the spare wheel and the tools required for wheel changing are located (refer to *'Breakdowns'* on page 42).

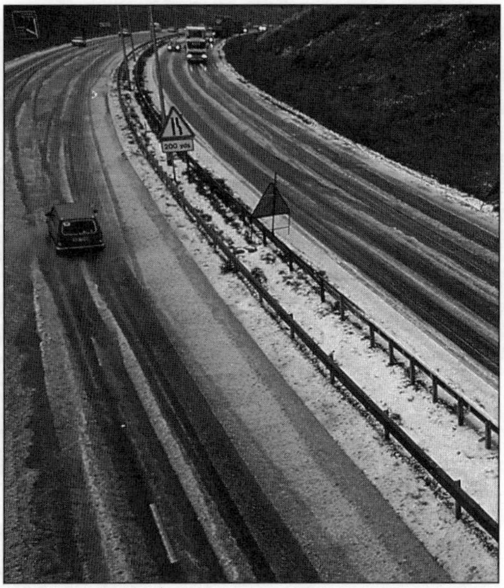

DRIVING IN BAD WEATHER

When driving in bad weather, always be prepared. Bad weather should never take you by surprise. Listen to a weather forecast: you should always be aware of the possibility of poor conditions on your intended journey.

Driving in bad weather requires more concentration, and is more tiring than driving in good weather conditions. Never allow yourself to be distracted by talkative passengers or loud music in the car and, if you feel tired, stop at the next opportunity and take a break.

Always look well ahead, so that you're aware of the condition of the road surface, and any obstacles; **slow down if necessary**.

The following advice is intended to help you to drive more safely in various bad weather conditions. However, above all, use common sense.

Rain

- Use dipped headlights in poor visibility.
- Slow down if visibility is poor or if there is a lot of water on the road surface.
- Keep a safe distance from the vehicle in front (stopping distances are doubled on a wet road surface).
- Be particularly careful after a long period of dry weather. Under these conditions, rain can make the road surface very slippery.
- Don't use rear foglights unless visibility is **seriously** reduced (generally less than 100 metres/300 feet). Foglights can dazzle drivers following behind, especially in motorway spray.

Fog

- Slow down. Fog is deceptive, and you may be driving faster than you think. Fog can also be patchy, and the visibility may suddenly be reduced. Always drive at a speed which allows you to stop in the distance you can see ahead.
- Use dipped headlights. Using main-beam headlights will usually reduce the visibility even further, as the fog will scatter the light.
- Use foglights (where they are fitted) if it's genuinely foggy (generally, where visibility is reduced to less than 100 metres/300 feet), and not just misty.
- Keep a safe distance from the vehicle in front.
- Use your windscreen wipers to clear moisture from the windscreen.

Snow

- Don't start a journey if there is any possibility that conditions may prevent you from reaching your destination. Listen to a weather forecast before setting off.
- Before starting a journey, clear **all** snow from the windscreen, windows and mirrors. Don't just clear a small area big enough to see through.
- Slow down.
- Keep a safe distance from the vehicle in front (stopping distances can be trebled or even quadrupled on a snow-covered or icy surface).
- Drive smoothly and gently. Accelerate gently, steer gently and brake gently.
- Don't brake and steer at the same time – this may cause a skid (refer to *'Skid control'* on page 52).
- When moving away from a standstill, or manoeuvring at junctions, etc, in a car with a manual gearbox use the highest possible gear that your car will accept to move away, and change up to a higher gear earlier than

usual. In a car with automatic transmission move the selector lever to prevent the transmission from using all the gears (usually position '2' – refer to *'Controls and equipment'* on page 23). This will provide more grip and will help to reduce wheelspin.

- Use main roads and motorways where possible. Major roads are likely to have been 'gritted' and are usually cleared before minor roads.
- Use dipped headlights in poor visibility.
- Don't use rear foglights unless visibility is **seriously** reduced (generally less than 100 metres/300 feet) – foglights can dazzle drivers following behind.

Ice and frost

- Follow the advice given for driving in snow.
- Be prepared for 'black ice'. Although you can't see 'black ice', reduced road noise from the tyres will usually tell you it's there.

Severe winter weather

The best advice in severe winter weather is to stay at home but, if you must drive your car, in addition to following the advice given for driving on snow and ice, there are a few additional pieces of advice which you should bear in mind before setting out on a journey.

- Make sure that you tell someone where you're going, and tell them roughly what time you're expecting to arrive at your destination, and what route you're taking.
- Keep a can of de-icer fluid, a scraper, a set of jump leads and a tow rope in the car at all times.
- Carry plenty of warm clothes and blankets.
- Make sure that you have a full tank of petrol before starting your journey. This will allow you to keep the engine running, without fear of running out of petrol, to provide warmth through the car's heating system should you be delayed by conditions, or worse still stuck.
- Pack some pieces of old sacking or similar material, which you can place under the driving wheels to give better traction if you get stuck.
- Carry a shovel, in case you need to dig yourself or someone else out of trouble.

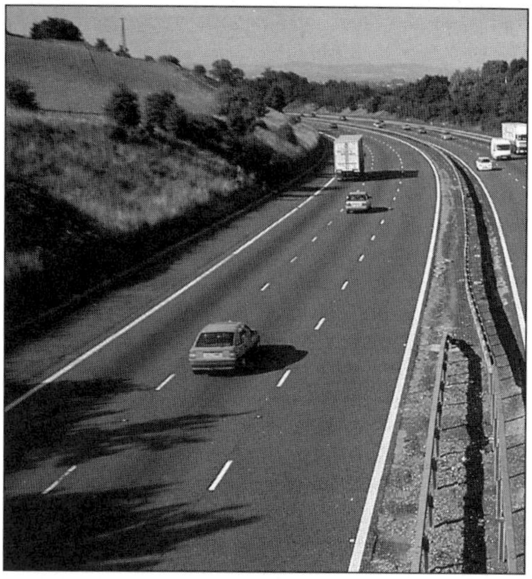

MOTORWAY DRIVING

Motorway driving requires a great deal of concentration and awareness. Motorways are generally busier than ordinary roads, and the traffic moves faster, so there is less time to react to any changes in road conditions ahead.

This Section covers the fundamental rules for safe motorway driving, and will help you to avoid many of the problems which occur on today's busy motorways. Remember that lack of common sense is probably the biggest cause of accidents on motorways.

Full rules and regulations for motorway driving can be found in 'The Highway Code'.

Joining and leaving a motorway

When you join a motorway, you will normally approach from a 'slip-road' on the left. You must give way to traffic already on the motorway. Watch for a safe gap in the traffic, and adjust your speed in the acceleration lane so that when you join the left-hand lane of the motorway you're already travelling at the same speed as the other traffic. Indicate before pulling onto the motorway. After joining the motorway, allow yourself some time to get used to the speed of the traffic before overtaking.

When you leave a motorway, indicate in plenty of time, and reduce your speed before you enter the slip-road – some slip-roads and link-roads between motorways have sharp bends which can only be taken safely by slowing down. Be very cautious immediately after leaving a motorway, as it can be difficult to judge speed after a long period of fast driving.

Rules for safe motorway driving

- **Concentrate and think ahead** – Always be prepared for the unexpected, and look well ahead. You should be aware of all the traffic in front and behind, not just the vehicle in front of you. If you're concentrating properly, nothing should take you by surprise on a motorway.
- **Always drive at a speed to suit the road conditions** – Don't break the speed limit, especially temporary speed limits which may apply to contra-flow systems or roadworks.
- **Slow down** in bad weather conditions. Driving too fast in fog and motorway spray is a major cause of motorway accidents.
- **Always keep a safe distance from the vehicle in front** – The closer you drive to the vehicle in front, the less chance you have of avoiding an accident if something happens ahead. Remember that you need more space in bad weather conditions.
- **Think** – If the vehicle ahead suddenly stops, do you have enough space to stop without hitting it?
- **Use your mirrors regularly** – It's just as important to be aware of what's happening behind you as it is in front.
- **Always signal your intentions clearly and in plenty of time** – Check your mirrors first, signal *before* you move, and change lanes smoothly and in plenty of time. Don't make any sudden moves which are likely to affect traffic approaching from behind.
- **Keep to the left** – The left-hand lane is *not* the slow lane, and you should drive in this lane whenever possible. You can stay in the middle lane when there are slower vehicles in the left-hand lane, but return to the left-hand lane when you've passed them. The right-hand lane is for overtaking only: it is *not* for driving at a constant high speed. If you use the right-hand lane, move back into the middle lane and then into the left-hand lane as soon as possible, but without cutting in.
- **Take note of direction signs** – You may need to change lanes to follow a certain route, in which case you should do so in plenty of time.
- **Stop as soon as practicable if you feel tired** – Driving on a motorway when feeling tired can be extremely dangerous. If necessary, wind down the window for fresh air. If you feel tired or drowsy, stop at the next service station, or turn off the motorway at the next junction and take a break before continuing your journey. You must not stop on the hard shoulder of a motorway other than in an emergency.
- **If you break down** – Refer to *'Breakdowns'* on page 41.

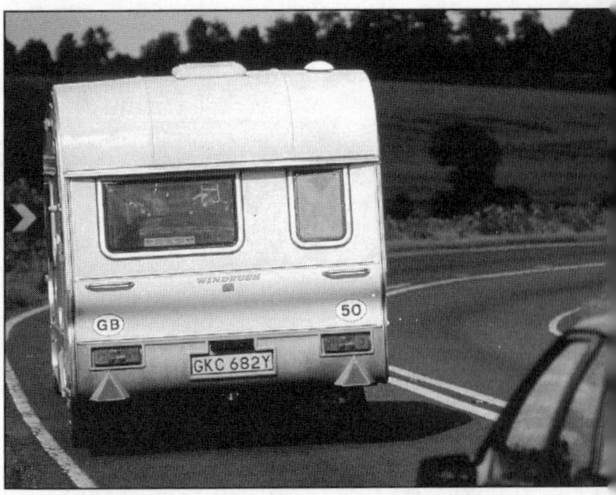

TOWING A TRAILER OR CARAVAN

When towing a trailer or a caravan, there are a few special points to bear in mind. There's more to towing a trailer or caravan than just simply bolting on a towbar and hitching up!

The law

Before using your car for towing, make sure that you're familiar with any special legislation which may apply, particularly if you're travelling abroad.

Make sure that you know the speed limits applicable for towing.

In some countries, including the United Kingdom, there is a legal requirement to have a separate warning light fitted in the car to show that the trailer/caravan direction indicator lights are working.

Always check on current regulations before you travel.

Before starting a journey

Before attempting to use your car for towing, there are one or two points which should be considered.

- **Make sure that your car can cope with the load which you're towing**
- **Don't exceed the maximum trailer or towbar weights for the car** – Refer to *'Dimensions and weights'* on page 11.
- **Engine** – Don't put unnecessary strain on your car's engine by trying to tow a very heavy load. Obviously, the smaller the engine, the less load the car can comfortably tow. Also bear in mind that the extra load on the engine when towing means that the engine's cooling system may no longer be adequate. Some manufacturers provide modified cooling system components for towing, such as larger radiators, etc, and if you intend to use your car for towing regularly, it may be worth enquiring about the availability and fitting of these components.
- **Suspension** – Towing puts extra strain on the suspension components, and also affects the handling of the car, since standard suspension components aren't usually designed to cope with towing. Heavy duty rear suspension components are available for most cars, and it's worth considering having these fitted if you intend to use your car for towing regularly. Special stabilisers are also available for fitting to most cars to reduce pitching and 'snaking' movements when towing.
- **Make sure that you can see behind the trailer/caravan using the car's mirrors** – Additional side mirrors with extended arms are available to fit most cars. The mirrors must be fitted with folding arms (so that they fold if hit), and should be adjusted to give a good view to the rear at all times. The mirrors can be removed when the car isn't being used for towing.
- **Make sure that the tyre pressures are correct** – Unless a light, unladen trailer is being towed, the car tyres should be inflated to their 'full load' pressures. Also make sure that where applicable the trailer or caravan tyres are inflated to their recommended pressure.
- **Make sure that the headlights are set correctly** – Check the headlight aim with the trailer/caravan attached, and if necessary adjust the settings to avoid dazzling other drivers.
- **Make sure that the trailer/caravan lights work correctly** – Make sure that the tail lights, brake lights, direction indicator lights and, where applicable, the reversing lights and fog lights all work correctly. Note that the additional load on the direction indicator circuit may cause the lights to flash at a rate slower than the legal limit, and in this case you may need to fit a 'heavy duty' flasher unit.
- **Make sure that the trailer/caravan is correctly loaded** – Refer to the manufacturer's recommendations for details of loading. As a general rule, distribute the weight so that the heaviest items are as near as possible to the trailer/caravan axle. Secure all heavy items so that they can't move.
  To provide the best possible control and handling of the car when towing, the manufacturers recommend an optimum noseweight for the trailer/caravan when loaded (refer to *'Dimensions and weights'* on page 11 for details). The noseweight can be measured using a set of bathroom scales as follows:
  Place a stout piece of wood between the trailer/caravan tow hitch cup and the scales platform, and read off the weight with the trailer/caravan level. If necessary, redistribute the load, to arrive as close as possible to the recommended noseweight. **Do not** exceed the maximum recommended noseweight.

Driving tips

Towing a trailer or caravan will obviously affect the handling of the car, and the following advice should be followed when towing.

- **If possible, avoid driving with an unladen car and a loaded trailer/caravan** – The uneven weight distribution will tend to make the car unstable. If this is unavoidable, drive slowly to allow for the instability.

- **Always drive at a safe speed** – The stability of the car and the trailer or caravan decreases as the speed increases. Always drive at a speed which suits the road and weather conditions, and always reduce speed in bad weather and high winds – especially when driving downhill. If the trailer or caravan shows any sign of 'snaking', reduce speed immediately – never try to stop 'snaking' by accelerating.
- **Always brake in good time** – If you're towing a trailer or caravan which has brakes, apply the brakes gently at first, then brake firmly. This will help to prevent the trailer wheels from locking. In cars with a manual gearbox, change into a lower gear before going down a steep hill so that the engine can act as a brake, and similarly, in cars with automatic transmission, move the selector lever to position '2', or '1' in the case of very steep hills.
- **Don't change to a lower gear unnecessarily** – Unless the engine is labouring, stay in as high a gear as possible to keep the engine revs as low as possible. This will help to avoid the engine overheating.

ALCOHOL AND DRIVING

By far the best advice on drinking and driving is **DON'T**.

You may feel fine, but it's a proven fact that even one small alcoholic drink will impair your driving to some extent.

Drinking alcohol has the following effects:

- **Reduces co-ordination**
- **Increases reaction time**
- **Impairs judgement of speed, distance and risk**
- **Encourages a false sense of confidence**

The risk of an accident increases sharply after drinking alcohol, and approximately one third of the total number of people killed in road accidents each year have blood alcohol levels above the legal limit for driving. Remember that you're putting other people as well as yourself at risk if you drive after drinking.

The legal limit for blood alcohol level in the UK is 80 milligrams per 100 millilitres. This doesn't correspond to any particular quantity of drink, as the amount of drink required to reach this level varies from person to person. The driving of many people who feel perfectly sober is seriously affected well below the legal limit.

The penalties for driving over the legal limit are severe, and can mean losing your driving licence, a heavy fine, or imprisonment. It's also important to realise that the laws abroad can be far more severe than in the UK, and some countries have a total ban on driving after drinking alcohol.

- **The safest course of action is not to drink and drive.**

SKID CONTROL

If you drive sensibly with due regard for the road conditions, you should never find yourself in a situation where your car is skidding. The following advice will help you to avoid situations which may cause a car to skid, and explains how to regain control of your car quickly should the need arise.

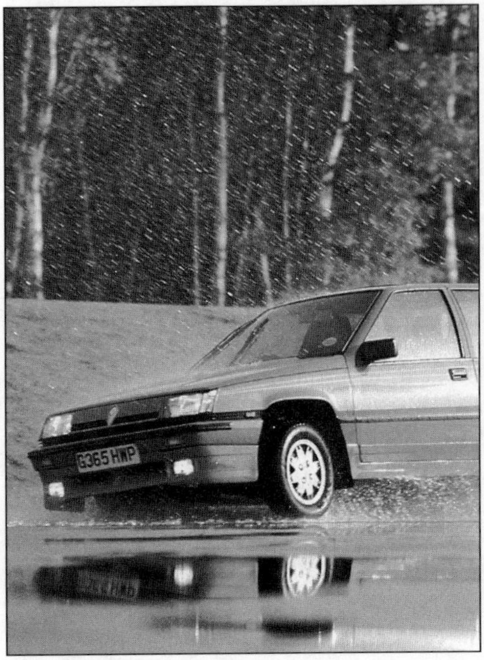

A skid is caused by one or a combination of the following:

- **Excessive speed in relation to the road conditions.**
- **Harsh or excessive acceleration.**
- **Sudden or excessive braking.**
- **Coarse or excessive steering.**

The most common basic cause of skidding is rough handling of the car's controls. Therefore the key to safe driving and preventing a skid is smooth, gentle handling of the car and its controls. Try to apply smooth pressure to the brake pedal, accelerator and steering wheel rather than just suddenly moving them a certain distance.

When a car is skidding, the following things happen:

- **The car is out of control. You can take action to regain control, but while skidding, the car can't be fully controlled.**
- **A car with the front wheels skidding can't be steered.**
- **A car with the rear wheels skidding is likely to spin round if any steering lock is applied.**
- **A car with all four wheels skidding will continue in a straight line in the direction it was travelling when the skid started, regardless of which way the car is pointing.**

Prevention is better than cure. When approaching a corner, reduce speed early by smooth progressive braking **in a straight line**. In a car with a manual gearbox, brake to an appropriate speed and select the correct gear for the corner. Turn into the corner early and smoothly, gently increasing the steering lock if necessary, and corner with your foot gently on the accelerator, so that the engine just 'pulls' the car through the corner, maintaining a constant speed. As you leave the corner, accelerate gently and smoothly.

If you follow the above advice, you should avoid finding yourself in a situation where your car is skidding. However, should you be unfortunate enough to experience skidding, the basic rule for skid control is to **remove the cause** of the skid. If you cause a skid by accelerating, braking or steering, **ease off**, and, when the skid stops, re-apply the accelerator, brake or steering control, but this time more gently and smoothly. If the front wheels are skidding, to regain steering control quickly, steer 'into the skid'. This is often misunderstood, and it basically means look in the direction you want to be facing, and steer in that direction – and be prepared to reduce the steering quickly if necessary when the wheels regain their grip.

Several organisations offer courses in skid control, using specially-equipped cars under carefully-controlled conditions. One of these courses could prove to be a very worthwhile investment, possibly helping you to avoid an accident.

ADVICE TO WOMEN DRIVERS

Unfortunately, it's a fact that women are more likely than men to be the subject of unwelcome attention when driving alone.

There's no reason to think that driving alone spells trouble, but it's a good idea to be aware of certain precautions which will help to avoid finding yourself in an unpleasant situation.

This Section aims to give advice which will help to reduce any risks when driving alone, and will help you to deal with the situation, should you be unfortunate enough to find yourself the subject of unwelcome attention.

Several organisations (some local police authorities, AA, etc) run courses especially for women drivers, in which subjects such as basic car maintenance and self defence, etc, are covered.

Sensible precautions

- **The car**

Make sure that you're familiar with your car.

Make sure that your car is regularly serviced. Refer to *'Regular checks'* on page 69, and make sure that all the checks described are carried out regularly. This will minimise the possibility of a breakdown.

Make sure that you know how to change a wheel, and make sure that the car jack is in good condition in case you have a puncture - refer to *'Breakdowns'* on page 42.

● The journey

If you're planning to undertake a particularly long or unfamiliar journey, the following advice may be helpful.

If you're travelling on an unfamiliar route, make a few notes before you set off, reminding yourself of the road numbers, where to turn, which junctions to use on motorways, etc. Try to stick to main roads where possible.Always carry a map.

Make sure that you have enough petrol for the journey. If you need to fill up during the journey, make sure that you do so in plenty of time, before the fuel level gets too low, and before petrol stations close if travelling at night.

If you think that your family or friends may be worried, you may want to 'phone someone at your destination before setting off to tell them that you're leaving, and tell them what time you expect to arrive. Similarly, when you arrive, you may want to 'phone someone at your starting point to confirm that you've arrived safely.

● Driving in traffic

Avoid attracting unnecessary attention.

Avoid 'jokey' stickers in car windows, which may encourage unwelcome attention.

Avoid eye contact with 'undesirables'.

If you're being followed, pull over and slow down, but **don't** stop. **Don't** drive to your home, but find a busy and well lit place. If the person following persists, blow your horn and flash your lights to attract attention.

If you're stopped by traffic or another vehicle, lock the doors and close the windows. **Don't** ram the other vehicle - damage to your car might prevent your escape.

● Leaving your car

Don't leave any clues that the car is being driven by a woman; make sure that any 'feminine' items are hidden from sight before leaving your car.

Refer to *'Car crime prevention'* on page 63 and take note of the advice given.

Try to park in a well-lit, preferably busy area.

If you park in a car park, try to park close to an exit, or close to the attendant's station. **Always** reverse into a parking space, so that you can drive away quickly if necessary after returning to your car.

Take note of any 'landmarks' so that you can find your car quickly when you return.

Always lock your car.

When you return to your car, walk with a group of people, if possible. Have the keys ready so that you don't have to spend unnecessary time outside your car searching for them, which may attract attention.

Before getting into your car, briefly check for forced entry, and look into the car for any suspicious signs. **Don't** get into the car if you notice anything suspicious.

● Breakdowns

Remember that you're more likely to be injured in an accident than a personal attack.

Refer to *'Breakdowns'* on page 41 and take note of the advice given but, in addition, bear in mind the following advice.

Always walk to 'phone for assistance, **don't** accept a lift. When you 'phone for assistance, mention that you're an unaccompanied woman.

If someone stops while you're 'phoning for help, give the operator details of the other vehicle's registration number and a brief description of the car and driver. If the driver approaches you, tell them that you have passed on his/her details to the police. If the driver's intentions are honourable, your reaction will be understood.

If you decide to stay with, but outside the car, leave the nearside door unlocked and slightly open, so that you can get inside quickly to lock yourself in if necessary.

If you decide to stay inside the car, sit in the passenger seat and lock the door - this will give the appearance that you're accompanied.

When help arrives, ask for some form of identification (even from a policeman) before giving any of your own details.

If someone offers assistance, tell them the police have been informed and are arranging recovery. If you have not yet contacted the police, consider asking the person to do so on your behalf, **but** if you're uncertain about the person's intentions, tell them that the police are aware and ask them to call the police again for you.

● **Accidents**

Keep calm.

Refer to *'Accidents and emergencies'* on page 33 and take note of the advice given but, in addition, bear in mind the following advice.

If you're bullied or shouted at, lock yourself in your car (if it's safe to do so), and wind the windows up. Communicate through a small gap at the top of the window.

If things get out of hand, refuse to talk to anyone except the police.

Self defence

This is a last resort and should not be used unless all else has failed.

There is no substitute for taking a properly supervised course in self-defence, but we aim to outline a few of the basic moves below.

If you are approached, act in a composed manner and use a soft tone.

In the event of an attack, stay calm - you can still safeguard yourself.

- **If you're held by one arm** - Use your free hand to grasp the attacker's thumb and twist the thumb sharply back towards the wrist.
- **If you're facing your attacker** - If your shoulders are held, thrust your hands/arms upwards and diagonally outwards to dislodge the attacker's grip.

  Use your knees or the blade of your hand to chop your attacker's groin, your feet to kick the shins, and your fingers to poke the eyes.
- **If you're attacked from behind** - Quickly lean forward, twisting your head sideways into the attacker to keep your airway (for breathing) clear. Often this will cause the attacker to lose balance.
- **If you've been pulled backwards already** - Turn your head as above, and chop hard with the blade of your hand or a clenched fist to the groin, or an elbow in the stomach.
- **If you've been forced to the floor** - Use your feet and legs to kick against the attacker's shins whilst swivelling your body to keep the attacker at bay.

Be ready to run as soon as the attacker's grip is released, and SCREAM!

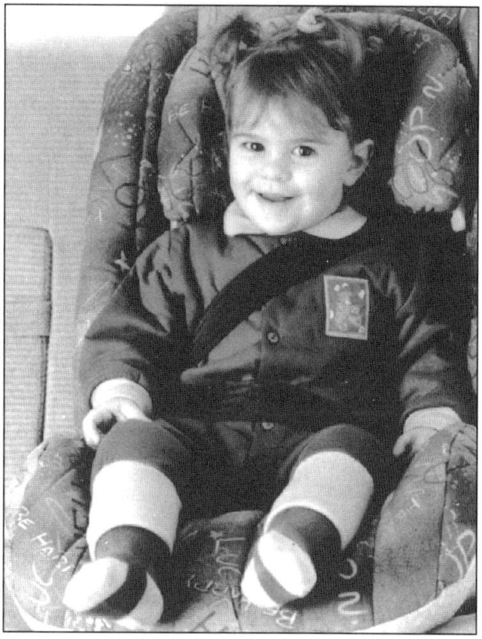

CHILD SAFETY

Every day, thousands of parents strap their offspring into child car seats, confident that they have done everything possible to protect their loved ones. However, a recent survey has shown that many young children are travelling in car seats which have been incorrectly fitted or are being incorrectly used, making them potentially dangerous should they be involved in an accident. The following advice will help you to make sure that you take every possible precaution to ensure the safety of your children when driving.

How to avoid unnecessary risks

- **Never allow young children to travel in a car unrestrained,** even for the shortest of journeys.
- **Never carry a child on an adult's lap or in an adult's arms.** Although you may feel that your baby is safer in your arms, this is not the case. An adult holding a child is far more likely to cause injury to the child than to give protection in the event of an accident.

- **Never rely solely on an adult seat belt to restrain a child,** and never sit a child on a cushion to enable a seat belt to fit properly.
- **Always strap young children into a properly designed child car seat** when carrying them in a car. The cost of a good car seat is a very small price to pay to save your child's life.

Choosing a child car seat

- It's vitally important to choose the correct type of car seat for your child. A wide range of child car seats is available, and it's worth spending some time looking at the various seats on the market before deciding on the most suitable seat for your particular requirements.
- Although age ranges are often given by the manufacturers, these should be taken as a rough guide. It's the weight of the child which is important; for example, a smaller than average baby could use a baby car seat for longer than a heavy baby of the same age.
- **Never** buy a secondhand child seat. This may sound like a ploy from the manufacturers to sell more seats, but all too often a secondhand seat is sold without the instructions, and sometimes there are parts missing. This often leads to secondhand seats being incorrectly fitted. A secondhand seat may have been damaged or weakened through carelessness or misuse, without necessarily showing any visible signs until it's put to the test in an accident!
- Your baby's first contact with the outside world is often on that first ride home from hospital, so make sure that you're prepared, and buy a car seat before your baby is born.
- Some seats are designed for babies from birth to a weight of around 22 pounds (10 kg), which for most babies is around nine months old. Usually, these first car seats are light and easy to transport through the use of a handle. This means that a sleeping baby can be carried from the car into the house without waking. Some baby seats come complete with a built-in headrest, which is very important for the early weeks when a baby's head needs to be supported.

  Certain seats can be fitted so that the baby faces the back of the car (ie rearward facing seats). This may be considered to improve safety, as the baby is supported across the back rather than purely by the harness, if the car is involved in a frontal impact. Combination type seats can then be used forward facing when the child reaches approximately nine months old.

  Other types of seat may be designed to accommodate children up to around 40 pounds (18 kg) or approximately four years old.

  Alternatively, some seats use the car's seat belts to hold both the child seat and the child, and these seats are obviously easier to fit. Make sure that this type of seat is fitted with a seat-belt lock, so that the seat belt cannot be pulled out of place or slackened. Another advantage of these seats is that they can easily be transferred from car to car.
- Try to choose a seat which has an easily adjustable harness, as this makes it easier to ensure that the harness fits the child securely for each trip. If the harness can be quickly loosened, it makes getting a struggling child in and out a little easier.

Using a child car seat

- Firstly, make absolutely sure that the seat is properly fitted in accordance with the manufacturer's instructions. If you're unsure about any of the fitting procedure, contact the manufacturer for advice.
- To hold a child securely, the harness must be reasonably tight. There should be just enough room to slide your flat hand under the strap. Children may be wearing bulky clothes one day, and thin clothes the next, so it is vital that the harness is adjusted before each journey to ensure a correct fit.
- If the seat is fitted using an adult's inertia reel seat belt, make sure that the seat is held firmly in position, and that the seat belt is securely locked to prevent it from loosening. Also, make sure that the seat belt buckle is not resting on the frame of the child seat. This is because the buckles are not designed to withstand the impact of a heavy child seat and, in an accident, could break open.

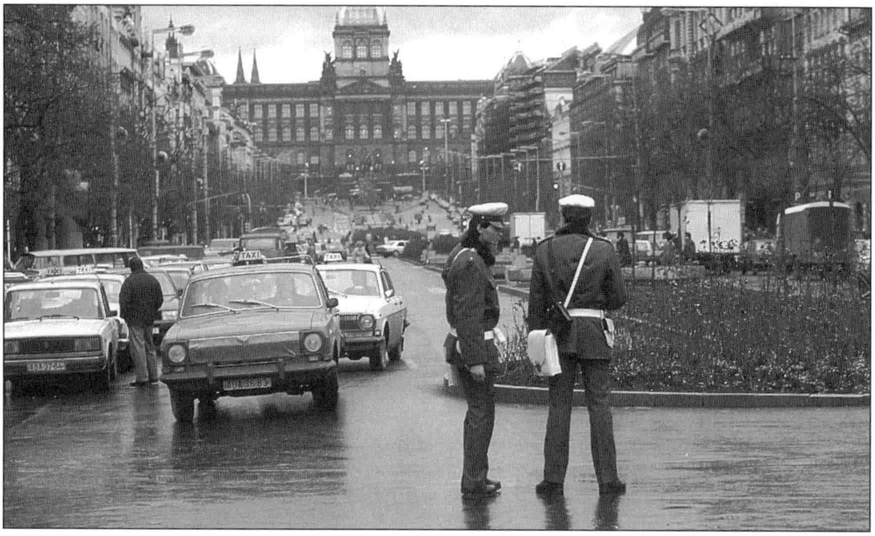

Driving abroad can be very different to driving in the UK. Besides the obvious differences, like climate and driving on the right-hand side of the road, various unfamiliar laws may apply, and it's advisable to prepare yourself and your car as far as possible before travelling.

This Section provides you with a guide which will help you to prepare for driving abroad, and will help you to avoid some of the pitfalls waiting for the unwary.

It may be worthwhile considering hiring a car abroad, rather than driving your own car. In this case, make sure that the insurance cover arranged suits your requirements, and make sure that a damage waiver is included (otherwise you will have to pay for any damage to the hire car).

Insurance

● Motoring

Make sure that you have adequate insurance cover for your car and your luggage.

Check on the legal requirements for insurance in the country you're visiting, and always inform your insurance company that you're taking your car abroad – they will be able to advise you of any special requirements.

Most car insurance policies automatically give the minimum legally-required cover for driving in EC countries, but if you require the same level of cover as you have in the UK, you will normally need to obtain a 'Green Card' (an internationally-recognised certificate of insurance) from your insurance company.

● Medical

It's always advisable to take out medical insurance for the car occupants. Not all countries have a free emergency medical service, and you could find yourself with a large unexpected bill in the event of yourself or one of your passengers being taken ill, or being involved in an accident (in some countries you may even have to pay for an ambulance).

NHS form E111 (available by filling in a form at a Post Office) entitles you to receive the same health care that residents receive in EC countries, but this is by no means comprehensive, and additional insurance cover is usually advisable.

● Breakdown

Recovery and breakdown costs can be far higher abroad than in the UK.

Most of the national motoring organisations (such as the AA and RAC) will be able to provide insurance cover which could save you a lot of inconvenience and expense should you be unfortunate enough to break down.

Documents

Always carry your passport, driving licence, car registration document, and insurance certificate (including 'Green Card' and medical insurance, where applicable).

Make sure that all the documents are valid, and that the car's road fund licence (tax) and MOT don't run out while you're abroad.

Before travelling, check with the authorities in the country you're visiting, in case any special documents or permits are required. You may need a visa to visit some countries, and an International Driving Permit (available from the AA or RAC) is sometimes required.

Driving laws

Before driving abroad, make sure that you're familiar with the driving laws in the country you're visiting, as there may be some laws which don't apply in the UK, and the penalties for breaking the law may be severe.

Fit a 'GB' plate to the back of your car, and make sure that it's displayed all the time you're abroad.

In some countries, you're legally required to carry certain items of safety equipment. These can include a first-aid kit, a warning triangle, a fire extinguisher, a set of spare bulbs/fuses, etc.

Remember that if you're visiting a country where you have to drive on the right-hand side of the road, you'll need to fit headlight beam deflectors or shields to avoid dazzling other drivers, or alternatively, it may be possible to have the headlight beams adjusted.

Make sure that you're familiar with the speed limits, and note that in some countries there is an absolute ban on driving after drinking *any* alcohol.

Servicing

Service your car before setting off on your trip, to reduce the possibility of any unexpected breakdowns.

Pay particular attention to the condition of the battery, windscreen wipers and tyres (including the spare), noting that the tyre pressures will probably have to be increased from their normal setting if the car is to be fully loaded. If you're travelling to a cold country, check the condition of the cooling system and the strength of the antifreeze.

Before setting off on your journey, refer to '*Regular checks*' on page 69, and carry out all the checks described. Check that the jack and wheel brace are in place in the car (refer to '*Breakdowns*' on page 42), and that the jack works properly.

Spares

In addition to the items which must be carried by law in the country you're visiting, it's a good idea to carry a few spares which may be difficult to obtain should you need them abroad (one of the national motoring organisations should be able to advise you). For example, you may want to carry clutch and throttle cable repair kits, as right-hand-drive components can be difficult to find outside the UK.

If your car uses a special oil, it's a good idea to take a pack with you.

It's also a good idea to carry a tow rope and a set of jump leads to help you out in case of a breakdown.

Fuel

The type and quality of petrol available varies from country to country, and it's a good idea to check on the availability of the correct petrol type before travelling (again, one of the national motoring organisations will be able to advise you). This is especially important if your car has a catalytic converter, as in this case you must only use unleaded petrol.

Find out what petrol pump markings to look for to give you the correct type and grade of petrol for your car.

Security

A foreign car packed with luggage is an inviting prospect for criminals, so refer to '*Car crime prevention*' on page 63, and don't take any chances.

Route planning

It's always a good idea to plan your approximate route before travelling. A vast number of maps and guides are available, or the AA and RAC can provide you with directions to your destination for a modest charge.

Bear in mind that in some countries, you'll have to pay tolls to use certain roads, and this can add unexpectedly to the cost of travelling.

What to carry when driving abroad

The following list provides a guide to the items which it is compulsory to use or carry, or it is strongly recommended that you carry in your car when driving in various European countries.

In the following table **'C'** indicates **'Compulsory'** and **'R'** indicates **'Recommended'.**

COUNTRY	HEADLAMP DEFLECTORS	GB STICKER	SEAT BELTS	WARNING TRIANGLE	FIRE EXTINGUISHER	FIRST AID KIT	SPARE BULBS
Austria	C	C	C	C	-	C	-
Belgium	C	C	C	C	C	-	-
Bulgaria	C	C	C	C	C	C	-
Czechoslovakia	C	C	C	C	-	C	C
Denmark	C	C	C	R	-	-	-
Eire	-	C	C	-	-	-	-
Finland	C	C	C	C	-	-	-
France	C	C	C	C	-	-	R
Germany	C	C	C	C	C	C	R
Greece	C	C	C	C	C	C	-
Holland	C	C	C	C	-	-	C
Hungary	C	C	C	C	-	-	C
Italy	C	C	C	C	-	-	R
Luxembourg	C	C	C	R	-	-	-
Norway	C	C	C	R	-	-	R
Poland	C	C	C	C	-	-	R
Portugal	C	C	C	C	C	-	-
Spain	C	C	C	C	-	-	C
Sweden	C	C	C	R	-	-	-
Switzerland	C	C	C	C	-	-	-
United Kingdom	-	-	C	-	-	-	-
Yugoslavia	C	C	C	C	-	C	C

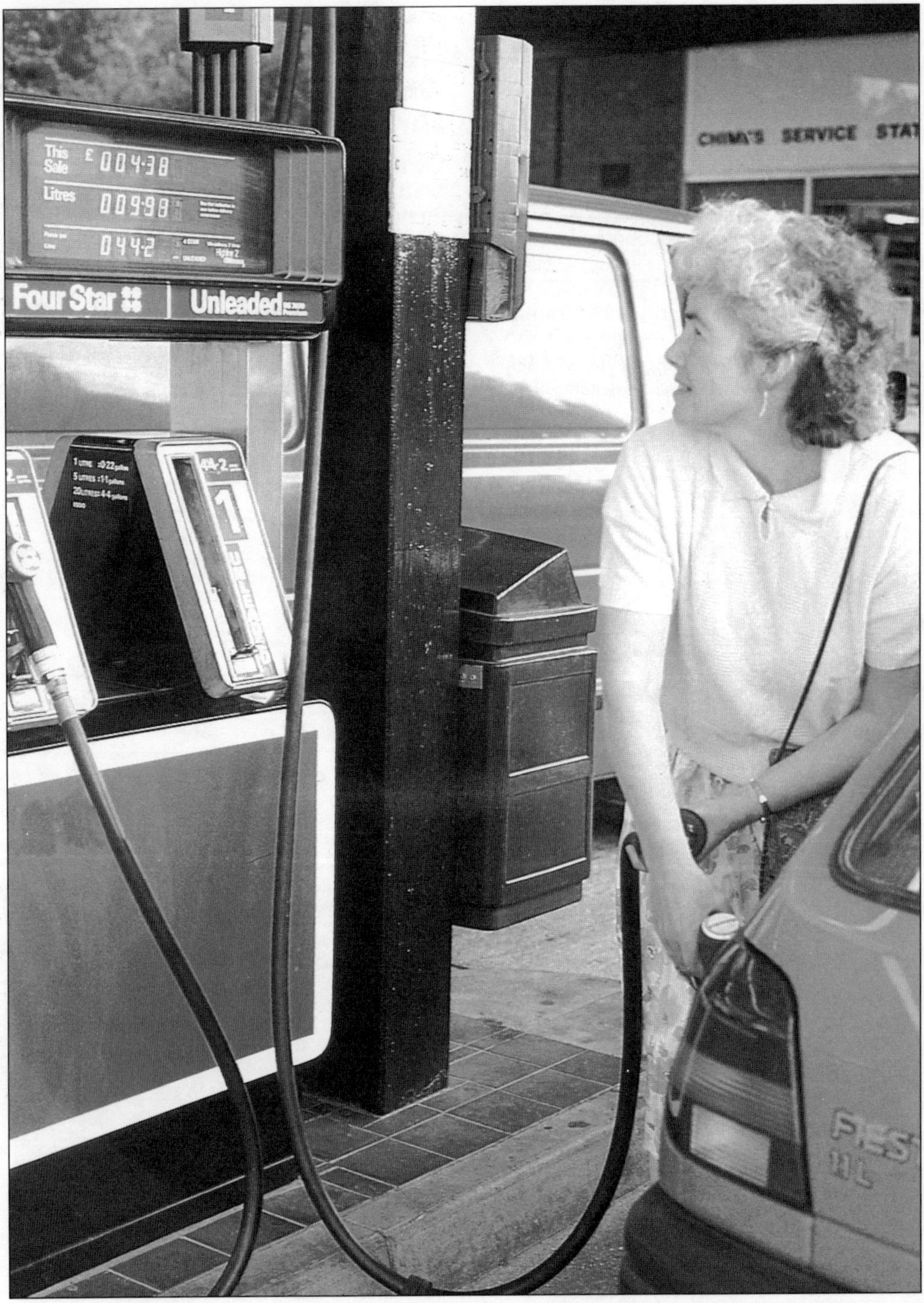
CHIMA'S SERVICE STAT
This Sale £ 004·38
Litres 0099.8
044·2
Four Star
Unleaded

ECONOMICAL DRIVING

Owning a car is always going to involve some expense, and the running costs can generally be divided into two main areas. The first concerns fixed costs which cannot be avoided, such as car tax and insurance (although obviously you can shop around for the best insurance quote). However, for most owners savings can be made in the second main area of expense, which covers fuel costs and servicing/maintenance bills.

It's surprisingly easy to reduce the amount of fuel used, simply by adapting your driving style to suit the prevailing conditions, and avoiding certain driving habits which tend to increase fuel consumption unnecessarily.

A large proportion of the average servicing bill is made up of garage labour time, money which can be saved by carrying out the work yourself. Refer to *'Servicing'* on page 77 for easy-to-follow instructions on how to carry out most servicing work. It's also worth bearing in mind that maintenance costs can be cut significantly by reducing unnecessary wear-and-tear on the car.

The following advice deals with the most significant causes of high fuel consumption and unnecessary wear-and-tear, and explains how to save money and reduce environmental pollution during everyday driving.

- **Don't warm the engine up with the car standing still** – Engine wear and pollution is at its highest when the engine is warming up, and the engine takes a long time to warm up when running at idle speed with the car stationary. To avoid excessive wear and pollution, drive off as soon as the engine starts, and don't use more 'revs' than necessary.
- **On cars with a manual choke, don't use the choke any longer than necessary** – Push the choke control fully in as soon as the engine will run smoothly without it. When the engine is running with the choke applied, extra fuel is being used and so the fuel consumption is increased, and more pollution is produced.
- **Avoid sudden full throttle acceleration** – Sudden acceleration increases fuel consumption, engine wear and pollution.
- **Don't drive at high engine speeds** – Minimum fuel consumption and pollution is achieved at low engine speeds and in the highest possible gear. Lower engine speed also means less noise and engine wear. For maximum economy, stay in as high a gear as possible for as long as possible, without making the engine labour.
- **Don't always drive at maximum speed** – Fuel consumption, pollution and noise increase rapidly at high speeds. A small reduction in speed (particularly during motorway driving) can significantly lower fuel consumption and pollution.
- **Look well ahead, and drive as smoothly as possible** – By looking well ahead you will be able to react to any change in road conditions in plenty of time, allowing you to brake and accelerate smoothly. Unnecessary or harsh acceleration and braking increases fuel consumption and pollution.
- **Where possible, avoid dense, slow-moving traffic** – In these conditions, more frequent braking, acceleration and gear changing are required, which increase fuel consumption and pollution.
- **Stop the engine during traffic hold-ups** – Obviously if your engine has stopped it doesn't use any fuel and there is no pollution.

- **Check the tyre pressures regularly** – Low tyre pressures increase the rolling resistance of the car, and therefore increase fuel consumption, as well as increasing tyre wear and causing handling problems.
- **Don't carry unnecessary luggage** – Weight has a significant effect on fuel consumption, especially in dense traffic where frequent acceleration is required.
- **Don't leave a roof rack fitted when not in use** – The extra air resistance increases fuel consumption.
- **Switch off any unnecessary electrical circuits as soon as possible** – Heated rear windows, foglights, heater blowers, etc, consume a considerable amount of electrical power. The engine must work harder to provide this power by driving the alternator, and the fuel consumption is therefore increased.
- **Check the fuel consumption regularly** – By doing this you will be able to notice any significant increase in fuel consumption, and any problem which may be causing it can be investigated before it develops into anything more serious.
- **Ensure that your car is serviced regularly** – This will ensure that the car operates as efficiently as possible, reducing fuel consumption and pollution.
- **If your car engine is suitable, use unleaded petrol** – This will reduce pollution. If in any doubt as to whether your car's engine is suitable for use with unleaded petrol, seek advice from the car's manufacturer, or from a recognised dealer.

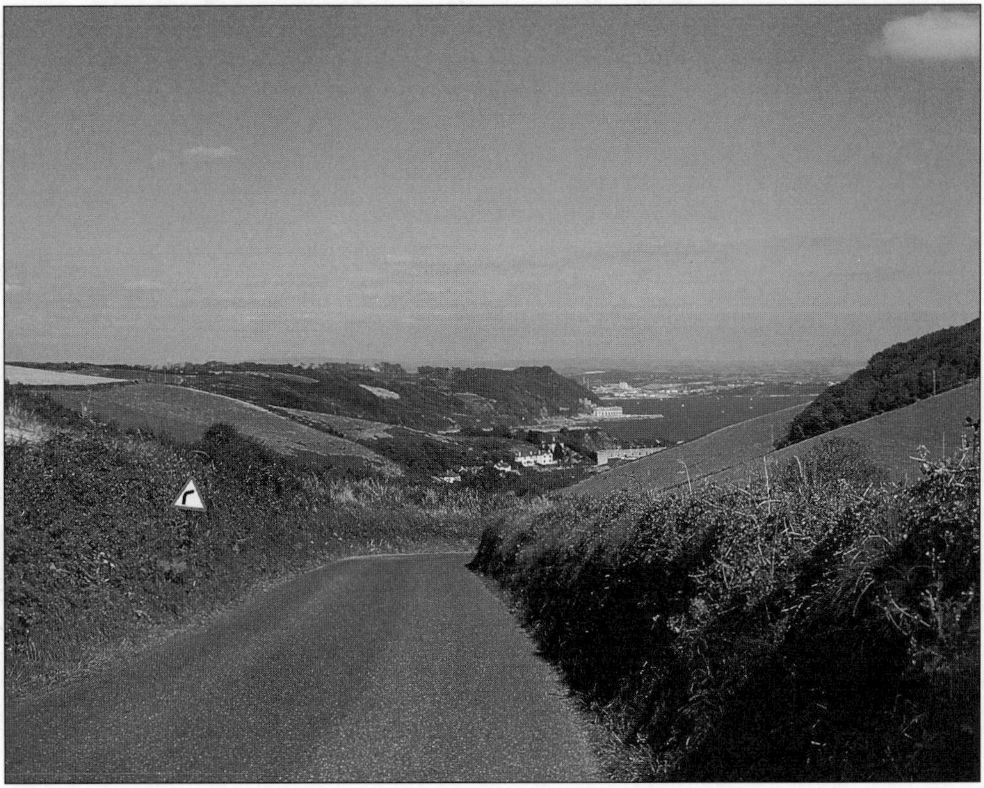

Crime against cars is a serious problem, and many owners suffer the consequences of theft or damage every year. The likelihood of your car becoming a target for criminals can be reduced by making it more difficult for your car to be broken into or stolen, and the following advice should prove helpful. Some of the points may seem obvious, but the majority of cars are broken into or stolen in a very short space of time with little force or effort required.

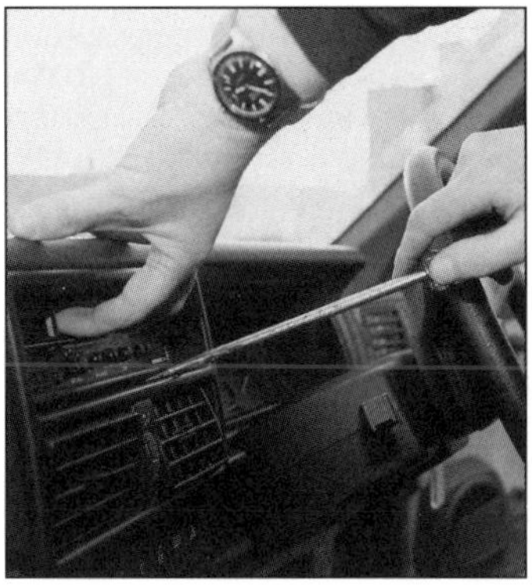

- **Always remove the ignition key** – even in a garage or driveway at home. Always make sure that the steering column lock is engaged after removing the key.
- **Always lock your car** – even in a garage or driveway at home. Where fitted, ensure that 'deadlocks' are engaged before leaving the car and, where applicable, don't forget to lock the fuel filler cover. Make sure that all the windows and the sunroof or folding roof, where applicable, are properly shut. If the car is in a garage, lock the garage. If your car is stolen or broken into while it's unlocked, your insurance company may not pay for the full value of loss or damage.
- **Never leave valuable items on display** – Even if you're only leaving your car for a few minutes, move anything that might be attractive to a thief (even a coat or briefcase) out of sight, and preferably take it with you or lock it safely in the boot. Don't leave valuable items (especially credit cards) in the glovebox. Don't leave your vehicle documents in the car (registration document, MOT certificate, insurance certificate, etc), as they could help a thief to sell it.
- **Park in a visible and (preferably) busy area** – This will deter thieves as they run a greater risk of being caught. If you're parking your car at night, try to leave it in a well-lit area.
- **Put your radio aerial down (where applicable) when parking** – Radio aerials can prove an attractive target for vandals.
- **Protect any in-car entertainment equipment** – The latest security-coded equipment won't work if someone tampers with it and disconnects it from the battery. Some equipment is specially designed so that you can remove the control panel or the entire unit, and take it with you when you leave the car.
- **Fit lockable wheel nuts (or bolts, as applicable)** – if your car is fitted with expensive alloy wheels. Alloy wheels are a favourite target for thieves.
- **Have your car windows etched with the registration number** – This will help to trace your car if it's stolen and the thieves try to change its identity. Other glass components such as sunroofs and headlamps can also be etched if desired. Many garages and specialists can provide this service, and it's possible to buy DIY glass etching kits from motor accessory shops if you prefer to tackle the job yourself.
- **Fit a vehicle immobiliser device** – Many different types are available, but the most common types consist of a substantial metal bar which can be locked in place between the steering wheel and the pedals to prevent the car from being driven.
- **Have an alarm fitted** – Many different types are available, and some are expensive, but they will deter thieves. Some alarms have built-in immobiliser devices to prevent the car from being driven. If you have an alarm fitted, remember to switch it on even if you're only leaving the car for a few minutes.

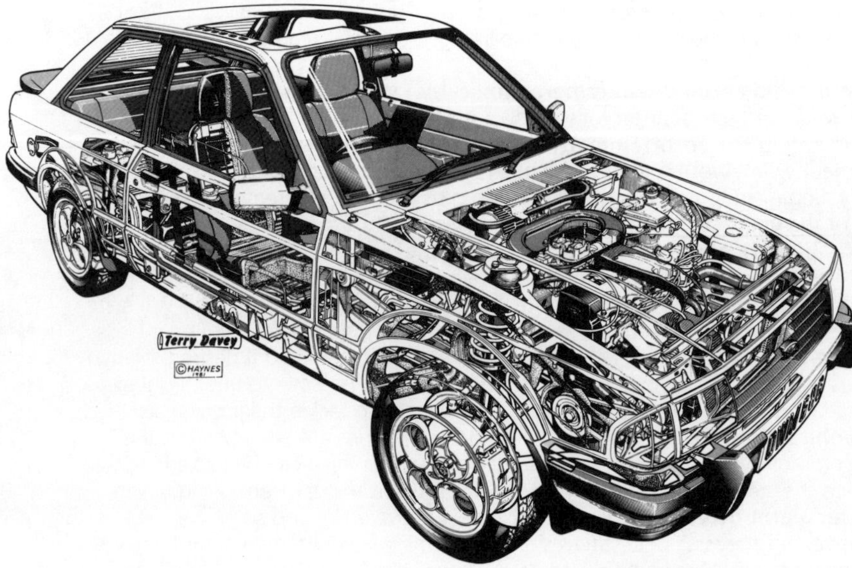
Terry Davey
©HAYNES

Lubricant and fluid capacities [Litres (Pints)]

Fuel tank capacity

Models up to May 1983	**40**	(8.8 gallons)
Models from May 1983	**48**	(10.6 gallons)

Engine oil

Quantity of oil required to bring level on dipstick from 'MIN' to 'MAX' mark	**1.0**	(1.8)

Engine oil capacity (for oil change)

OHV engines	**3.25**	(5.7)
CVH engines:		
Carburettor models up to July 1982	**3.75**	(6.6)
Carburettor models from July 1982	**3.50**	(6.2)
Fuel injection models	**3.85**	(6.8)

Coolant capacity (for coolant change)

1.1 litre OHV engine	**6.7**	(11.8)
1.1 litre CVH engine:		
With small radiator	**6.2**	(11.0)
With large radiator	**7.2**	(12.6)
1.3 litre OHV engine	**7.1**	(12.5)
1.3 litre CVH engine:		
Models up to 1986	**7.1**	(12.5)
Models from 1986	**7.6**	(13.3)
1.4 litre CVH engine	**7.6**	(13.3)
1.6 litre CVH engine:		
Models up to 1986	**6.9**	(12.1)
Models from 1986	**7.8**	(13.7)

Contact breaker points [mm (in)]

Points gap

Bosch distributor	**0.40** to **0.50**	(0.016 to 0.020)
Lucas distributor	**0.40** to **0.59**	(0.016 to 0.023)

Spark plugs

Type	Motorcraft	Champion
OHV engines	**AGRF 22**	**RS9YCC** or **RS9YC**
CVH engines:		
Carburettor models	**AGPR 22C**	**RC7YCC** or **RC7YC**
Fuel injection models (except RS Turbo)	**AGPR 12C**	**C6YCC** or **RC6YC**
RS Turbo models	**AGPR 901C1**	**C59C**

Electrode gap [mm (inches)**]**

Motorcraft plugs:		
All models except RS Turbo	**0.75**	(0.030)
RS Turbo models	**1.00**	(0.040)
Champion plugs:		
RS9YCC, RC7YCC and **C6YCC** plugs	**0.80**	(0.032)
RS9YC, RC7YC, RC6YC and **C59C** plugs	**0.70**	(0.028)

Tyre pressures – cold [bar (lbf/in^2)]

Note: *The following is intended as a guide only. Manufacturers frequently change tyre pressure recommendations, and it is suggested that a Ford dealer is consulted for latest recommendations.*

Escort Models	Front	Rear
Up to 3 occupants:		
145 SR 13 tyres (models up to 1986)	**1.8** (26)	**1.8** (26)
145 SR 13 tyres (models from 1986)	**1.6** (23)	**2.0** (29)
155 SR or TR 13 tyres (manual gearbox models)	**1.6** (23)	**2.0** (29)
155 SR or TR 13 tyres (automatic transmission models)	**1.8** (26)	**2.0** (29)
175/70 SR or HR 13 tyres	**1.8** (26)	**1.8** (26)
175/65 HR 14 tyres	**1.6** (23)	**2.0** (29)
185/60 HR 13 tyres	**1.8** (26)	**1.8** (26)
185/60 HR 14 tyres	**1.6** (23)	**2.0** (29)
195/50 VR 15 tyres	**1.8** (26)	**1.8** (26)
Fully laden:		
All except 195/50 VR 15 tyres	**2.0** (29)	**2.4** (33)
195/50 VR 15 tyres	**1.8** (26)	**2.0** (29)

Orion models		
Up to 3 occupants:		
All except models with 155 SR or TR 13 tyres and automatic transmission, and 1600E models	**1.6** (23)	**2.0** (29)
Models with 155 SR or TR 13 tyres and automatic transmission, and 1600E models	**1.8** (26)	**2.0** (29)
Fully laden (all models)	**2.0** (28)	**2.3** (33)

Recommended lubricants and fluids

Component/system	Lubricant/fluid type and specification	Duckhams recommendation
ENGINE	Multigrade engine oil, viscosity range SAE 10W/30 to 20W/50	Duckhams QXR, QS, Hypergrade Plus or Hypergrade
COOLING SYSTEM	55% clean water and 45% antifreeze to Ford specification SSM-97B-9103-A	Duckhams Universal Antifreeze and Summer Coolant
BRAKE SYSTEM	Brake fluid to Ford specification SAM-6C 9103-A	Duckhams Universal Brake and Clutch Fluid
MANUAL GEARBOX	Hypoid gear oil, viscosity SAE 80EP to Ford specification SQM-2C 9008-A	Duckhams Hypoid 80
AUTOMATIC TRANSMISSION	**Early type conventional transmission** Automatic transmission fluid to Ford specification SQM-2C 9010-A or ESP-M2C 138-CJ	Duckhams Uni-Matic
	Later type conventional transmission (black dipstick) and CTX transmission Automatic transmission fluid to Ford specification ESP-M2C 166-H	Duckhams Uni-Matic

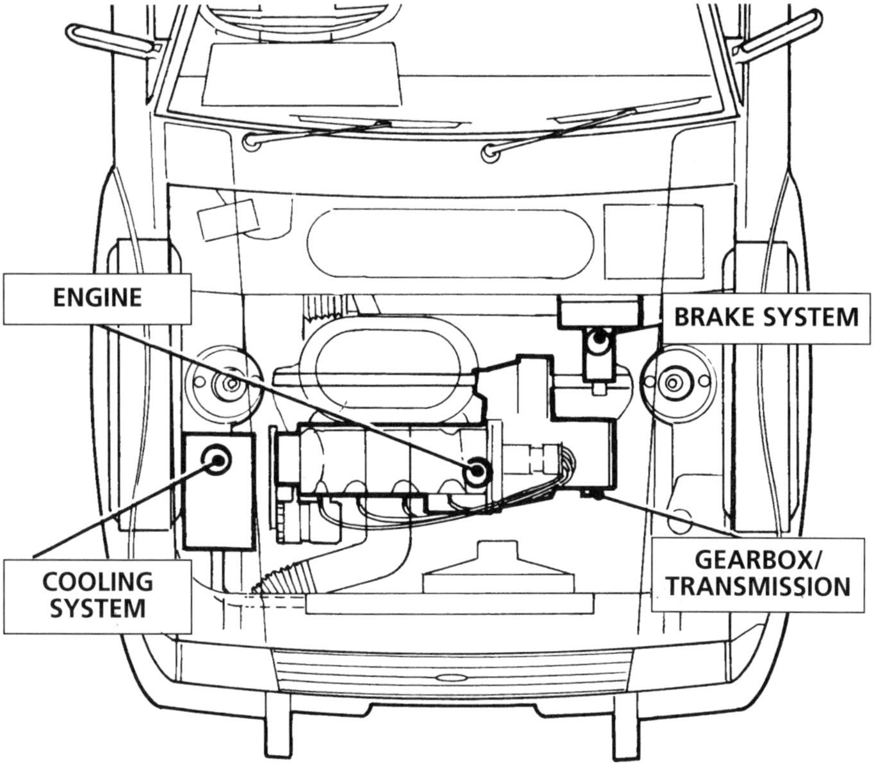

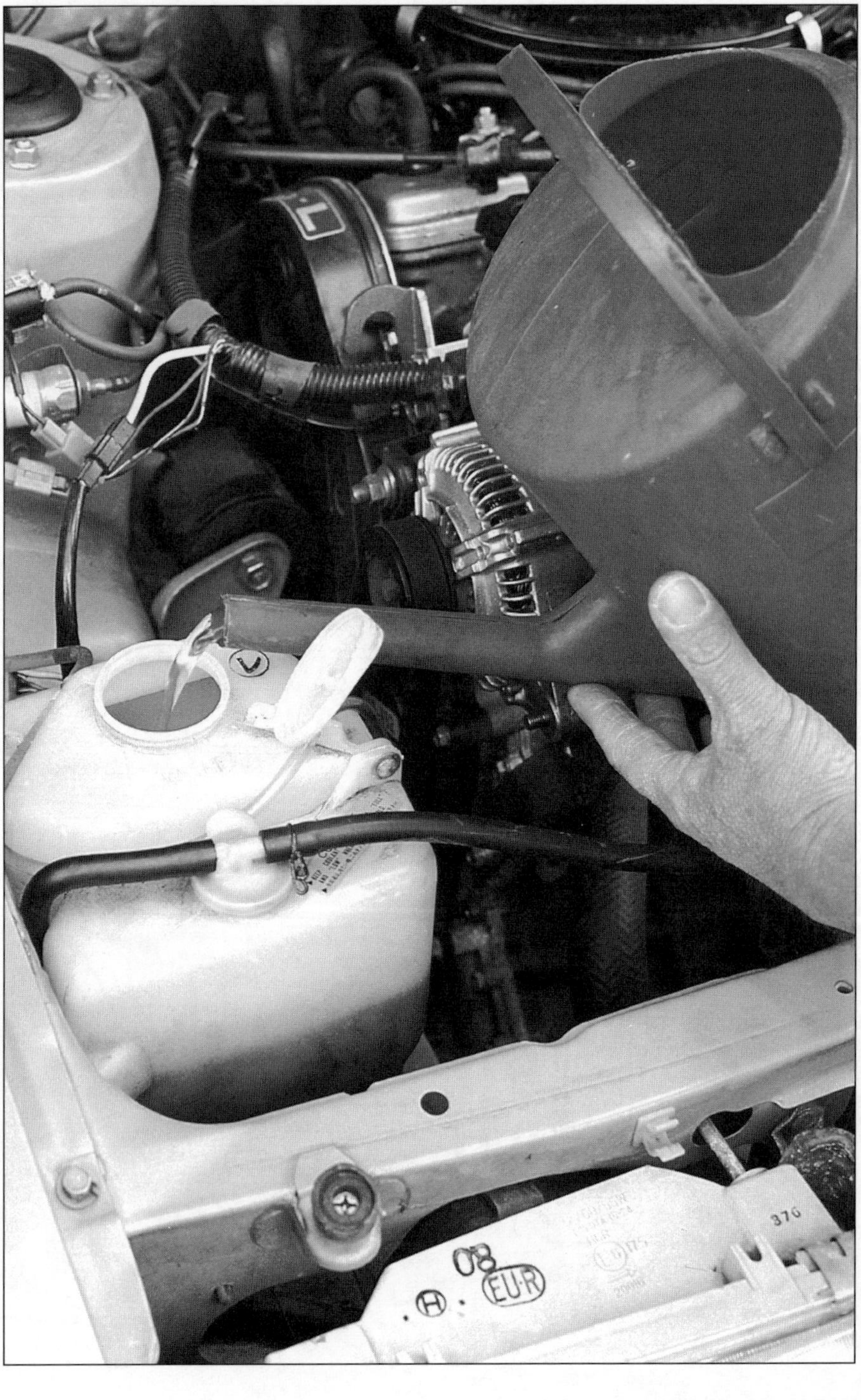
08
EU-R
376

To ensure that your car is reliable and safe to drive, there are one or two essential checks which are so simple that they're often ignored. These checks only take a few minutes, and could save you a lot of inconvenience and expense. It's a good idea to carry out these checks once a week, and certainly before you start off on a long journey. This Section explains how to carry out the checks, and what to do if things aren't quite as they should be.

Whenever you're carrying out checks or servicing jobs, safety must always be the first consideration, and you should bear in mind the advice given in the *'Safety first!'* notes on page 82 before proceeding.

CHECKS

The following checks should be carried out regularly. The checks are explained in more detail in the following pages.

- *Check the oil level*
- *Check the coolant level*
- *Check the brake fluid level*
- *Check the tyres*
- *Check the washer fluid level*
- *Check the battery electrolyte level (where applicable)*
- *Check the wipers and washers*
- *Check the lights*
- *Check for fluid leaks*

ITEMS REQUIRED WHEN CARRYING OUT CHECKS

When carrying out the regular checks, it's a good idea to have the following items close-to-hand. You won't always need all the items, but it's as well to have them available just in case.

● *Small quantity of clean rag* ● *Tyre pressure gauge and foot pump* ● *Small screwdriver (for removing stones from tyres)* ● *Pin (for adjusting washer nozzles)* ● *1.0 litre pack of engine oil (of the correct type - see* ***'Service specifications'*** *on page 67)* ● *Small quantity of coolant solution (made up from approximately 55% clean water and 45% antifreeze)* ● *Small container of brake fluid (must be an airtight container)* ● *Washer fluid additive* ● *Small quantity of distilled water - for models fitted with batteries which require topping up*

Note: *For details of how to identify OHV and CVH engines, refer to* ***'Servicing'*** *on page 90.*

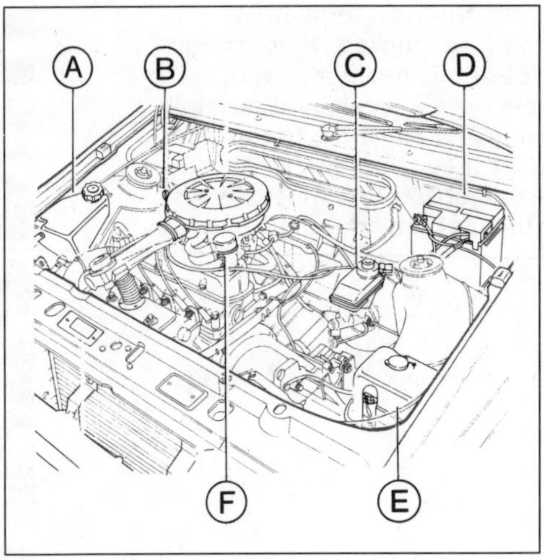

▲ *Typical engine compartment – OHV engine models (CVH engine models similar)*
A *Coolant expansion tank*
B *Oil level dipstick*
C *Brake fluid reservoir*
D *Battery*
E *Washer fluid reservoir*
F *Oil filler cap*

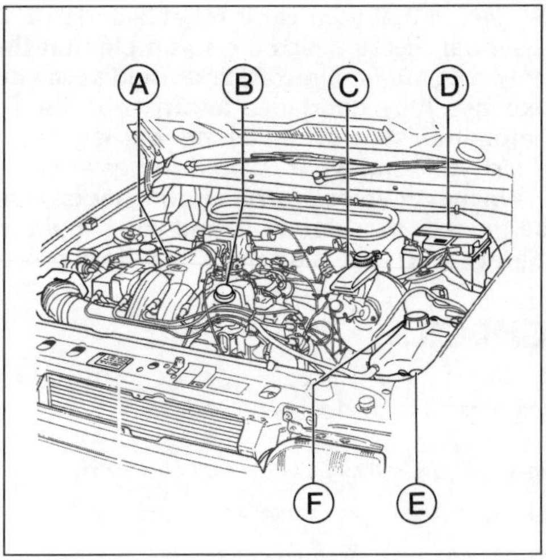

▲ *Typical engine compartment – later 1.6 litre fuel injection models (except RS Turbo) from August 1989 approx*
A *Oil level dipstick*
B *Oil filler cap*
C *Brake fluid reservoir*
D *Battery*
E *Washer fluid reservoir*
F *Coolant expansion tank*

Checking oil level

To check the oil level, the car should be standing on level ground, and the engine should have been stopped for at least five minutes.

Open the bonnet, and look for the oil dipstick, which is at the back of the engine on the right-hand side (when viewed from the driver's seat). Pull out the dipstick and wipe it clean (with a clean non-fluffy cloth), then slowly push it back into its tube and pull it out again. On some models, an oil level sensor is fitted to the dipstick so, where applicable, take care not to damage the wires when moving the dipstick. Note the oil level, which should never be allowed to drop below the 'MIN' mark.

If the oil needs topping up, pull the oil filler cap from the top of the engine, and top up to the 'MAX' mark on the dipstick. Note that the amount of oil required to raise the level on the dipstick from the 'MIN' to the 'MAX' mark is approximately 1.0 litre (1.75 pints). Always try to use the same type and make of oil, and take care not to overfill. Mop up any oil which might have been spilt, and make sure that the oil filler cap is correctly refitted.

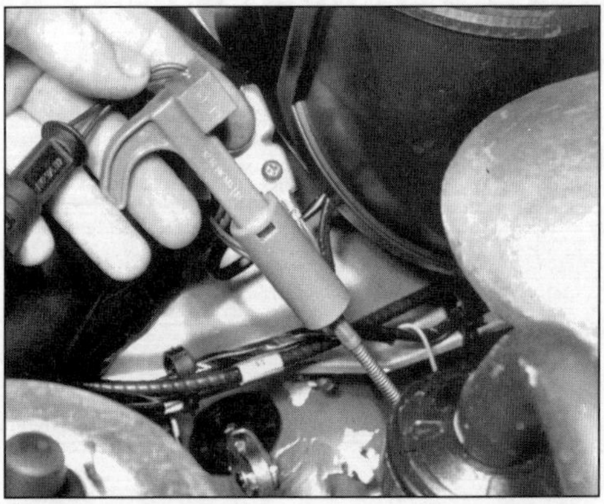

▲ *Removing the engine oil level dipstick (model with oil level sensor)*

If the oil needs to be topped up regularly, check for leaks, and if necessary seek advice.

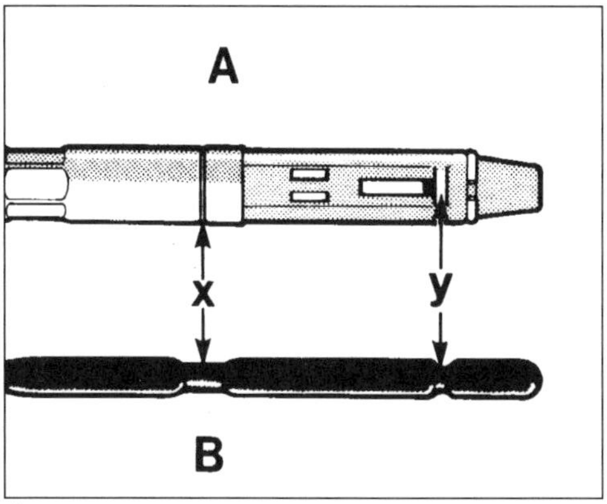

▲ *Engine oil level dipstick markings (markings may vary depending on model)*
A Dipstick with oil level sensor
B Standard dipstick
x Maximum oil level
y Minimum oil level

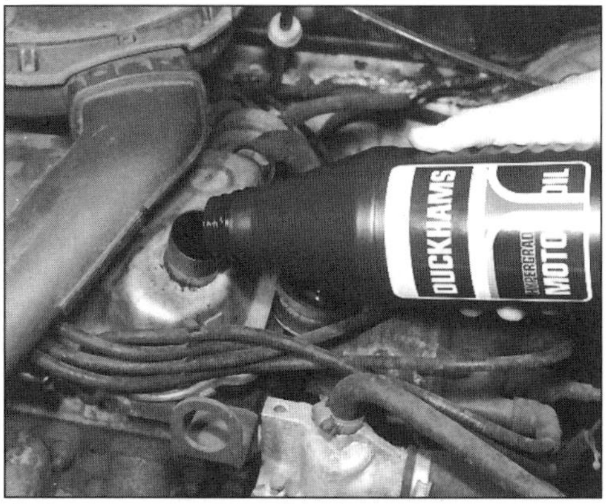

▲ *Topping up the engine oil level*

Checking coolant level

The coolant level can be checked visually by checking the level in the expansion tank when the engine is **cold**. The level should be between the 'MIN' and 'MAX' marks on the side of the tank.

If topping up is necessary, first the cooling system pressure cap must be removed.

Topping up should always be done with the engine cold, but if it does prove necessary to remove the cooling system pressure cap with the engine hot for any reason, take care to

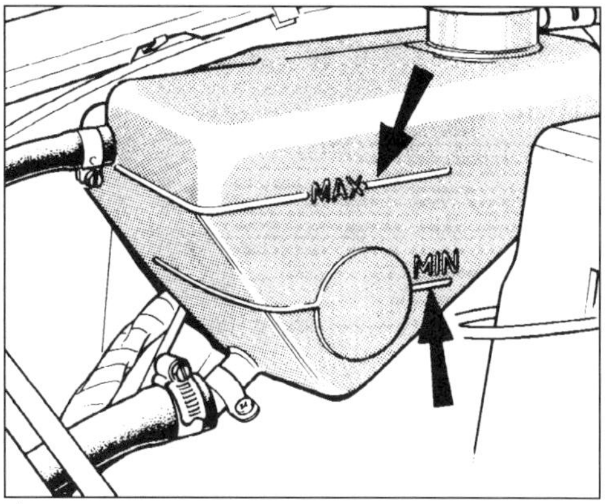

▲ *Coolant level markings (arrowed) on expansion tank*

avoid scalding. Place a thick rag over the cap, and loosen the cap slowly in stages to gradually release the pressure in the system.

On early models, the pressure cap may be located either on the expansion tank or on the thermostat housing, depending on model. Where the pressure cap is fitted to the thermostat housing, a simple 'lift' type cap will be fitted to the expansion tank. Note that the thermostat housing is located at the right-hand end of the engine on OHV engines, and at the left-hand end of the engine on CVH engines (when viewed from the driver's seat). To remove the pressure cap, slowly turn it anti-clockwise until it reaches its stop. Wait until any pressure in the system has escaped, then press the cap down and turn it further in an anti-clockwise direction. Release the downward

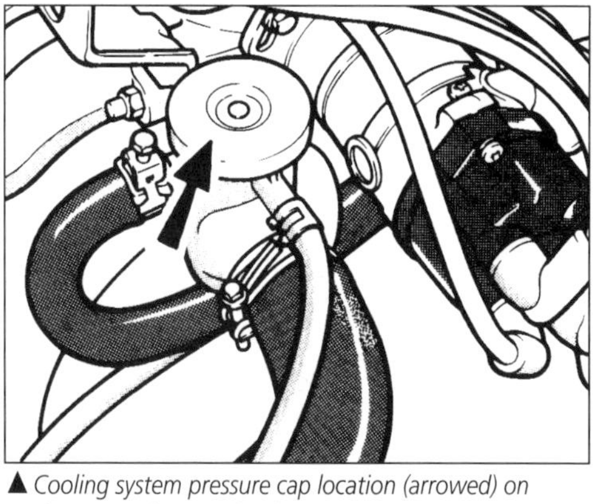

▲ *Cooling system pressure cap location (arrowed) on thermostat housing (early CVH engine model)*

pressure slowly and remove the cap. Now lift up the filler cap on the expansion tank.

On later models, a screw type pressure cap is fitted to the expansion tank and the cap on the

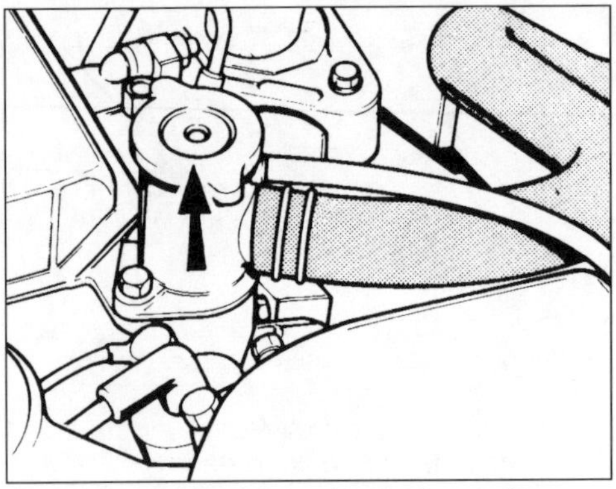

▲ *Cooling system pressure cap location (arrowed) on thermostat housing (early OHV engine model)*

thermostat housing is omitted. On these models, slowly unscrew the cap a quarter of a turn, wait for the pressure in the system to be released, then remove the cap.

Coolant should be added through the expansion tank. Topping up should always be done with a mixture of water and antifreeze to the same strength as the mixture already in the system. Although plain water can be used, it's unwise to make it a habit, as the strength of the antifreeze in the main system will gradually be diluted. If there's any doubt about the strength of the coolant mixture, it's better to add too much antifreeze than not enough.

Normally, topping up will rarely be required, and if the need for regular topping up arises, it will probably be due to a leak somewhere in the system. Leaks are most likely to occur from the radiator or the various hoses. If no leaks can be found, it's possible that there's an internal fault in the engine, such as a crack in the cylinder head, or a blown cylinder head gasket, but in this case it's best to seek specialist advice. It's important to note that because of the different types of metals used in the engine, it's vital to use antifreeze with suitable anti-corrosion additives all year round. **Never** use plain water to fill the whole system.

Checking brake fluid level

Note: *Refer to* ***'Safety first'*** *on page 82 for special precautions which should be taken when handling brake fluid.*

Although a low brake fluid level warning light is fitted, the fluid level should be checked visually whenever the oil and coolant levels are checked. The level should be up to the 'MAX' mark on the side of the reservoir, but it will fall slightly as the brake friction material wears. The fluid level must **never** be allowed to drop below the 'MIN' mark.

If topping up is required, always use the correct type of fluid, which should always be stored in a full, air-tight container. Don't top up using fluid which has been stored in a partly

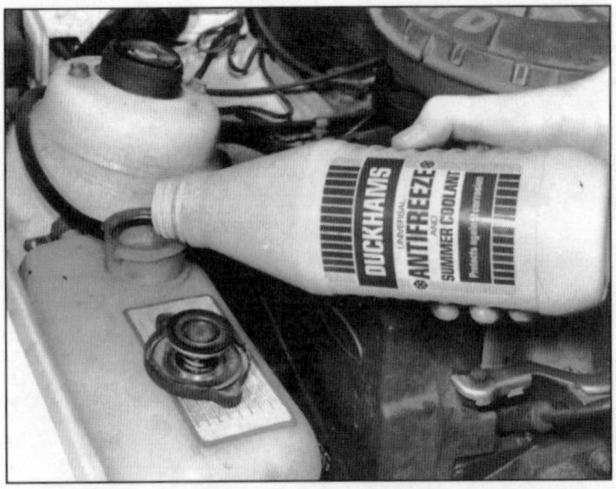

▲ *Topping up the coolant level through the expansion tank*

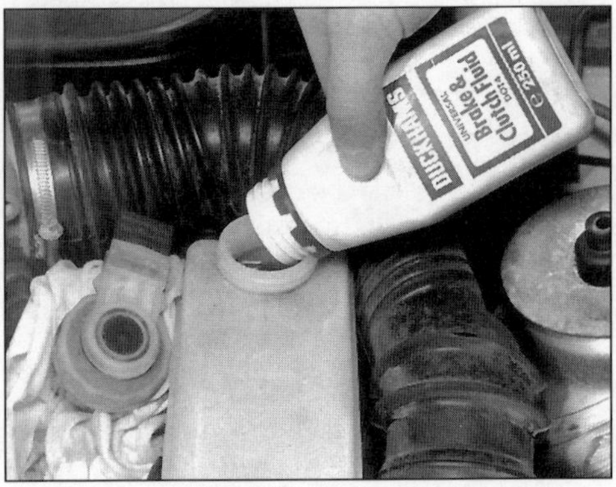

▲ *Topping up the brake fluid level*

full container, as it will have absorbed moisture from the air which can reduce its performance.

Topping up should hardly ever be required unless there's a leak somewhere in the hydraulic system. If a leak is suspected, the car should not be driven until the braking system has been thoroughly checked. **Never** take any risks where brakes are concerned.

Checking tyres

It's extremely important to carry out regular checks on the tyres to make sure that the pressures are correct, and that the tyres are not damaged. The tyres are the only part of the car in contact with the road, and so their condition will affect the steering and general handling of the car, and therefore its safety.

To check tyre pressures accurately, the tyres must be cold, which means that the car must not have been driven recently. Note that it can make a noticeable difference to the tyre pressures if the car has been standing out in the sun. This can be very noticeable when one side of the car is in the sun, and the other side is in shadow.

Note that the recommended tyre pressures vary depending on the size of tyres fitted – refer to '*Service specifications*' on page 66. The size of the tyre (eg 155 SR 13) is clearly marked on the tyre sidewall, although the style of the tyre size marking may vary depending on the tyre manufacturer – consult a Ford dealer or a tyre specialist for further details of tyre size markings and the latest pressure recommendations.

If the tyres are being checked after the car has been driven, for example when filling up with petrol during a journey, the pressures are bound to be higher than specified. It's best to simply check that the pressures in the two front

Shoulder wear | **Centre wear** | **Uneven wear** | **Toe wear**

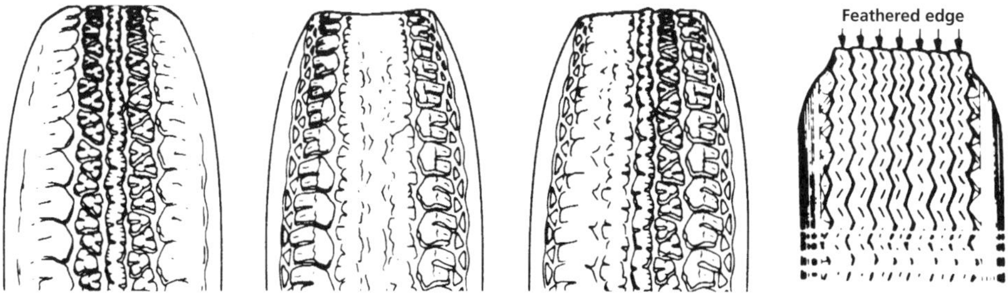

Shoulder wear

Probable cause:
Underinflation (wear on both sides)
Action: Check and adjust pressure

Probable cause:
Incorrect wheel camber (wear on one side)
Action: Repair or renew suspension parts

Probable cause:
Hard cornering
Action: Reduce speed

Centre wear

Probable cause:
Overinflation
Action: Measure and adjust pressure

Uneven wear

Probable cause:
Incorrect camber or castor
Action: Repair or renew suspension parts

Probable cause:
Malfunctioning suspension
Action: Repair or renew suspension parts

Probable cause
Unbalanced wheel
Action: Balance tyres

Probable cause:
Out-of-round brake disc/drum
Action: Machine or renew disc/drum

Toe wear

Probable cause:
Incorrect toe setting
Action: Adjust front wheel alignment

▲ *Tyre wear patterns and causes*

tyres are equal, and similarly for the two back tyres (remember that the specified pressure for the rear tyres may be different to the front). Never let air out of the tyres of a car which has been driven to bring the pressures down to that specified (unless the tyre pressures have been increased for a fully loaded car, and the load has just been reduced).

When checking the tyre pressures, don't forget to check the spare!

With the tyres properly inflated, run your fingers around the edge of the tyre to check for any cuts and bulges in the tyre walls. Ideally, the car should be jacked up to visually check the tyres all round but, alternatively, the car can be moved backwards and forwards to enable you to check all round the tread. Check all round the tread for cuts, and remove any debris, such as small stones and broken glass, using a screwdriver or similar tool. Any large items such as nails which have penetrated the surface of the tyre should be left in the tread (to identify the location of the damage) until the tyre has been repaired. Refer to *'Breakdowns'* on page 42, for details of how to fit the spare wheel.

Also check the tyre treads for wear. Uneven wear across one particular tyre may be due to a fault with the suspension or steering. By law, the tread depth must be at least 1.6 mm (0.06 in) throughout a continuous band comprising the central three-quarters of the width of the tyre tread around the full circumference of the tyre.

If you find that any of the tyres is excessively worn or damaged, obtain a new tyre as soon as possible. It's a good idea to try and stick to one type of tyre if possible, rather than mixing several different makes on the car. Generally, you'll find that it's much cheaper to buy tyres from a tyre specialist, rather than an ordinary garage. Make sure that when you buy a new tyre you have the wheel balanced, otherwise you might find that the new tyre causes vibration when driving.

Checking washer fluid level

The windscreen washer fluid reservoir is located at the front left-hand side of the engine compartment (when viewed from the driver's seat).

On early models with a tailgate washer system, the tailgate washer fluid reservoir is located behind a panel at the left-hand side of the boot, or in the spare wheel well on some Estate models.

On later models, the tailgate washer and windscreen washer systems share the same reservoir in the engine compartment.

On certain RS Turbo models, and cars fitted with headlamp washers, the fluid reservoir is located under the left-hand front wing, and the reservoir cap is fitted with a dipstick to check the fluid level.

If topping up is necessary, pull the cap from the reservoir, and top up as necessary with clean water. A suitable washer fluid additive will keep the glass free from smears, and will prevent the fluid freezing in winter.

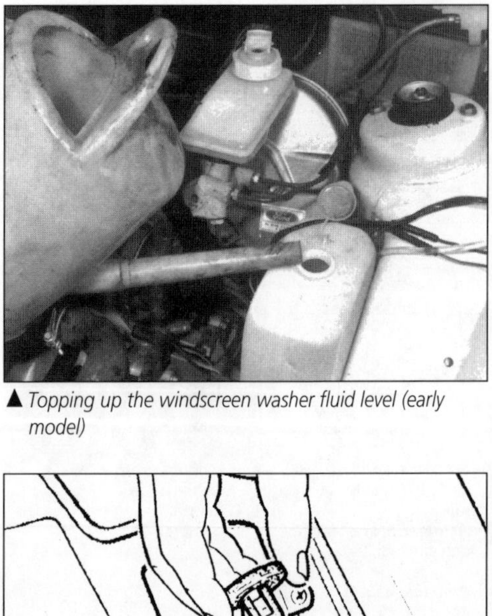

▲ *Topping up the windscreen washer fluid level (early model)*

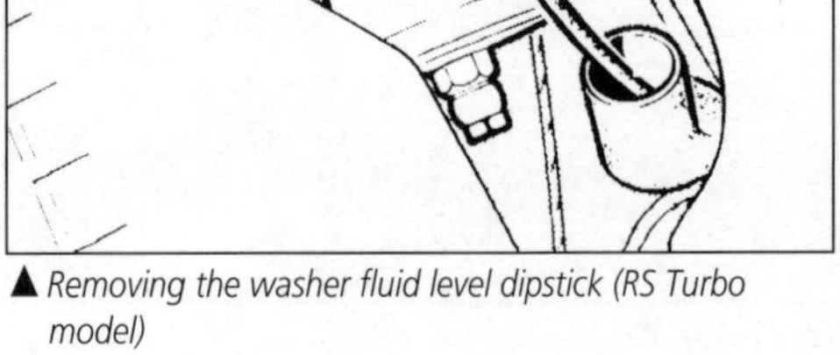

▲ *Removing the washer fluid level dipstick (RS Turbo model)*

Checking battery electrolyte level

From approximately 1982, Ford cars have been fitted with a maintenance-free battery during production. The maintenance-free battery is 'sealed for life', and does not require topping up with distilled water. A maintenance-free battery is usually clearly marked, and there will be no removable covers to enable topping up.

On early models with a standard or low maintenance type battery, or on later models where the battery has been replaced by one of this type from another source, the electrolyte level should be checked as follows.

The battery is located at the rear left-hand side of the engine compartment (when viewed from the driver's seat). Remove the caps or the cover from the top of the battery, and check the level of the electrolyte fluid (with some types of battery you can see the fluid level through the battery case). The level should be just above the tops of the metal plates inside the battery, or in some cases up to a mark on the battery case.

If necessary, add distilled water (not ordinary tap water) to each cell to bring the level just above the tops of the battery plates or up to the marks, as applicable. With some types of battery, distilled water is added to a trough in the top of the battery until all the filling slots are full, and the bottom of the trough is just covered. On completion, refit the caps or cover, and carefully wipe up any drops of water that were spilt.

Topping up should hardly ever be required, and the need for frequent topping up indicates that the battery is being overcharged due to a fault in the charging circuit – seek advice from someone suitably qualified if this is the case.

Checking wipers and washers

Check all the wipers and washers to make sure that they're working properly. Don't allow the wipers to work on dry glass for too long, as it will strain the motor. If necessary, the washer nozzles can be adjusted using a pin inserted into the end of the nozzle. If you're adjusting the windscreen washer nozzles, remember to aim them fairly high on the windscreen, as the airflow will usually deflect the spray down when the car is moving.

Over a period of time, the wiping action of the wiper blades will deteriorate, causing smearing of the glass. The rubber may also crack, particularly at the edges of the blades. When this happens, the blades must be renewed. This is a straightforward job, and is accomplished as follows:

Pull the wiper arm away from the glass, against the spring pressure, until the arm clicks into position. Press the small retaining clip on the blade, then slide the blade out of the hooked part of the arm. The blade can be renewed complete, or the rubber insert can be renewed as follows:

The rubber is held in the arm by a metal spring clip at one end. Slide back the rubber from the end of the blade, then squeeze the spring clip and pull it from the blade. The

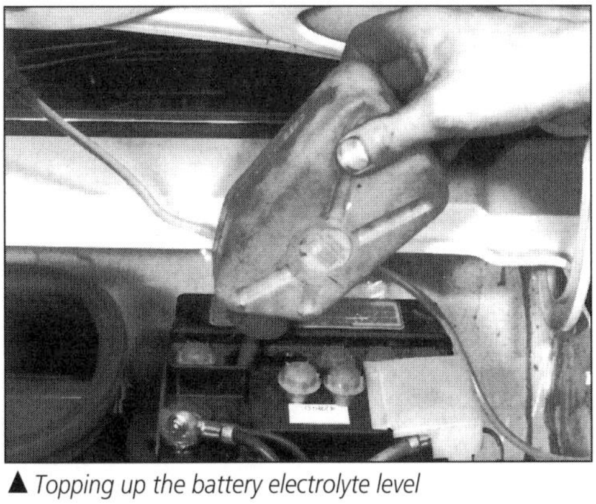

▲ *Topping up the battery electrolyte level*

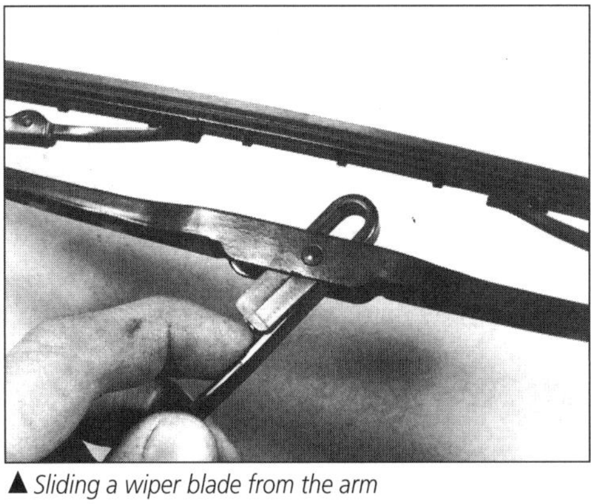

▲ *Sliding a wiper blade from the arm*

rubber can now be slid from the end of the blade. Fit the new rubber and/or the blade by reversing the removal operations.

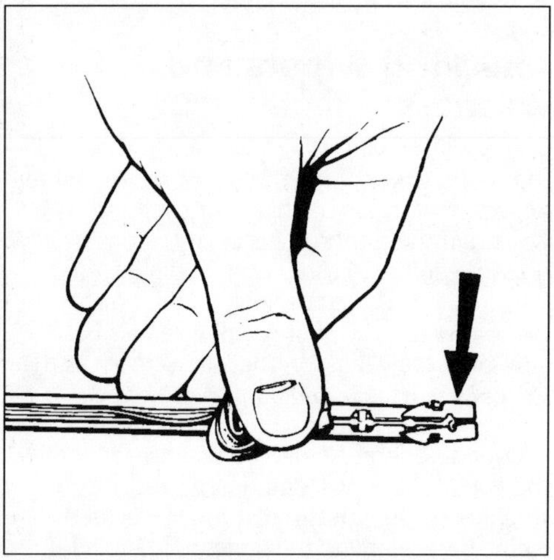

▲ *Sliding back the wiper blade rubber to expose the spring clip (arrowed)*

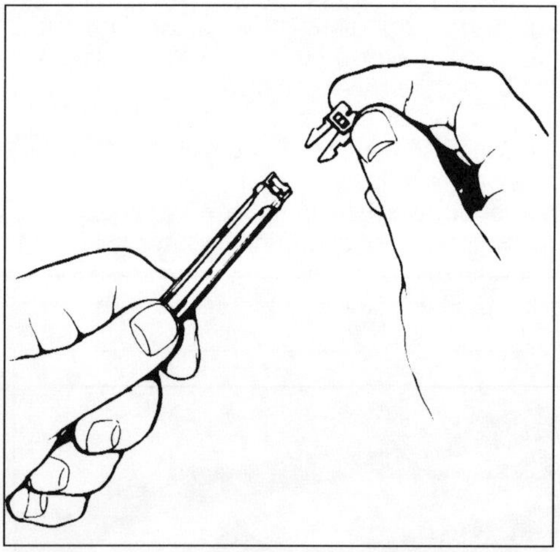

▲ *Removing the spring clip from the wiper blade*

Checking lights

Switch on all the lights and check that they're working. Don't forget to check the direction indicators and the brake lights (the ignition must be switched on to check these), either with the help of an assistant, or by looking for the reflection in a suitable window or door etc.

Check that the direction indicators work with the brake lights on, and that the brake lights work with the tail lights on. Some faults may cause the various rear lights to interact, which can be dangerous.

If any of the bulbs need renewing, refer to *'Bulb, fuse and relay renewal'* on page 113. Any other problems are likely to be caused by a faulty switch, or loose or corroded connections (especially earth connections), and it's best to seek advice to solve these.

Checking for fluid leaks

Check the ground where the car is normally parked for any stains or spots of fluid which may have been caused by fluid leaking from the car.

Open the bonnet, and make a quick check of all the hoses and pipes, and the surfaces of all the components in the engine compartment. If there's any sign of leaking fluid, try to find the source of the leak and seek advice if necessary. It can be difficult to identify leaking fluids, but if there's obviously a major leak, or if you suspect even a slight brake fluid or petrol leak, don't drive the car until the problem has been investigated by someone suitably qualified.

Regular servicing will ensure that your car is reliable and safe to drive, and could save you a lot of money in the long run. Many of the unexpected expenses which can crop up if things go wrong with your car can be avoided by carrying out regular servicing.

A significant proportion of the average garage servicing bill (well over 50% in many cases) is made up of labour costs, so obviously a lot of money can be saved by carrying out the work yourself. You'll find that most of the servicing jobs are very straightforward, and you don't need to be a mechanical genius to 'have a go' yourself. Don't be put off when you look under your bonnet; there are surprisingly few items which require frequent attention, and most of those which do are easily accessible without the need for anything more than basic tools. You'll discover that DIY servicing can be very rewarding, and will help you to understand what makes your car 'tick'.

The following chart lists all the servicing tasks recommended by the car manufacturer, and details of how to carry out the necessary work can be found in the subsequent pages. A few of the jobs require more extensive knowledge, or the use of special tools, and detailed explanation is beyond the scope of this Handbook. These more complicated tasks are identified on the chart, and details can be found in our Owners Workshop Manual for your particular model. Even if you decide to have the work done by a garage, the chart will enable you to check that the necessary work has been carried out.

Whenever you're carrying out servicing, safety must always be the first consideration, and you should read through the *'Safety first!'* notes on page 82 before proceeding any further.

ENGINE COMPARTMENT
Check all components for fluid leaks, corrosion or deterioration

ENGINE
Check engine oil level

Renew engine oil and filter

On OHV engines remove and clean oil filler cap

On OHV engines check valve clearances

On CVH engines renew timing belt

COOLING SYSTEM
Check coolant level

Renew coolant

FUEL AND EXHAUST SYSTEMS
Renew air cleaner filter element

On CVH engines renew crankcase emission control filter

On RS Turbo models check tightness of exhaust manifold nuts

Check idle speed and mixture settings

On RS Turbo models check tightness of turbocharger-to-exhaust manifold nuts

On fuel-injected engines renew fuel filter

IGNITION SYSTEM
Clean distributor cap (where applicable), coil and HT leads

Lubricate distributor (where applicable)

Check contact breaker points gap (where applicable)

On RS Turbo models renew spark plugs

On all models except RS Turbo renew spark plugs

Renew contact breaker points (where applicable)

Check ignition timing (where applicable)

MANUAL GEARBOX
Check gearbox oil level

AUTOMATIC TRANSMISSION
Check transmission fluid level

Check downshift linkage

Note: *In addition to the tasks listed in the table, Ford specify that on models fitted with CTX type automatic transmission, the transmission fluid should be renewed every 24 000 miles (40 000 km) or 1 year, whichever comes first. This job should be referred to a Ford dealer.*

REGULAR **Weekly**	**6000 miles** (10 000 km) **6 months**	**12 000 miles** (20 000 km) **1 year**	**24 000 miles** (40 000 km) **2 years**	**36 000 miles** (60 000 km) **3 years**
■	■	■	■	■
■	■	■	■	■
	■	■	■	■
	■	■	■	■
		□	□	□
				□
■	■	■	■	■
			■	
			■	
			■	
	□	□	□	□
	□	□	□	□
		□	□	□
			□	
	■	■	■	■
	■	■	■	■
	■	■	■	■
	■	■	■	■
		■	■	■
		■	■	■
	□	□	□	□
		■	■	■
		■	■	■
	□	□	□	□

Items marked □ are considered to be beyond the scope of this Handbook, and details can be found in the Owners Workshop Manual for your car (OWM 686 for Escort models, or OWM 1009 for Orion models).

BRAKING SYSTEM

Check brake fluid level

Check front disc pad friction material thickness

Check rear brake shoe friction material thickness

Inspect all components for leaks, deterioration and wear

Renew brake fluid

SUSPENSION AND STEERING

Check tyres for condition and pressure

Check tightness of roadwheel bolts

Check shock absorbers for fluid leaks

Inspect roadwheels for damage

Check all components for security, damage and wear

Check security of front suspension lower arm balljoint

Check wheel bearings for wear

Check front wheel alignment

INTERIOR AND BODYWORK

Check seat belts

Inspect paintwork and bodywork

Check and lubricate all door, tailgate/boot and bonnet release components

ELECTRICAL SYSTEM

Check washer fluid level

Check battery electrolyte level (where applicable)

Check wipers and washers

Check operation of all lights and electrical equipment

Check condition and adjustment of alternator drivebelt

CAR UNDERSIDE

Check all components for fluid leaks, corrosion or deterioration

ROAD TEST

Check instruments and electrical equipment

Check steering, suspension and general handling

Check engine, clutch (where applicable), gearbox and driveshafts

Check braking system

REGULAR Weekly	6000 miles (10 000 km) 6 months	12 000 miles (20 000 km) 1 year	24 000 miles (40 000 km) 2 years	36 000 miles (60 000 km) 3 years
■	■	■	■	■
	□	□	□	□
	□	□	□	□
				□
				□
■	■	■	■	■
	■	■	■	■
		■	■	■
		■	■	■
	□	□	□	□
	□	□	□	□
		□	□	□
			□	
	■	■	■	■
	■	■	■	■
		■	■	■
■	■	■	■	■
■	■	■	■	■
■	■	■	■	■
■	■	■	■	■
	■	■	■	■
	■	■	■	■
		■	■	■
		■	■	■
		■	■	■
		■	■	■

Items marked □ are considered to be beyond the scope of this Handbook, and details can be found in the Owners Workshop Manual for your car (OWM 686 for Escort models, or OWM 1009 for Orion models).

SAFETY FIRST!

Professional motor mechanics are trained in safe working procedures. No matter how enthusiastic you may be about getting on with the job you have planned, take time to read this Section. Don't risk an injury by failing to follow the simple safety rules explained here. The following is a guide to encourage you to be 'safety conscious' as you work on your car.

Essential points

ALWAYS use a safe system of supporting your car when working underneath it. The car's own jack (or a single hydraulic jack) is never sufficient. Once you've raised the car you should use a safe means of holding it up. Axle s ands, ramps or substantial wooden blocks are good; concrete blocks and bricks may crack or disintegrate and should not be used. Make sure that you locate the supports where you know the car won't collapse and where they can't slip.

ALWAYS loosen wheel nuts and other 'high torque' nuts or bolts (as applicable for the task to be carried out) before jacking up your car, or it may slip and fall.

ALWAYS make sure that your car is in **Neutral** or in **Park** (in the case of automatic transmission), and that the handbrake is securely on before trying to start the engine.

UNLESS the engine is cold, **ALWAYS** cover the cooling system's pressure (expansion tank) cap with several thicknesses of cloth before trying to remove it. Release the pressure slowly or the coolant may escape suddenly and scald you.

ALWAYS wait until the engine has cooled down before draining the engine (and/or transmission) oil, or the coolant. Oil or coolant that is very hot may scald you. If you can touch the engine sump/transmission/radiator (as applicable) without discomfort, the engine has probably cooled sufficiently to avoid scalding.

ALWAYS allow the engine to cool before working on it. Many parts of the engine become very hot in normal operation and you may burn yourself badly.

ALWAYS keep brake fluid, antifreeze and other similar liquids away from your car's paintwork as it may damage the finish (or remove the paint altogether).

ALWAYS keep toxic fluids, such as fuel, brake and transmission fluids and antifreeze off your skin, and never syphon them by mouth.

ALWAYS wear a mask when doing any dusty work, or where spraying is involved, especially when doing body repair and brake jobs.

ALWAYS clean up oil and grease spills – someone may slip and be injured.

ALWAYS use the right tool for the job. Spanners and screwdrivers which don't fit properly are likely to slip and cause injury.

ALWAYS get help to lift and handle heavy parts – it's never worth risking an injury.

ALWAYS take time over the jobs you take on. Plan out what you must do, and make sure that you have the right tools and spare parts. Follow the recommended steps, and check over the job once you're finished. Leave 'short-cuts' to the experts.

ALWAYS wear eye protection when using power tools such as drills, sanders and grinders, when using a hammer, and when working beneath your car.

ALWAYS use a barrier cream on your hands when doing dirty jobs, especially when in contact with fuel, oils, greases, and brake and transmission fluids. It will help protect your skin against infection and will make the dirt easier to remove later. Make sure that your hands aren't slippery. The use of a suitable specialist hand cleaner will make dirt and grease easier to remove without causing infection or damage to skin. Long term or regular contact with used oils and fuel can be a health hazard.

ALWAYS keep loose clothing and long hair out of the way of any moving parts.

ALWAYS take off rings, watches, bracelets

and neck chains before starting work on your car, especially the electrical system.

ALWAYS make sure that any jacking equipment or lifting tackle you use has a safe working load which will cope with what you intend to do, and use the equipment exactly as recommended by the manufacturers.

ALWAYS keep your work area tidy, someone may trip or slip on articles left lying around and be injured.

ALWAYS get someone to check up on you from time to time if you're working on the car alone to make sure that you're alright.

ALWAYS do the work in a logical order, and check that you've put things back together properly and that everything is tightened as it should be.

ALWAYS keep children and animals away from an unattended car, and from the area where you're working.

ALWAYS park cars with catalytic converters away from materials which may burn, such as dry grass, oily rags, etc, if the engine has recently been run. Catalytic converters reach extremely high temperatures, and any such materials close by may catch fire.

REMEMBER that your safety, and that of your car and other people rests with you. If you are in any doubt about anything, get specialist advice and help right away.

IF in spite of these precautions you injure yourself – get medical help immediately.

Asbestos

Some parts of your car, such as brake pads and linings, clutch linings and gaskets contain asbestos and you should take appropriate precautions to avoid inhaling dust (which is hazardous to health) when working with them. If in doubt, assume that they **do** contain asbestos.

Fire

Remember at all times that petrol is highly flammable. Never smoke, or have any kind of naked flame around, when working on the car. But the risk doesn't end there – a spark caused by an electrical short-circuit, by two metal surfaces contacting each other, by careless use of tools, or even by static electricity built up in your body under certain conditions, can ignite petrol vapour, which in a confined space is highly explosive.

If a fuel leak is suspected, try to find the cause and seek advice as soon as possible, and never risk fuel leaking onto a hot engine or exhaust. Catalytic converters (where fitted) run at extremely high temperatures, and therefore can be an additional fire hazard – observe the precautions outlined previously in this Section.

It's recommended that a fire extinguisher of a type suitable for fuel and electrical fires is kept handy in the garage or workplace at all times.

Never try to extinguish a fuel or electrical fire with water.

Fumes

Certain fumes are highly toxic and can quickly cause unconsciousness and even death if inhaled to any extent, especially if inhalation takes place through a lighted cigarette or pipe. Petrol vapour comes into this category, as do the vapours from certain solvents such as trichloroethylene. Any draining or pouring of such fluids should be done in a well ventilated area.

When using cleaning fluids and solvents, read the instructions carefully. Never use materials from unmarked containers – they may give off poisonous vapours.

Never run a car engine in an enclosed space such as a garage. Exhaust fumes contain carbon monoxide which is extremely poisonous; if you need to run the engine, always do so in the open air or at least have the rear of the car outside the workplace. Although cars fitted with catalytic converters produce far less toxic exhaust gases, the above precautions should still be observed.

If you're fortunate enough to have the use of an inspection pit, never run the engine while the car is standing over it; the fumes, being heavier than air, will concentrate in the pit with possibly lethal results.

The battery

Never short across the two poles of the battery! (A battery is shorted by connecting the two terminals directly to each other, and this can happen accidentally when working under the bonnet with metal tools.) The heavy discharge caused will create 'gassing' of hydrogen from the battery and this is highly explosive. Shorting across a battery may also cause sparks and the combination can cause the battery to explode with potentially lethal results. A conventional battery will normally be giving off a certain amount of hydrogen all the time, so for the same reasons given above, never cause a spark or allow a naked flame close to it.

Batteries which are sealed for life require special precautions which are normally outlined on a label attached to the battery. Such precautions usually relate to battery charging and jump starting from another vehicle (for details of jump starting refer to *'Breakdowns'* on page 45).

If possible, loosen the filler plugs or cover when charging the battery from an external source. Don't charge at an excessive rate or the battery may burst. Special care should be taken with the use of high charge-rate boost chargers to prevent the battery from overheating.

Take care when topping up and when carrying the battery. The battery contains dilute sulphuric acid which is very corrosive. It will burn and may cause long-term damage if in contact with skin, eyes or clothes. Similarly, corrosive deposits around the battery terminals may be harmful.

Always wear eye protection when cleaning the battery to prevent the corrosive deposits from entering your eyes.

Mains electricity and electrical equipment

When using any electrical equipment which works from the mains, such as an electric drill or inspection light, always ensure that the appliance is correctly connected to its plug and that, where necessary, it's properly earthed. Always use an RCD (Residual Current Device, a safety device incorporating a circuit breaker) when using mains electrical equipment. Don't use such appliances in damp conditions, and take care not to create a spark or apply excessive heat close to fuel or fuel vapour. Also make sure that the appliances meet the relevant national safety standards.

Ignition HT voltage

A severe electric shock can result from touching certain parts of the ignition system, such as the spark plug HT leads, when the engine is running or being cranked, particularly if components are damp or the insulation is faulty. Where an electronic ignition system is fitted, the HT voltage is much higher than that used in a contact breaker system, and could prove fatal, especially to wearers of cardiac pacemakers.

Disposing of used engine oil

Used engine oil is a hazard to health and the environment, and should be disposed of safely and cleanly. Most local authorities provide a disposal site which will have a special tank for waste oil. If in doubt, contact your local council for advice on where you can dispose of oil safely – there may be a local garage who will allow you to use their specialised oil disposal tank free of charge. Remember that it's not just the oil which causes a problem, but empty containers, old oil filters, and oily rags, so these should be taken to your local disposal site too.

Do not under any circumstances pour engine oil down a drain, or bury it in the ground.

Jacking and vehicle support

The jack provided with the car is designed for emergency wheel changing, and should not be used for servicing and overhaul work. Instead, a more substantial workshop jack (trolley jack or similar) should be used. Whichever type is used, it's essential that additional safety support is provided by means of axle stands designed for this purpose. Never use makeshift means such as narrow wooden blocks or piles of house bricks, as these can easily topple or, in the case of bricks, disintegrate under the weight of the car. Further information on the correct positioning of the jack and axle stands is provided at the end of this Section.

If you don't need to remove the wheels, the use of drive-on ramps is recommended. Ensure that the ramps are correctly aligned with the wheels, and that the car is not driven too far along them so that it promptly falls off the other end or tips the ramps.

JACK AND AXLE STAND POSITIONS

When using a trolley jack or other type of workshop jack, to raise the front of the car, the jack head should be placed under the centre of the front lower body crossmember, with a shaped block of wood between the jack head and the crossmember to act as an insulator.

To raise the rear of the car, the head of the jack should be placed under the right-hand

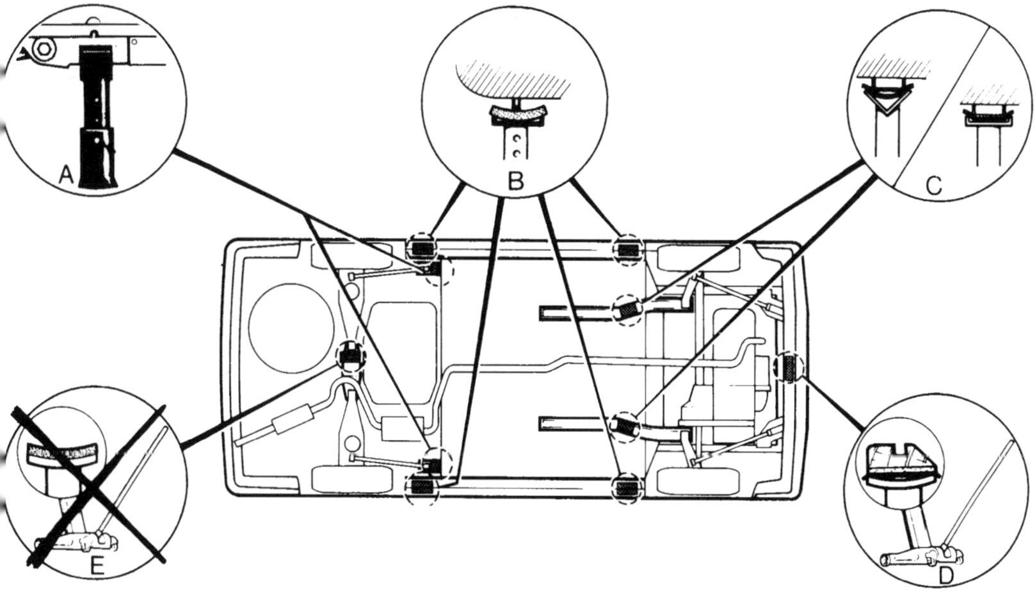

▲ *Jacking and support points on car underside*
- ***A*** *Axle stand positions (rear)*
- ***B*** *Axle stand positions under sills (with wooden or rubber pads)*
- ***C*** *Axle stand positions (front)*
- ***D*** *Trolley jack position for raising front of car (use shaped wooden block as shown on pre-1986 models)*
- ***E*** *Trolley jack position for raising rear of car (not to be used on fuel injection models up to approximately August 1989)*

rear suspension lower arm mounting bracket, with a rubber pad between the jack head and the bracket to act as an insulator (**Note:** *On fuel injection models up to approximately August 1989, this jack location **must not** be used due to the fuel pump location*). Provided only one side of the rear of the car is to be raised, the jack can be positioned under the spring seat on the suspension lower arm.

Axle stands should only be located under the double-skinned sections of the side members at the front of the car, or under the members to which the tie-bars are attached at the rear of the car. Axle stands can also be placed under the sill jacking points.

BUYING SPARE PARTS

When buying spare parts such as an oil filter, or an air filter, make sure that the correct replacement parts are obtained for your particular car. Many changes are made during the production run of any car, and when ordering spare parts, it will usually be necessary to know the year the car was built, the model type (eg 'L' or 'XR3') and engine size, and in some cases the Vehicle Identification Number (VIN). The VIN is stamped on a metal plate attached to the body panel above the radiator in the engine compartment, and usually appears on the Vehicle Registration Document.

All of the components required for servicing will be available from an official Ford dealer, but most parts should also be available from good motor accessory shops and motor factors.

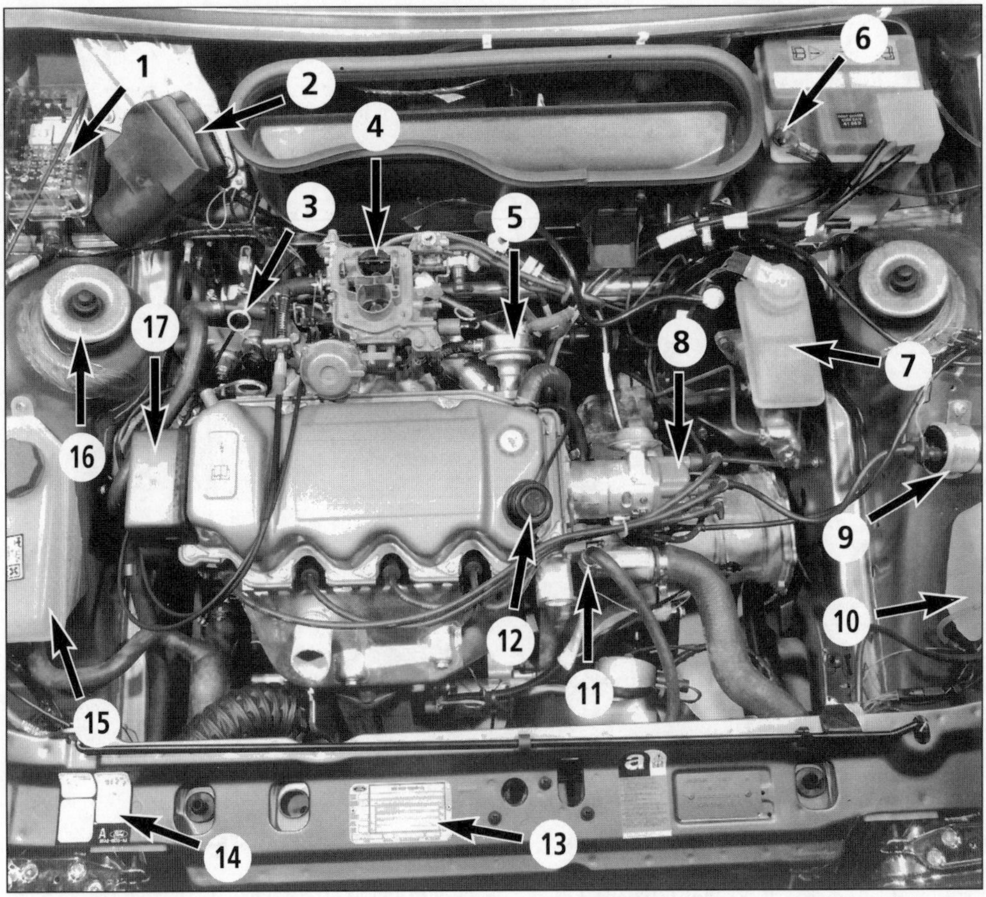

▲ *Underbonnet component locations on a 1986 1.4 litre CVH engine Escort model (air cleaner removed for clarity) – Orion similar*

- ***1*** *Fusebox*
- ***2*** *Windscreen wiper motor*
- ***3*** *Engine oil level dipstick*
- ***4*** *Carburettor*
- ***5*** *Fuel pump*
- ***6*** *Battery earth terminal*
- ***7*** *Brake fluid reservoir*
- ***8*** *Distributor*
- ***9*** *Ignition coil*
- ***10*** *Washer fluid reservoir*
- ***11*** *Cooling system thermostat housing*
- ***12*** *Oil filler cap*
- ***13*** *Vehicle Identification Number plate*
- ***14*** *Engine tuning decal*
- ***15*** *Cooling system expansion tank*
- ***16*** *Suspension strut top mounting*
- ***17*** *Camshaft drivebelt cover*

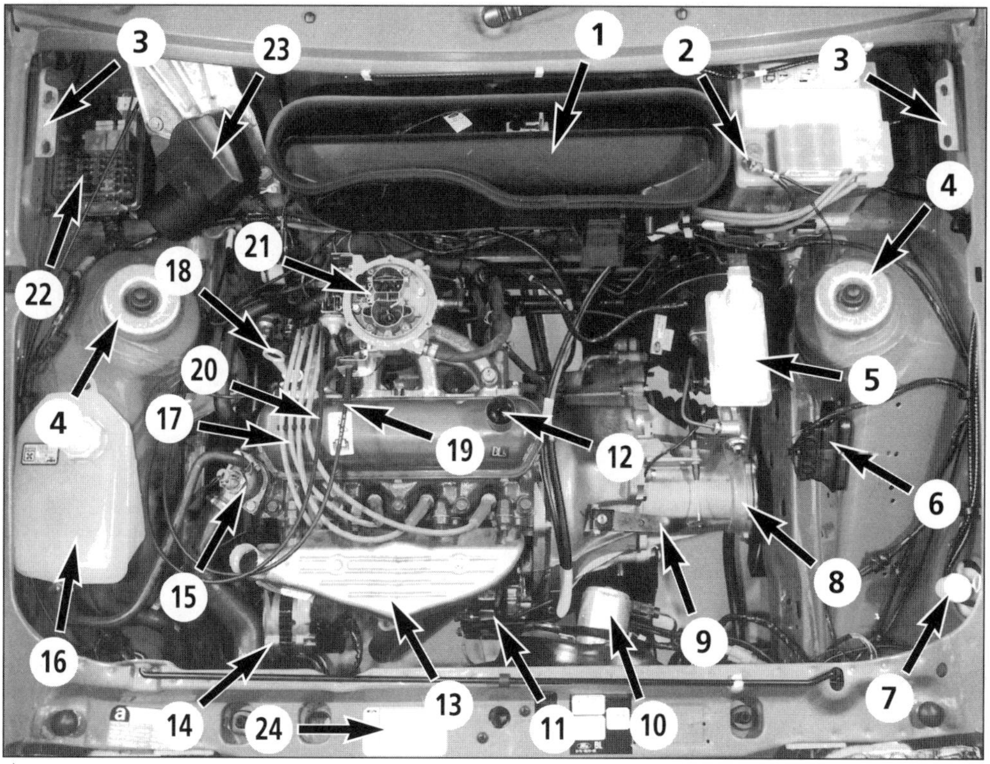

▲ *Underbonnet component locations on a 1989 1.3 litre OHV engine Escort model (air cleaner removed for clarity) – Orion similar*

1 *Interior ventilation air inlet duct*
2 *Battery earth terminal*
3 *Bonnet hinge*
4 *Suspension strut top mounting*
5 *Brake fluid reservoir*
6 *Ignition system electronic module*
7 *Washer fluid reservoir filler cap*
8 *Gearbox housing*
9 *Clutch release lever*
10 *Cooling fan motor*
11 *Starter motor*
12 *Engine oil filler neck (cap removed)*
13 *Exhaust manifold hot air shield*
14 *Alternator*
15 *Cooling system thermostat housing*
16 *Cooling system expansion tank*
17 *Spark plug HT leads*
18 *Engine oil level dipstick*
19 *Choke cable*
20 *Throttle cable*
21 *Carburettor*
22 *Fusebox*
23 *Windscreen wiper motor*
24 *Vehicle Identification Number plate*

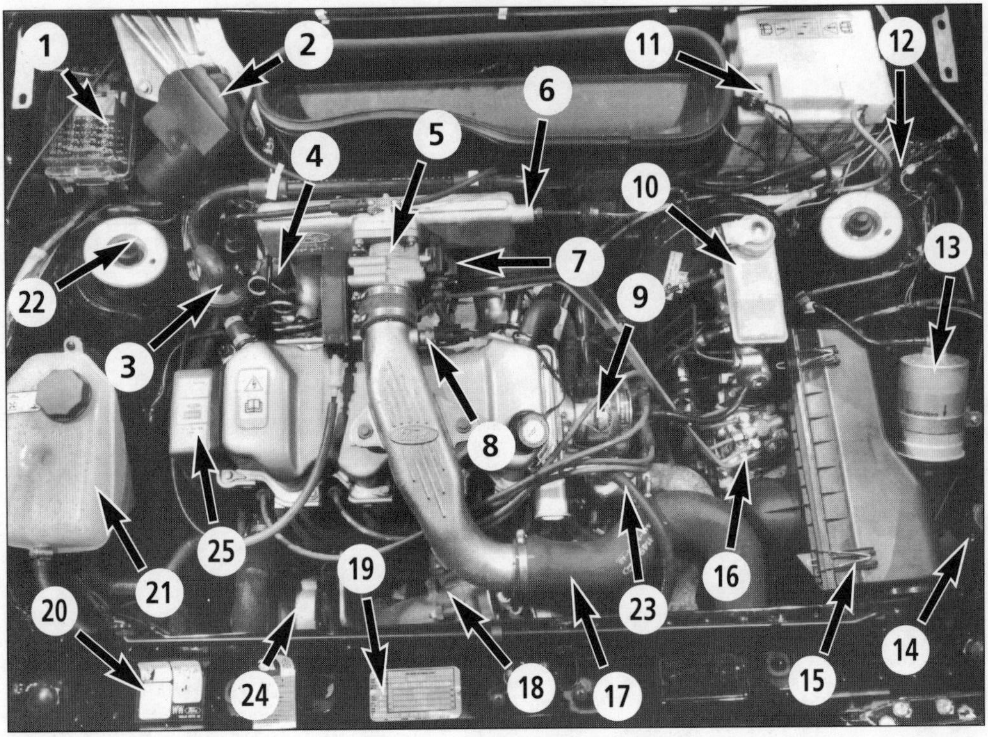

▲ *Underbonnet component locations on a 1986 Escort RS Turbo model*

1 *Fusebox*
2 *Windscreen wiper motor*
3 *Crankcase emission control filter*
4 *Engine oil level dipstick*
5 *Throttle housing*
6 *Inlet manifold*
7 *Throttle position sensor (fuel injection system)*
8 *Charge air temperature sensor (fuel injection system)*
9 *Distributor*
10 *Brake fluid reservoir*
11 *Battery earth terminal*
12 *Ignition coil*
13 *Fuel filter*
14 *Washer fluid reservoir filler cap*
15 *Air cleaner*
16 *Fuel distributor (fuel injection system)*
17 *Intake air hose*
18 *Turbocharger*
19 *Vehicle Identification Number plate*
20 *Engine tuning decal*
21 *Cooling system expansion tank*
22 *Suspension strut top mounting*
23 *Cooling system thermostat housing*
24 *Alternator*
25 *Camshaft drivebelt cover*

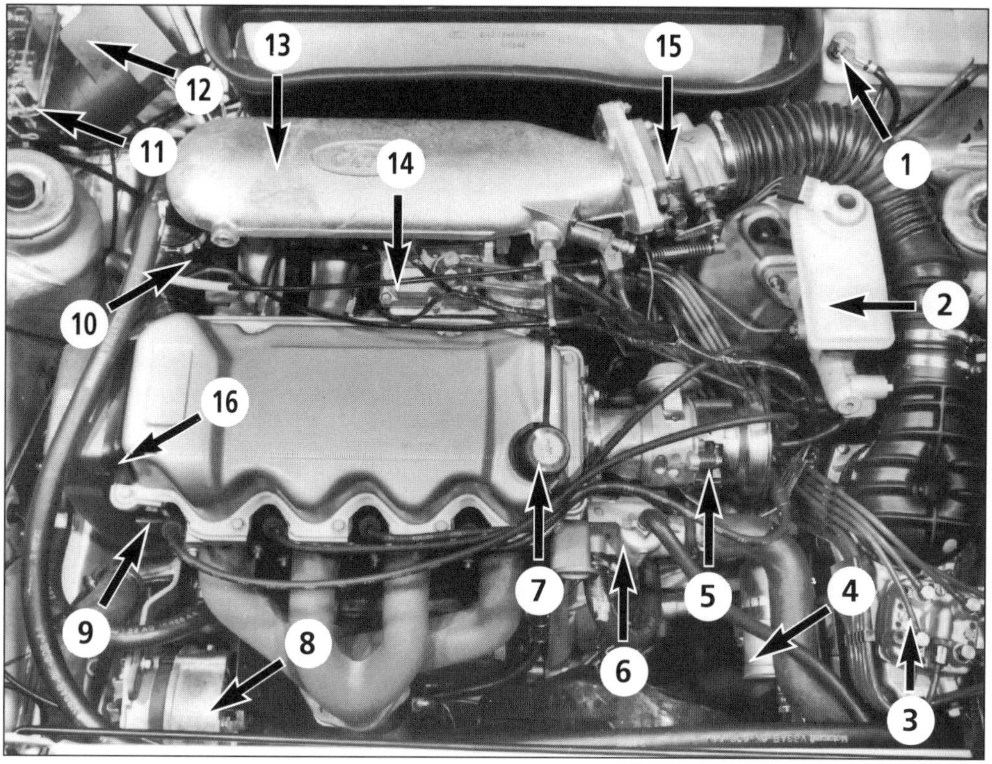

▲ *Underbonnet component locations on a 1984 1.6 litre CVH fuel injection engine Orion model – XR3i similar*

1 Battery earth terminal
2 Brake fluid reservoir
3 Fuel distributor (fuel injection system)
4 Fuel filter
5 Distributor
6 Cooling system thermostat housing
7 Oil filler cap
8 Alternator
9 Engine coolant pump
10 Crankcase emission control filter
11 Fusebox
12 Windscreen wiper motor
13 Plenum chamber (fuel injection system)
14 Warm-up regulator (fuel injection system)
15 Throttle housing
16 Camshaft drivebelt cover

SERVICE TASKS

The following pages provide easy-to-follow instructions to enable you to carry out the regular service tasks recommended by the manufacturer.

Identifying CVH and OHV engines

To identify a CVH (Compound Valve angle, Hemispherical combustion chambers) engine, look at the right-hand end of the engine (when viewed from the driver's seat). CVH engines have a moulded plastic cover on the end of the engine which covers the camshaft drivebelt. If there's no plastic cover, then the engine is an OHV (overhead valve) type.

Every 250 miles (400 km) or weekly

Refer to *'Regular checks'* on page 69 and carry out all the checks described.

Every 6000 miles (10 000 km) or 6 months – whichever comes first

ENGINE COMPARTMENT

Check all hoses and pipes, and the surfaces of all components for signs of fluid leakage, corrosion or deterioration

If there's any sign of leaking fluid, try to find the source of the leak and seek advice if necessary. It can be difficult to identify leaking fluids, but if there's obviously a major leak, or if you suspect even a slight brake fluid or petrol leak, don't drive the car until the problem has been investigated by someone suitably qualified.

Check all rubber or fabric hoses for signs of cracking, damage due to rubbing on other components, and general deterioration. It's sensible to have any suspect hoses renewed as a precaution against possible failure.

Check for obvious signs of corrosion on metal pipes, hose clips, and component joints, which may indicate a fluid leak. Any badly corroded components should be cleaned and, if necessary, renewed. Pay particular attention to metal fluid pipes, and have them renewed if they're badly pitted or corroded.

ENGINE

Renew the engine oil and filter

Note: *The following items will be required for this task:*

- *A suitable quantity of engine oil of the correct type – refer to* ***'Service specifications'*** *on page 67*
- *New oil filter (of the correct type for your particular car)*
- *New oil drain plug sealing washer (depending on the condition of the old one)*
- *Suitable container to catch the old oil as it drains (make sure that the capacity of the container is larger than the oil capacity of the engine – refer to* ***'Service specifications'*** *on page 65)*
- *Oil filter wrench – for removal of old oil filter*
- *Small quantity of clean rag*
- *Suitable spanner or socket to fit oil drain plug*

The oil should be drained when the engine is warm, immediately after a run. If you can touch the engine sump without discomfort, the oil has probably cooled sufficiently to avoid scalding. Ideally, the front of the car should be jacked up to improve access. If the front of the car is to be raised, apply the handbrake, then jack up the front of the car and support it securely on axle stands (refer to *'Jacking and vehicle support'* on page 84 for details of where to position the jack and axle stands).

Position a suitable container under the engine sump to catch all the oil.

Remove the oil filler cap from the top of the engine, then working under the car, unscrew the drain plug from the rear of the engine sump using a suitable spanner or a socket. Oil will be released before the drain plug is removed completely, so take precautions against scalding, as the oil will be hot.

Allow the oil to drain for at least 15 minutes.

Check the condition of the oil drain plug sealing washer and renew it if necessary.

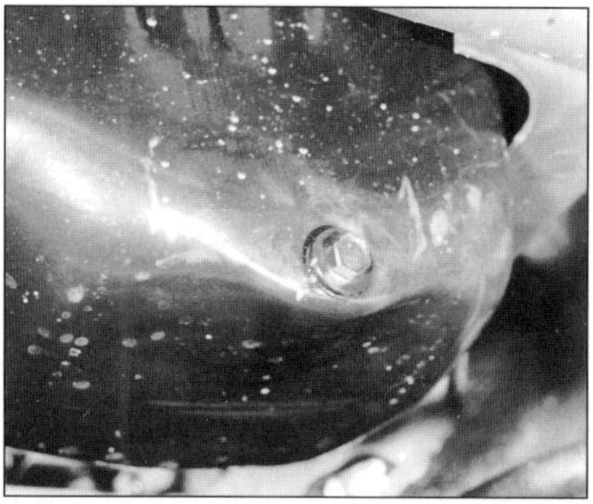

▲ *Engine oil drain plug (CVH engine)*

When the oil has finished draining, clean the drain plug, washer, and the mating face of the sump, then refit and tighten the drain plug.

Position a suitable container under the oil filter at the rear of the engine, and unscrew the filter using a suitable oil filter wrench to loosen it. Be prepared for the spillage of warm oil.

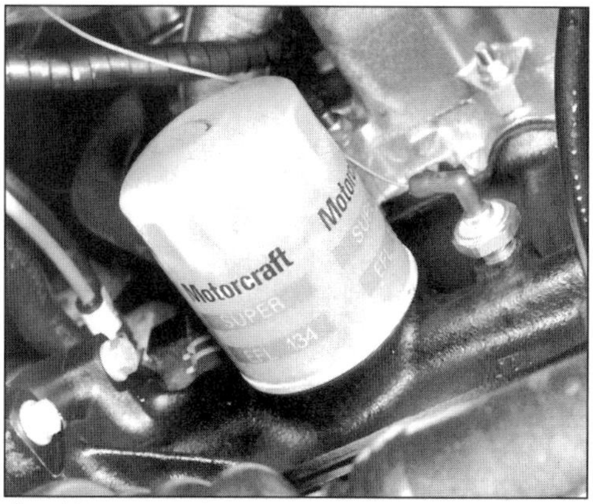

▲ *Oil filter viewed from underneath the car (CVH engine)*

Wipe clean the oil filter mounting flange on the engine. Smear a little clean engine oil on the sealing ring of the new oil filter, then screw the filter onto the engine, and tighten it *by hand only*. If no instructions are provided with the filter, tighten it until the sealing ring touches the mounting face on the engine, then tighten it a further three-quarters of a turn.

Where applicable, lower the car to the ground and, with the car parked on level ground, fill the engine with the correct quantity and grade of oil through the filler on top of the engine. Fill until the level reaches the 'MAX' mark on the dipstick.

Make sure that the oil filler cap is fitted on completion.

When the engine is started, there may be a delay before the oil pressure warning light goes out, as the engine lubrication system fills with oil.

Run the engine and check for leaks from the filter and the drain plug, then stop the engine and check the oil level. Refer to *'Regular checks'* on page 70 for details of how to check the oil level.

Dispose of the old engine oil safely (refer to *'Safety first!'* on page 84). **Don't** pour it down a drain.

On OHV engines remove and clean the oil filler cap

Remove the oil filler cap from the top of the engine, and disconnect the hose(s).

Carefully clean the inside of the cap, taking care not to damage the filter gauze, where applicable (the cap can be cleaned using paraffin, but dry it thoroughly before refitting).

At the same time, check the O-ring seal at the bottom of the filler cap, and renew it if it's damaged or worn.

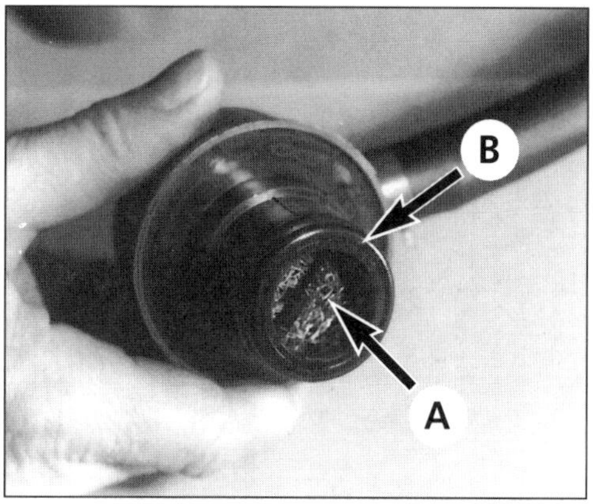

▲ *Oil filler cap on later OHV engine*
A *Filter gauze*
B *O-ring seal*

COOLING SYSTEM

Check the coolant level and top up if necessary

Refer to *'Regular checks'* on page 71.

IGNITION SYSTEM

Clean the distributor cap (where applicable), coil and HT leads

Remove the distributor cap, which may be secured with spring clips or screws (some later models have a distributorless ignition system, in which case ignore the references to the distributor cap).

Thoroughly clean the cap inside and out with a dry lint-free cloth.

Examine the inside of the distributor cap, and if any of the four HT lead contacts inside the cap appear badly burnt or pitted, or if there are any signs of hairline cracks in the plastic, renew the cap.

Make sure that the carbon contact in the centre of the cap is not excessively worn, that it's free to move, and that it protrudes from its holder – if not, renew the cap.

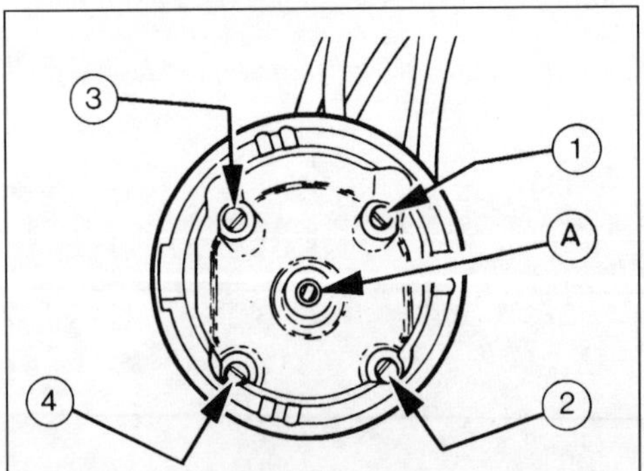

▲ *HT lead contacts inside distributor cap* ***(1, 2, 3*** *and* ***4)****, and carbon centre contact* ***(A)***

Disconnect the HT leads from the coil, distributor cap, and the spark plugs, noting their precise locations.

Wipe the coil clean and check the contacts on the coil, distributor cap, and the ends of the HT leads for corrosion.

Carefully clean away any corrosion, and wipe the leads clean over their entire length before refitting.

Make sure that the HT leads are refitted in their correct firing order, as noted before removal.

On models with a contact breaker points distributor, lubricate the distributor

Remove the distributor cap, and wipe clean the cam on the distributor shaft which operates the contact breaker points.

Apply a trace of high melting point grease to each of the four cam lobes (the highest points of the cam, which open the contact breaker points). The grease is best applied using the tip of a screwdriver or a similar tool.

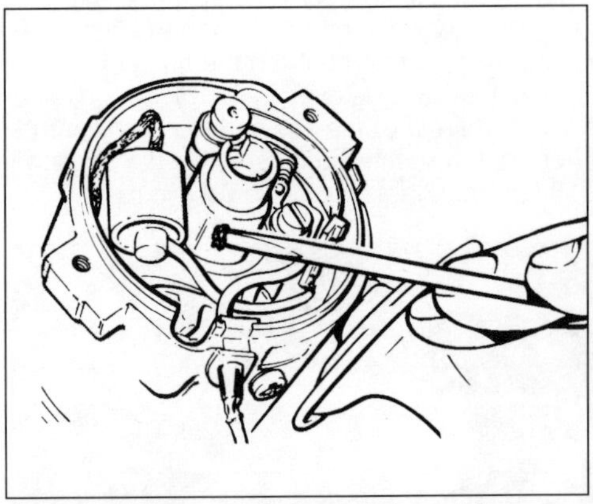

▲ *Applying grease to a distributor shaft cam lobe*

On OHV engine models, apply two drops (no more) of light oil to the felt pad at the top of the distributor shaft.

On models with a contact breaker points distributor, check and, if necessary, adjust the points gap

Note: *A set of feeler gauges and (on automatic transmission models) a suitable spanner to fit the crankshaft pulley bolt will be required for this check*

Remove the distributor cap, then pull the rotor arm from the distributor shaft.

Using a screwdriver, gently prise the contact breaker points open to examine the condition of the contact faces.

If the contacts are rough, pitted, or

excessively dirty, the points should be renewed as described in the *'12 000 miles (20 000 km)'* service Section on page 96.

Assuming that the points are in good condition, the gap between the two contact faces should be checked and if necessary adjusted. This can be done using feeler gauges as follows, although it's preferable to use the more accurate 'dwell angle' method described in the Owners Workshop Manual.

To check the points gap using feeler gauges, turn the crankshaft until the heel of the contact breaker arm is resting on the peak of one of the four lobes on the distributor shaft cam, and the points are fully open.

On cars with a manual gearbox, the crankshaft can be turned by engaging 3rd gear

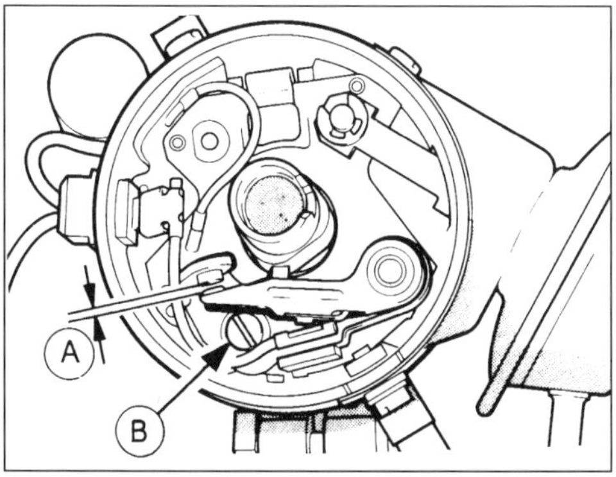

▲ *Contact breaker points gap (**A**), and adjustment screw (**B**) – Bosch distributor*

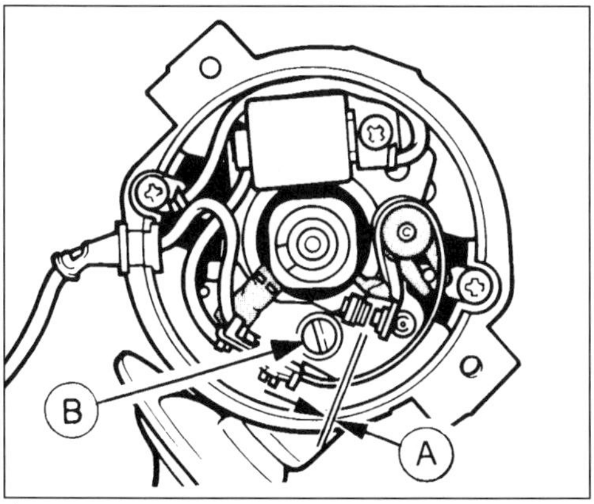

▲ *Contact breaker points gap (**A**), and adjustment screw (**B**) – Lucas distributor*

and pushing the car; on automatic transmission models it will be necessary to turn the crankshaft by means of a suitable spanner on the crankshaft pulley bolt. The crankshaft pulley bolt is located at the bottom right-hand side of the engine (when viewed from the driver's seat), in the centre of the engine pulley which carries the alternator drivebelt (the lower pulley on OHV type engines).

Select a feeler gauge of thickness equal to the specified points gap (refer to *'Service specifications'* on page 65), and slide it between the two contact faces. The feeler gauge should be a firm sliding fit.

If adjustment is required, slacken the points retaining screw slightly, so that the fixed point can just be moved to give the required gap.

The easiest way of moving the fixed point is to engage a screwdriver in the slot on the end of the fixed point, and lever against the corresponding slot or pips on the distributor baseplate.

After adjustment, tighten the retaining screw and recheck the gap.

Refit the rotor arm and the distributor cap.

On RS Turbo models, renew the spark plugs

Refer to the procedure for spark plug renewal given in the *'12 000 miles (20 000 km)'* service Section on page 96.

SUSPENSION AND STEERING

Check the tyres for damage, tread depth and uneven wear

Refer to *'Regular checks'* on page 73.

Check and if necessary adjust the tyre pressures

Refer to *'Regular checks'* on page 73.

Check the tightness of the roadwheel bolts

Using the wheel brace (refer to *'Changing a wheel'* Section on page 42), check that the bolts cannot be turned easily using reasonable force. Do not overtighten the bolts.

INTERIOR AND BODYWORK

Check the seat belt webbing for cuts and damage, and check the seat belt operation

If any of the seat belt webbing is damaged, frayed or worn, the relevant seat belt(s) must be renewed.

Check that all inertia reel seat belts can be pulled smoothly from their retractors, and that they return smoothly, unassisted.

Check that the locking mechanism works correctly by sharply tugging the seat belt webbing.

If a seat belt retractor or locking mechanism appears to be faulty, the relevant seat belt should be renewed.

Carefully inspect the paintwork for damage and the bodywork for corrosion

Touch up any minor stone chips, and have any corroded areas repaired before the damage becomes serious.

For details of how to treat minor paint scratches, refer to *'Bodywork and interior care'* on page 111.

ELECTRICAL SYSTEM

Check the operation of all lights, electrical equipment and accessories

Refer to *'Fault finding'* on page 127 if any problems are discovered.

If any of the bulbs need to be renewed, refer to *'Bulb, fuse and relay renewal'* on page 113.

Check the condition and adjustment of the alternator drivebelt

Note: *If the drivebelt requires adjustment, a suitable spanner or socket will be required to fit the alternator mounting and adjuster link bolts*

Examine the drivebelt for signs of cracking, obvious wear, or contamination, and renew it if necessary (note that on OHV engines, the belt also drives the engine coolant pump).

To check the tension of the belt, press down on the belt midway between the alternator and water pump pulleys on OHV engines, or midway between the alternator and crankshaft pulleys on CVH engines.

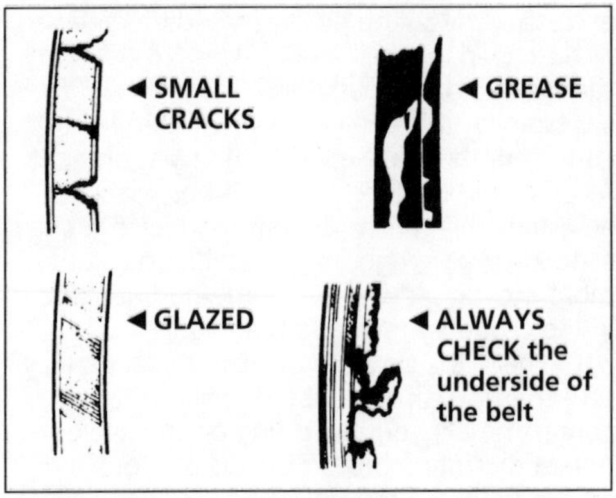

▲ *Examine the alternator drivebelt for signs of wear, deterioration or contamination*

The deflection of the belt should be approximately 10 mm (0.4 in) under moderate finger pressure.

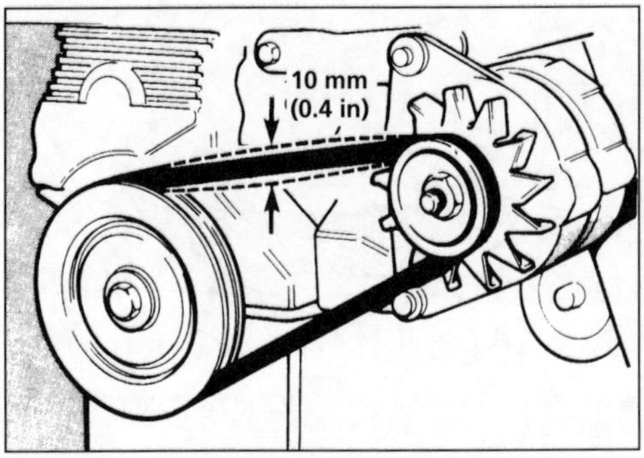

▲ *Alternator drivebelt tension checking point (CVH engine)*

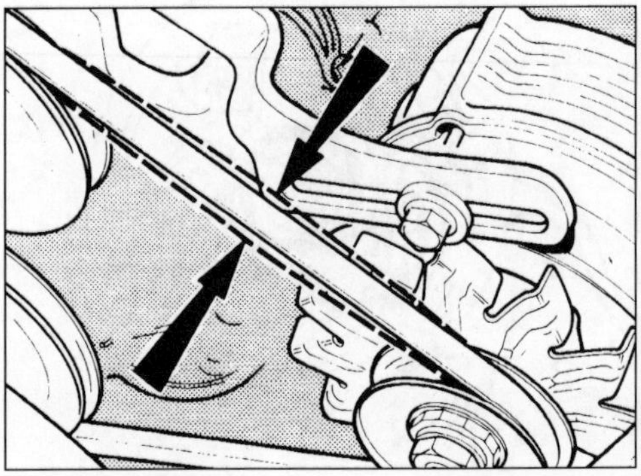

▲ *Alternator drivebelt tension checking point (OHV engine)*

To adjust the tension, slacken the alternator mounting bolts and the adjuster link bolts, and move the alternator towards or away from the engine as necessary to give the correct tension.

Once the tension is correct, tighten the adjuster link-to-alternator bolt, adjuster link-to-engine bolt, and the alternator front and rear mounting bolts in that order.

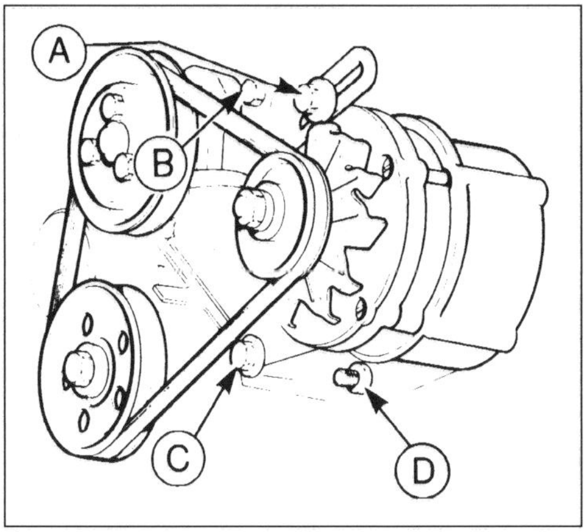

▲ *Alternator mounting and adjuster link bolts (OHV engine)*
***A** Adjuster link-to-alternator bolt*
***B** Adjuster link-to-engine bolt*
***C** and **D** Alternator mounting bolts*

To renew the belt, slacken all four mounting and adjuster bolts, and move the alternator towards the engine to remove the belt.

Fit the new belt, then pull the alternator away from the engine until the belt is fairly tight, and tighten the adjuster link-to-alternator bolt.

Tension the belt as described previously.

If a new belt has been fitted, the tension should be rechecked after the engine has run for approximately ten minutes.

CAR UNDERSIDE

Check all hoses and pipes, and the surfaces of all components for signs of fluid leakage, corrosion, damage or deterioration

Refer to 'Engine compartment' checks at the beginning of the *'6000 miles (10 000 km)'* service Section on page 90.

In addition, check the exhaust system and the fuel tank for any sign of damage or serious corrosion (light surface rust is to be expected).

Check the exhaust mountings to make sure that they're secure.

Check the visible suspension and steering components for obvious signs of damage or wear.

Check the driveshafts for obvious signs of distortion or damage.

Pay particular attention to the driveshaft and steering gear rubber gaiters, which should be renewed if they're split, or if there are any obvious signs of lubricant leakage.

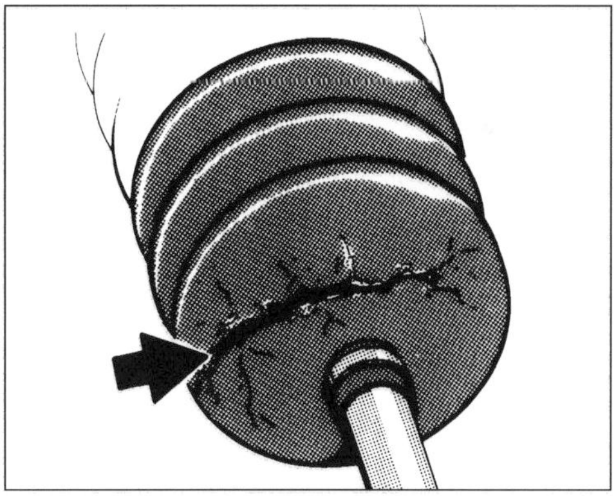

▲ *Check the driveshaft and steering gear rubber gaiters for splits (arrowed)*

ADDITIONAL TASKS

Note that as well as the tasks described in the preceding paragraphs, the additional tasks given in the *'Service schedule'* chart on page 78 should be carried out every 6000 miles (10 000 km) or 6 months – whichever comes first. These tasks require more detailed explanation, or the use of special tools, and are considered beyond the scope of this Handbook. For details of these additional tasks, refer to the Owners Workshop Manual.

Every 12 000 miles (20 000 km) or 1 year – whichever comes first

In addition to all the items in the *'6000 miles (10 000 km)'* service on page 90, carry out the following.

IGNITION SYSTEM

Renew the spark plugs

Note: *Ensure that the correct type of new spark plugs is obtained for your particular car. A suitable spark plug spanner and a spark plug gap adjustment tool, or a set of feeler gauges will be required for this task.*

The spark plugs must be renewed with the engine *cold*.

Mark the spark plug HT leads to make sure that they're refitted in their correct positions, then pull the leads from the spark plugs. Pull on the rubber insulators at the ends of the leads, not on the leads themselves.

Before removing the spark plugs, brush any grit from the area around the plug recesses to avoid it dropping into the engine as the plugs are removed.

Using a spark plug spanner, unscrew the spark plugs and remove them from the engine.

Before fitting the new plugs, the electrode gap must be set as follows (refer to *'Service specifications'* on page 66 for the correct electrode gap).

Measure the gap between the electrodes using a spark plug gap adjustment tool, or a feeler gauge.

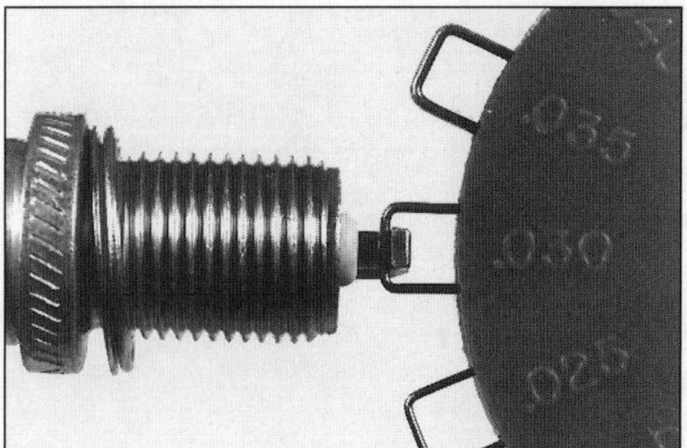

▲ *Checking a spark plug gap using a suitable tool*

If adjustment is required, carefully bend the **outer** electrode until the correct gap is obtained. **Never** try to bend the centre electrode.

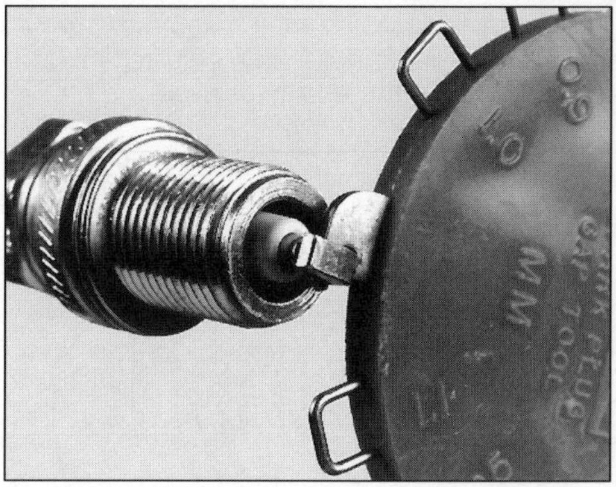

▲ *Adjusting a spark plug gap using the correct tool*

Make sure that the plug threads and the seating areas in the cylinder head are clean, and apply a little light oil to the plug threads. Screw the plugs in by hand initially.

Using the spark plug spanner, tighten the plugs until initial resistance is felt, then tighten by a further one sixteenth of a turn for the taper seat type plugs fitted to OHV engines, or one quarter of a turn for the washer type plugs fitted to CVH engines. **Do not** overtighten the plugs.

Refit the spark plug HT leads in their correct positions as noted before removal, making sure that they are a secure fit over the ends of the plugs.

On contact breaker points distributors renew the contact breaker points

Note: *Ensure that the correct type of new contact breaker points are obtained for your particular car*

Remove the distributor cap, then pull the rotor arm from the distributor shaft.

Disconnect the wiring from the contact breaker points. On Bosch type distributors the wiring can simply be pulled from the spade connector. On Lucas type distributors, the contact breaker spring arm must be eased out of the plastic insulator, and the wiring must be slid from the hooked end of the spring arm.

Unscrew the contact breaker points retaining screw, and withdraw the points from the distributor. Take care not to drop the screw and washer into the distributor. If possible use a magnetic screwdriver, or hold the screw on the end of the screwdriver using a blob of grease.

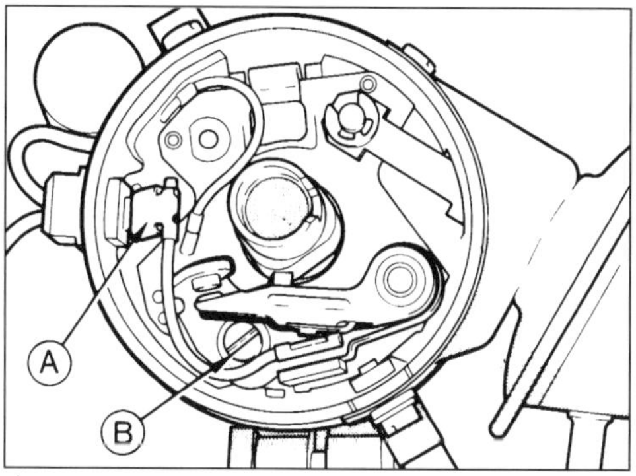

▲ *Contact breaker points renewal (Bosch distributor)*
A *Wiring connector*
B *Contact breaker points retaining screw*

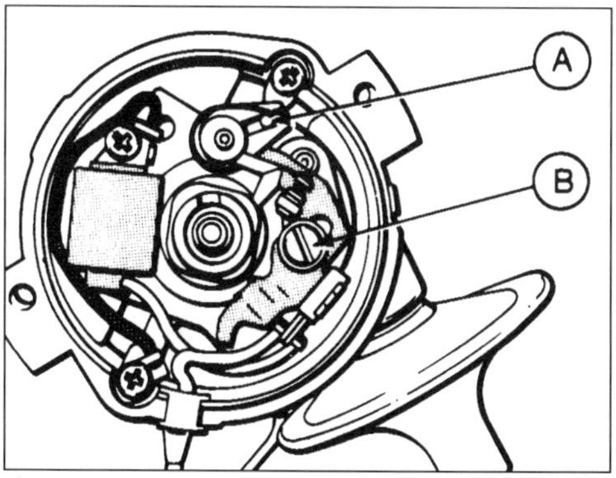

▲ *Contact breaker points renewal (Lucas distributor)*
A *Contact breaker points cam and distributor baseplate peg*
B *Contact breaker points retaining screw*

Wipe clean the cam on the distributor shaft which operates the contact breaker points, then apply a trace of high melting point grease to each of the four cam lobes.

On OHV engine models, apply two drops (no more) of light oil to the felt pad at the top of the distributor shaft.

New contact breaker points are usually supplied coated with a protective film. This should be wiped from the points before fitting, using a cloth moistened with methylated spirit.

Locate the new contact breaker points in the distributor, and lightly tighten the retaining screw. On the Lucas type distributor, make sure that the cam at the end of the contact breaker points is engaged with the peg on the distributor baseplate, and that both washers are fitted to the retaining screw.

Reconnect the wire, then adjust the points gap as described in the *'6000 miles (10 000 km)'* service Section on page 92.

MANUAL GEARBOX

Check and if necessary top up the gearbox oil level

Note: *A suitable spanner or socket, or on later models a Torx or Allen key (depending on model), will be required to remove and refit the oil filler plug*

With the car on level ground, wipe around the filler plug which is located at the front of the gearbox casing. Unscrew the plug using a suitable spanner, or a Torx or Allen key, as applicable, on later models. The plug can be reached from above or below the car.

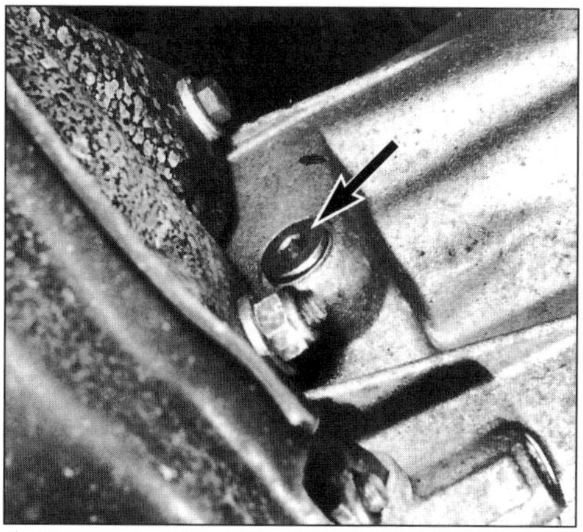

▲ *Allen type gearbox oil level plug (arrowed)*

Locate the aluminium build code tag, which is secured to one of the upper gearbox housing bolts, and note the gearbox part number stamped on the tag.

If the last letter of the part number suffix is a 'D', the oil level must be maintained between 5 and 10 mm (0.2 and 0.4 in) below the lower edge of the filler plug hole.

If the last letter of the part number suffix is an 'E', the oil level must be maintained between 0 and 5 mm (0 and 0.2 in) below the lower edge of the filler plug hole.

To make level checking easier, a dipstick can be made from a thin rod bent at right-angles and having marks on one 'leg' made with a file at 5 mm (0.2 in) intervals.

Rest the unmarked leg on the lower edge of the filler plug hole, with the marked end immersed in the oil.

Remove the dipstick, read off the oil level and top up if necessary using the specified grade of oil (refer to *'Service specifications'* on page 67).

Refit and tighten the filler plug on completion.

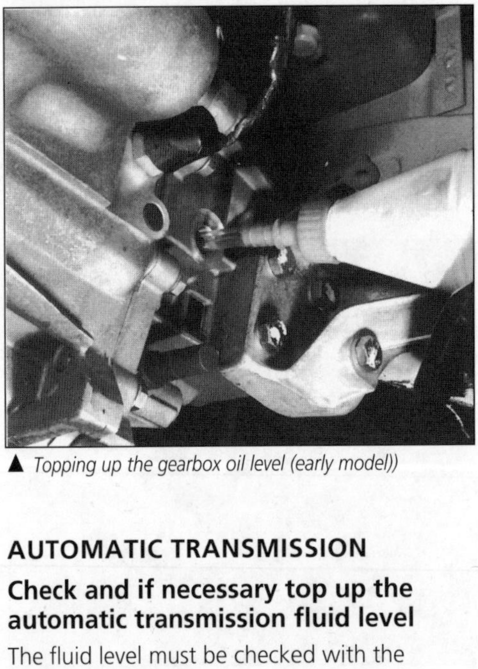

▲ *Topping up the gearbox oil level (early model))*

AUTOMATIC TRANSMISSION

Check and if necessary top up the automatic transmission fluid level

The fluid level must be checked with the engine and transmission at normal operating temperature, preferably after a short journey.

Park the car on level ground, then apply the handbrake.

With the engine running at its normal idle speed, apply the brake pedal, while moving the transmission selector lever through the full range of positions three times then back to the **P** position.

Allow the engine to idle for a further minute.

With the engine still idling, pull out the automatic transmission fluid level dipstick (located at the front left-hand side of the engine compartment when viewed from the driver's seat) and wipe it dry with a clean lint-free rag.

Fully insert the dipstick, then withdraw it again and check the fluid level, which should be between the 'MAX' and 'MIN' marks.

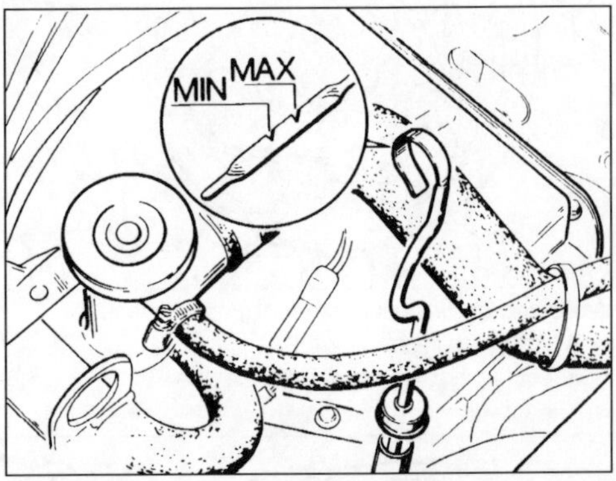

▲ *Automatic transmission fluid level dipstick location and level markings*

If topping up is necessary, use only the specified fluid type (refer to *'Service specifications'* on page 67). On later models with a conventional automatic transmission (not a CTX type), an improved type of Ford fluid is used. If the Ford specification fluid is to be used for topping up, it's necessary to identify the transmission so that the correct fluid can be obtained. The later type of transmission is identified by having a black dipstick, stating the fluid specification and type. **Under no circumstances must the later type of Ford fluid be used in the early type transmission, and vice versa.**

Top up by pouring the fluid through the dipstick tube. Take care not to overfill, the level **must not** exceed the 'MAX' mark.

If there's a need for regular topping up, it's likely that there's a fluid leak, and the problem should be referred to a Ford dealer.

SUSPENSION AND STEERING

Check the front and rear shock absorbers for fluid leaks

Check around the body of each shock absorber for signs of dampness which may be due to fluid leakage.

If any fluid is noticed, seek advice, and if necessary renew the shock absorber.

Inspect the roadwheels for damage

Check around both the outside and inside edges of each roadwheel for signs of damage or distortion, and make sure that any wheel balance weights are secure with no obvious signs that any are missing.

If there is any evidence of damage to a wheel, seek advice immediately, and if necessary renew the wheel.

If a wheel balance weight is obviously missing, some vibration can be expected whilst driving, and the wheel should be rebalanced.

BODYWORK

Lubricate all hinges, door locks, and the bonnet release mechanism

Use general purpose light oil for the door locks, and a suitable general purpose grease for the hinges and bonnet release mechanism.

Don't use an excess of lubricant which may find its way onto other components, or the clothing of the car's occupants.

Check the operation of all door, tailgate/boot, bonnet release and window regulator components

If any of the components prove to be faulty, seek advice. Have the problem fixed as soon as possible, and without delay if the problem is likely to affect the car's security and/or safety (faulty lock, window which can't be closed etc).

ROAD TEST

Check the operation of all instruments and electrical equipment

Make sure that all instruments read correctly, and switch on all electrical equipment in turn to check that it functions properly.

Check for any abnormalities in the steering, suspension, handling or road feel

Drive the car and check that there are no unusual vibrations or noises.

Check that the steering feels positive, with no excessive 'sloppiness', or roughness, and check for any suspension noises when cornering and driving over bumps.

Check the performance of the engine, clutch (where applicable), gearbox and driveshafts

Listen for any unusual noises from the engine, clutch and gearbox.

Make sure that the engine runs smoothly when idling, and that there's no hesitation when accelerating.

Check that, where applicable, the clutch action is smooth and progressive, that the drive is taken up smoothly, and that the pedal travel is not excessive. Also listen for any noises when the clutch pedal is depressed.

On manual gearbox models, check that all gears can be engaged smoothly without noise and that the gear lever action is not abnormally vague or 'notchy'.

On automatic transmission models, make sure that all gearchanges occur smoothly without snatching and without an increase in engine speed between changes. Check that all the gear positions can be selected with the car at rest. If any problems are found, they should be referred to a Ford dealer.

Listen for a metallic clicking sound from the front of the car as the car is driven slowly in a circle with the steering on full lock. Carry out this check in both directions. If a clicking noise is heard, this indicates wear in a driveshaft joint, in which case seek advice and renew the joint if necessary.

Check the operation and performance of the braking system

Make sure that the car does not pull to one side when braking, and that the wheels do not lock prematurely when braking hard.

Check that there's no vibration through the steering when braking.

Check that the handbrake operates correctly without excessive movement of the lever, and that it holds the car stationary on a slope.

ADDITIONAL TASKS

Note that as well as the tasks described in the preceding paragraphs, the additional tasks given in the *'Service schedule'* on page 78 chart should be carried out every 12 000 miles (20 000 km) or 1 year – whichever comes first. These tasks require more detailed explanation, or the use of special tools, and are considered beyond the scope of this Handbook. For details of these additional tasks, refer to the Owners Workshop Manual.

Every 24 000 miles (40 000 km) or 1 year – whichever comes first

CTX TYPE AUTOMATIC TRANSMISSION

Renew the automatic transmission fluid

Refer to a Ford dealer.

Every 24 000 miles (40 000 km) or 2 years – whichever comes first

In addition to the items in the *'12 000 miles (20 000 km)'* service on page 96 and *'6000 miles (10 000 km)'* service on page 90, carry out the following.

COOLING SYSTEM

Renew the coolant

Note: *The following items will be required for this task:*

- *A suitable quantity of coolant solution (made up from approximately 55% clean water and 45% antifreeze)*
- *Suitable container to catch the old coolant as it drains*
- *Suitable spanner or socket to fit the cylinder block drain plug (where applicable)*
- *A suitable screwdriver to fit the radiator drain plug or radiator hose clip(s), as applicable*

Draining the system

The coolant should be drained with the engine cold.

Set the heater temperature control inside the car to the fully hot position.

Remove the cooling system pressure cap. Refer to the *'Checking coolant level'* procedure on page 71 for details of the cap location and type.

Check to see if a drain plug is fitted to the lower left-hand side of the radiator (when viewed from the driver's seat).

If so, position a suitable container underneath the radiator, making sure that the container is big enough to hold all the coolant, then unscrew the drain plug and allow the coolant to drain.

If no drain plug is fitted, position the container beneath the radiator bottom hose connection, then slacken the hose clip, release the hose, and allow the coolant to drain.

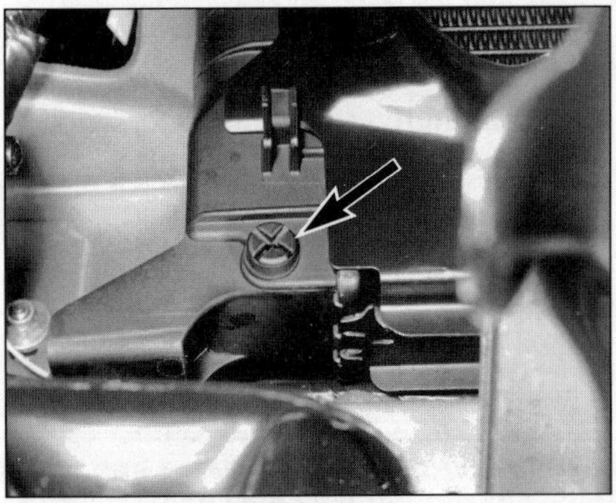

▲ *Radiator drain plug (arrowed)*

A cylinder block drain plug is also fitted to certain models, on the forward facing side of the engine, towards the gearbox end. Where a drain plug is fitted, reposition the container, then unscrew the plug and allow the remaining coolant in the cylinder block to drain into the container.

If rust or sludge is evident in the coolant which has been drained, the cooling system should be flushed to remove any further contamination from the engine and radiator.

If the coolant drained is clean, then the cooling system can be refilled as described later in this Section.

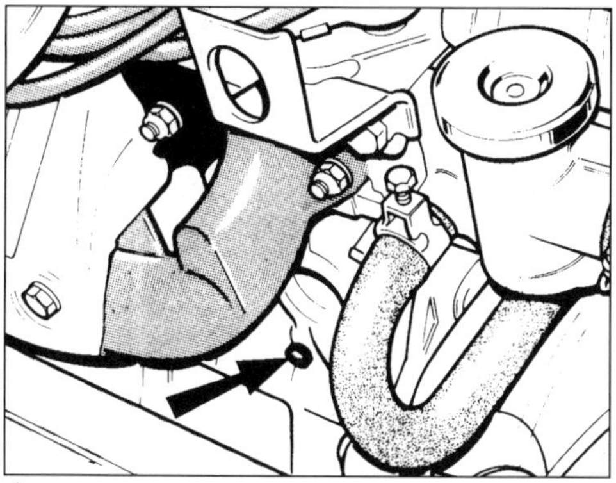

▲ *Cylinder block drain plug location (arrowed) – CVH engine*

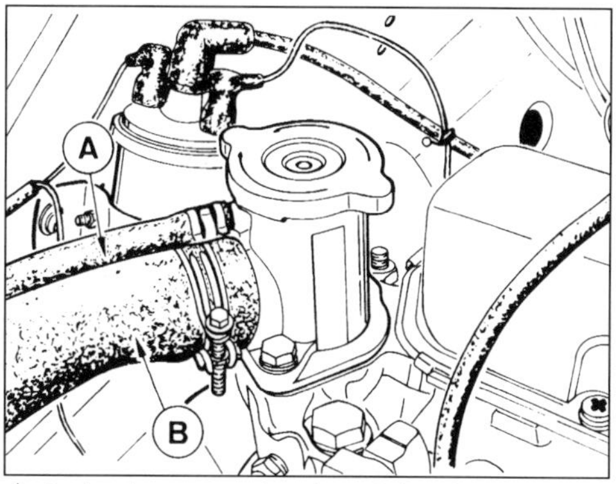

▲ *Coolant hose connections (**A** and **B**) at thermostat housing (OHV engine)*

Flushing the system

Note: *A new thermostat housing gasket will be required for this task*

To flush the cooling system, first the thermostat must be removed.

On OHV engines the thermostat is located in a housing at the right-hand end of the engine, and on CVH engines the thermostat is located in a housing at the left-hand end of the engine (when viewed from the driver's seat).

Slacken the clips and disconnect the coolant hoses from the thermostat housing.

Disconnect the wiring from the radiator fan switch which is located in the thermostat housing.

Unscrew the securing bolts (two on OHV engines and three on CVH engines), and remove the thermostat housing cover. If it's stuck, tap it gently with a soft-faced mallet or similar tool (Don't use a metal-faced hammer).

On OHV engines the thermostat can now be lifted from its location in the cylinder block. If the thermostat is stuck in position, don't lever it out, but cut around the edge with a sharp knife.

On CVH engines, the thermostat is retained in the thermostat housing cover, and there is no need to remove it once the cover has been removed from the engine.

Insert the end of a garden hose into the thermostat housing in the cylinder block, and flush the system through using cold water.

Continue flushing until clean water flows from the disconnected radiator bottom hose or radiator drain plug, and cylinder block drain plug, as applicable.

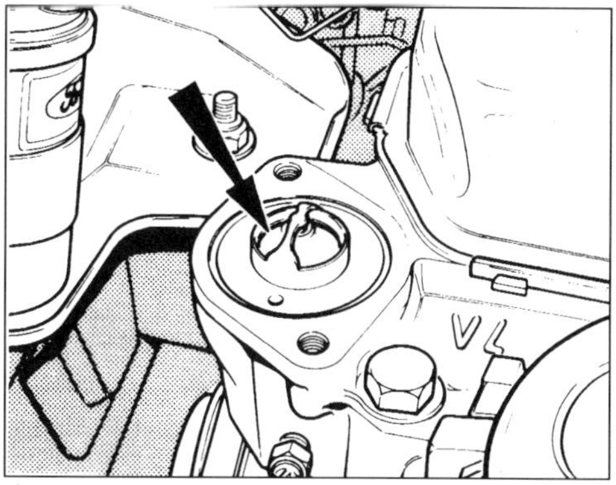

▲ *Thermostat (arrowed) with housing cover removed (OHV engine)*

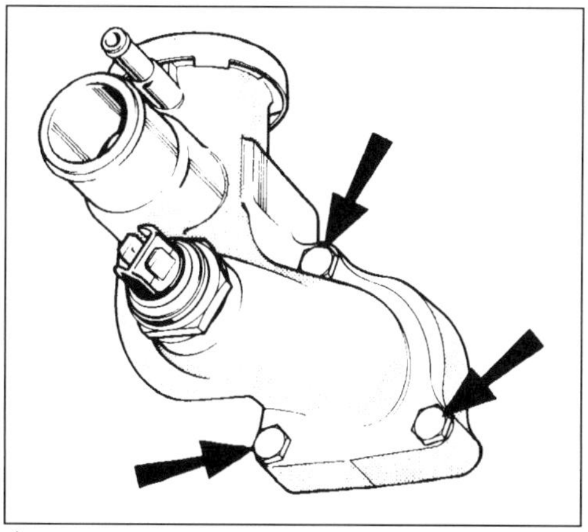

▲ *Thermostat housing cover securing bolts (arrowed) CVH engine*

If it seems that the system is particularly badly contaminated, and flushing does not appear to be solving the problem, seek advice, as it may be possible to clean the radiator using a proprietary cleaning compound.

When flushing is complete, refit the thermostat.

Carefully remove all traces of old gasket from the faces of the thermostat housing and cover, then refit the cover using a new gasket, and tighten the securing bolts.

Reconnect the hoses and the wiring, and tighten the hose clips.

Refilling the system

Reconnect the radiator bottom hose and tighten the clip, or refit and tighten the radiator drain plug, and the cylinder block drain plug, as applicable.

A solution of 55% clean water and 45% antifreeze should be used to fill the system all year round. It's important to note that because of the different types of metals used in the engine, it's vital to use antifreeze with suitable anti-corrosion additives all year round. **Never** use plain water to fill the whole system. If there's any doubt about the strength of the coolant mixture, it's better to add too much antifreeze than not enough.

On early models with a pressure cap on the thermostat housing, the system should be filled slowly through the thermostat housing filler neck until the coolant is nearly overflowing. Wait a few moments for trapped air to escape, then add more coolant. Repeat this procedure until the level does not drop, then refit the pressure cap. Pour coolant into the expansion tank until the level reaches the 'MAX' mark, then refit the cap.

On later models with a screw type pressure cap on the expansion tank, fill the system slowly through the expansion tank until the level reaches the 'MAX' mark. Wait a few moments for trapped air to escape, then add more coolant. Repeat this procedure until the level does not drop any more, then refit the pressure cap.

On all models, start the engine and run it to normal operating temperature, then check that the heater works, and switch off the engine.

Once the engine has cooled, squeeze the hoses and check for air locks (it should be possible to feel coolant in all the hoses).

If the heater failed to give warm air, there may be an air lock in the heater, in which case the air can be forced out by squeezing the heater hoses (which run to the bulkhead at the back of the engine compartment).

If necessary, air can be removed from a hose by loosening a hose clip, and squeezing the hose until all the air is forced out (obviously some coolant will be forced out too).

Recheck the coolant level and carry out any final topping up to the expansion tank.

FUEL AND EXHAUST SYSTEMS

Renew the air cleaner filter element

Note: *Ensure that the correct type of new filter element is obtained for your particular car*

Carburettor models and 1.4 litre fuel injection models

The air cleaner is located on the top of the carburettor/fuel injection unit (as applicable) at the rear of the engine.

Unscrew and remove the air cleaner cover retaining screws or bolts as applicable.

Where applicable, release the cover retaining clips around the side of the air cleaner body, then remove the cover and lift out the air cleaner element. (On some fuel injection models it may be necessary to unscrew two nuts before the element can be removed.)

Wipe out the inside of the air cleaner body and the cover, then place the new element in position. Refit the cover using a reversal of the removal procedure.

▲ *Unscrewing air cleaner cover retaining screws (carburettor model)*

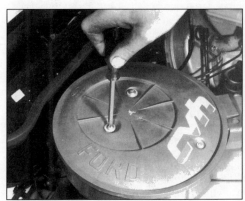

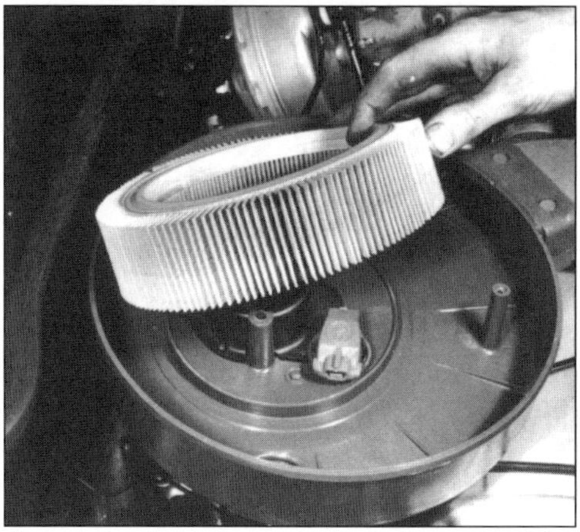

▲ *Removing the air cleaner element (carburettor model)*

1.6 litre fuel injection models (except RS Turbo) up to August 1989 (approx)

Note: *A new sensor unit-to-air cleaner cover gasket may be required for this task (depending on the condition of the old one)*

The air cleaner is located at the front left-hand side of the engine compartment (when viewed from the driver's seat).

Loosen the clamp screw on the metal band securing the air ducting to the sensor unit on top of the air cleaner.

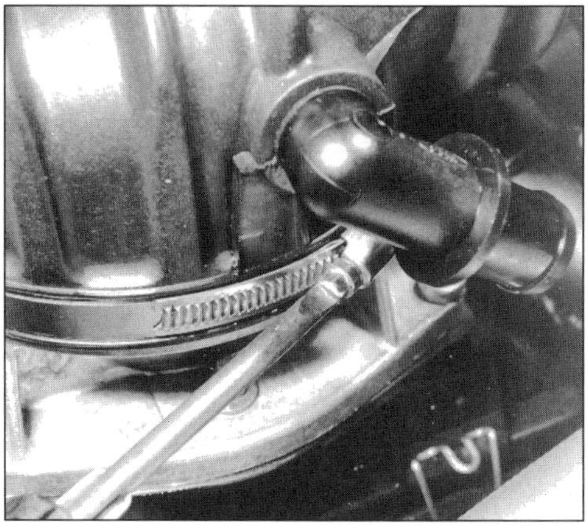

▲ *Loosening the air ducting metal band securing screw – fuel injection models (except RS Turbo) up to August 1989 (approx)*

Carefully pull the hose from the connector on the side of the air ducting, then lift the air ducting to one side out of the way.

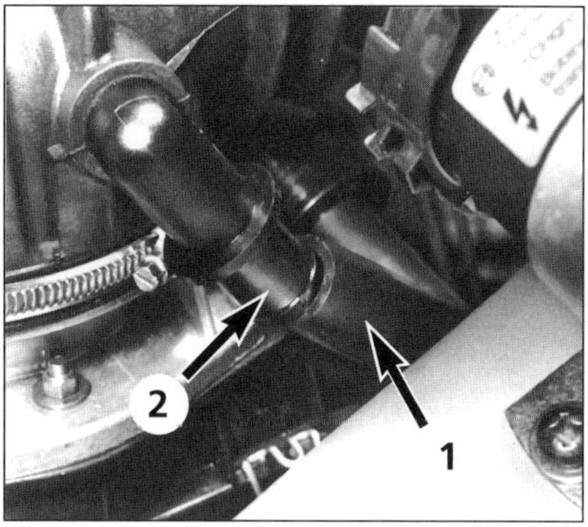

▲ *Pull the hose (**1**) from the connector (**2**) on the side of the air ducting – fuel injection models (except RS Turbo) up to August 1989 (approx)*

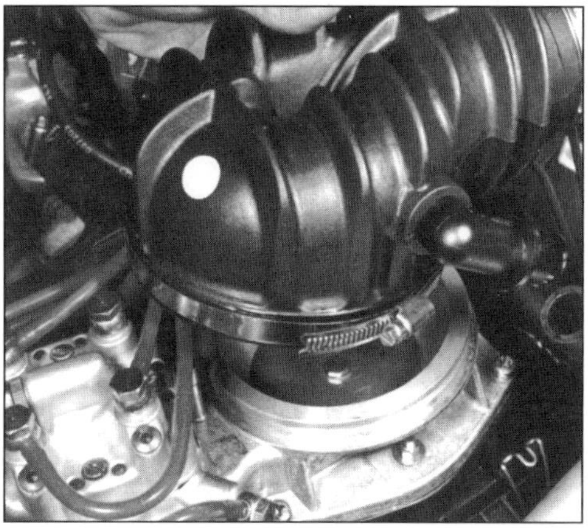

▲ *Lifting the air ducting away from the sensor unit – fuel injection models (except RS Turbo) up to August 1989 (approx)*

Unscrew and remove the six screws securing the sensor unit to the air cleaner cover, but leave the sensor unit in position for the moment.

Release the clips securing the air cleaner cover to the air cleaner body, then carefully pull the hose from the front of the air cleaner cover.

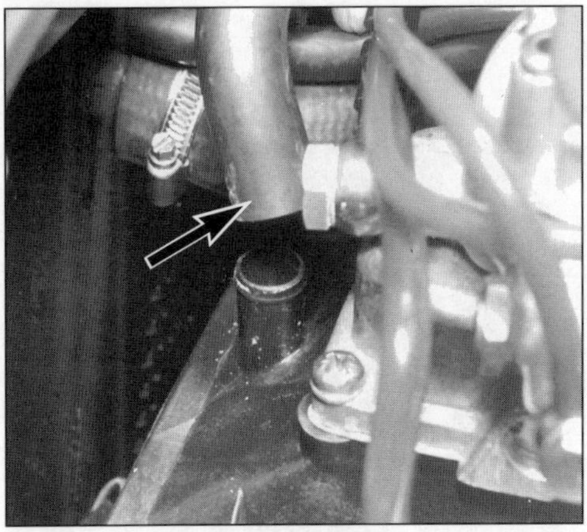

▲ *Pull the hose (arrowed) from the front of the air cleaner cover – fuel injection models (except RS Turbo) up to August 1989 (approx)*

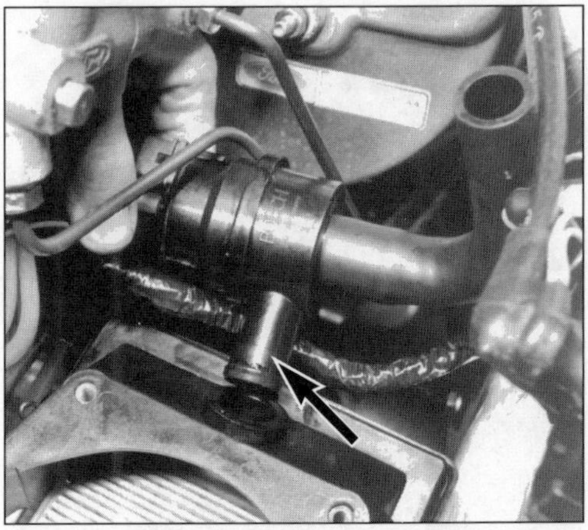

▲ *Pull the valve (arrowed) from the rear of the air cleaner cover – fuel injection models (except RS Turbo) up to August 1989 (approx)*

Carefully lift the sensor unit clear, together with its gasket, and pivot it back out of the way. Take care not to damage the sensor unit, as it's a delicate instrument.

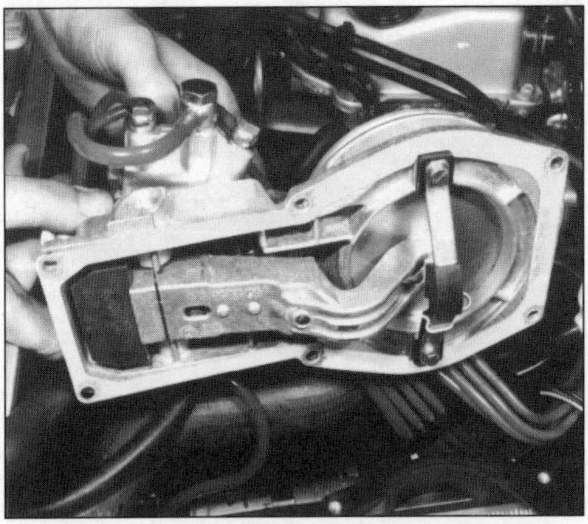

▲ *Lifting the sensor unit clear – fuel injection models (except RS Turbo) up to August 1989 (approx)*

Carefully pull the valve from the rear of the air cleaner cover, then lift out the cover, and remove the air cleaner element from the casing.

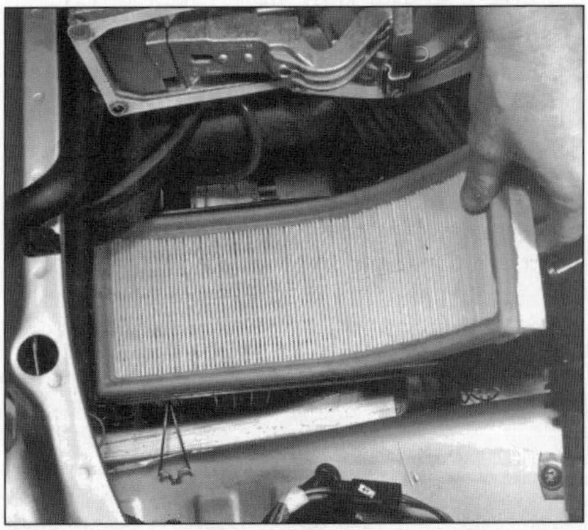

▲ *Removing the air cleaner element – fuel injection models (except RS Turbo) up to August 1989 (approx)*

Wipe out the inside of the air cleaner casing and the cover, then place the new element in position. Refit the components using the reverse of the removal procedure. When fitting the sensor unit in position on the air cleaner cover, check that the gasket is in good condition and aligned correctly. If necessary renew the gasket.

Check that all the connections are secure on completion.

1.6 litre fuel injection models (except RS Turbo) from August 1989 (approx)

The air cleaner is located at the front right-hand side of the engine compartment (when viewed from the driver's seat).

Disconnect the wiring plug and the hose from the valve on the air cleaner cover.

Release the cover retaining clips, and withdraw the cover and the element.

Wipe out the inside of the air cleaner casing and the cover, then place the new element in position. Refit the components using the reverse of the removal procedure.

Check that all the connections are secure on completion.

RS Turbo models

The air cleaner is located at the front left-hand side of the engine compartment (when viewed from the driver's seat).

Unscrew and remove the two bolts securing the air cleaner assembly to the top of the sensor unit, then remove the air cleaner assembly.

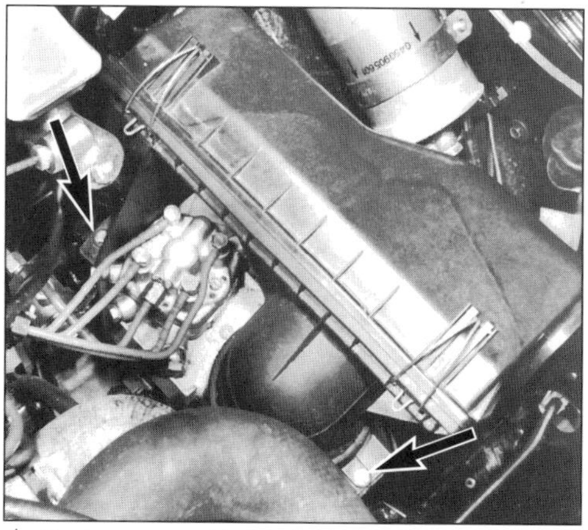

▲ *Air cleaner assembly securing bolts (arrowed) – RS Turbo models*

Release the air cleaner cover retaining clips, then lift off the cover and remove the filter element.

Wipe out the inside of the air cleaner casing and the cover, then place the new element in position, and refit the components using the reverse of the removal procedure.

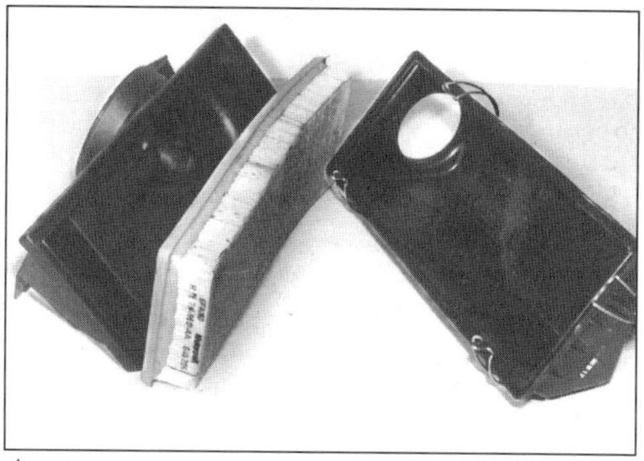

▲ *Lift off the air cleaner cover and remove the element – RS Turbo models*

On CVH engines renew the crankcase emission control filter (where fitted)

Note: *Ensure that the correct type of new filter is obtained for your particular car*

Carburettor models

Where fitted, the filter is located in the underside of the air cleaner body.

To renew the filter, disconnect the hoses from the filter, noting their locations, then pull the filter from the air cleaner.

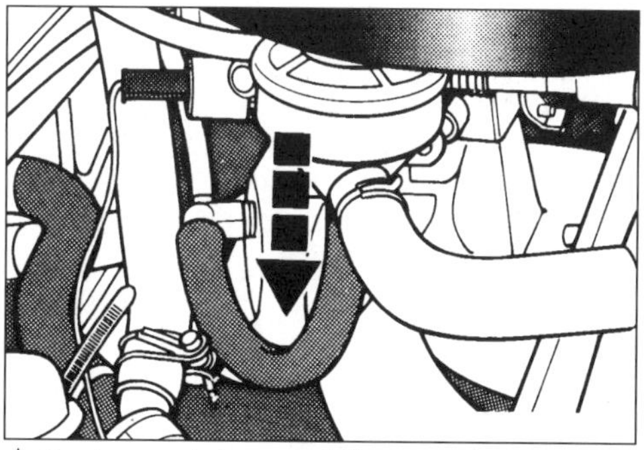

▲ *Crankcase emission control filter renewal (carburettor model)*

Make sure that the sealing grommet is in position in the air cleaner body, before pushing the new filter into position and reconnecting the hoses in their correct positions.

Fuel injection models

On fuel injection models, the filter is positioned on the right-hand side of the engine compartment (when viewed from the driver's seat). Various types of filter have been fitted, but they can all be removed in the same way by disconnecting the hoses from the valve body, noting the hose locations. On some early models, it may be necessary to detach the filter from a support bracket.

Make sure that hoses are reconnected in their correct positions.

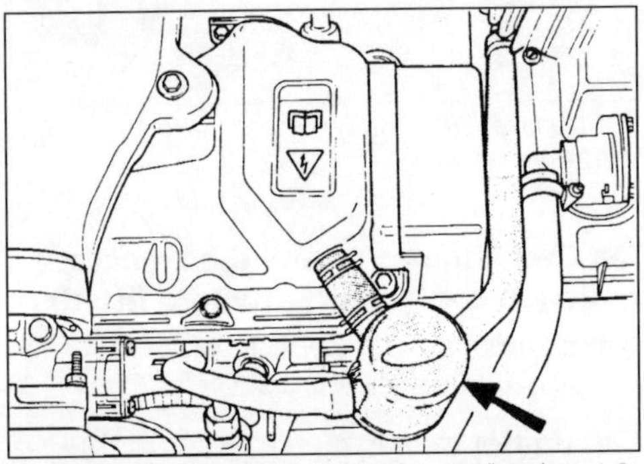

▲ *Crankcase emission control filter (arrowed) on later 1.6 litre fuel injection (non-RS Turbo) model*

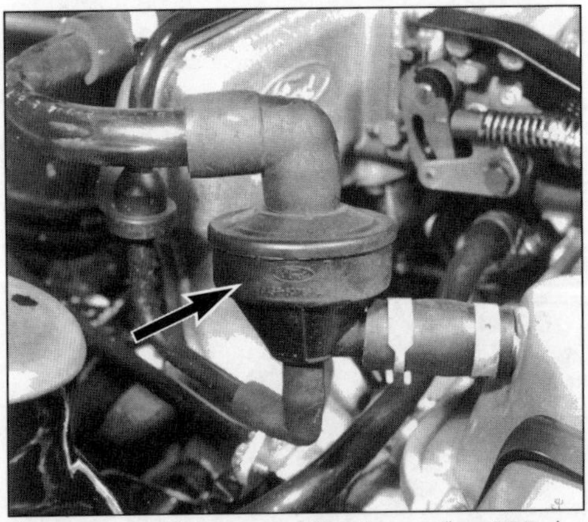

▲ *Crankcase emission control filter (arrowed) on RS Turbo model*

ADDITIONAL TASKS

Note that as well as the tasks described in the preceding paragraphs, the additional tasks given in the *'Service schedule'* chart on page 78 should be carried out every 24 000 miles (40 000 km) or 2 years – whichever comes first. These tasks require more detailed explanation, or the use of special tools, and are considered beyond the scope of this Handbook. For details of these additional tasks, refer to the Owners Workshop Manual.

Every 36 000 miles (60 000 km) or 3 years – whichever comes first

In addition to the items listed in the previous services, the additional tasks given in the *'Service schedule'* chart on page 78 should be carried out every 36 000 miles (60 000 km) or 3 years – whichever comes first. These tasks require more detailed explanation, or the use of special tools, and are considered beyond the scope of this Handbook. For details of these additional tasks, refer to the Owners Workshop Manual.

SEASONAL SERVICING

If you carry out all the procedures described in the previous Section, at the recommended mileage or time intervals, then you'll have gone a long way towards getting the best out of your car in terms of both performance and long life. In spite of this, there are always other areas, not dealt with in regular servicing, where neglect can spell trouble.

A little extra time spent on your car at the beginning and end of every winter will be well worthwhile in terms of peace of mind and prevention of trouble. The suggested tasks which follow have therefore been divided into Spring and Autumn Sections – but it's always a good idea to do them more frequently if you feel able.

Autumn

COOLING SYSTEM

Check the radiator and all hoses for signs of deterioration or damage

Refer to *'Engine compartment'* on page 90.

Check the strength of the coolant solution

This can be done using a coolant hydrometer, which should be available from most motor accessory shops and motor factors.

The hydrometer will give an indication of the amount of antifreeze in the system, and should be used exactly in accordance with the manufacturer's instructions.

The strength of the solution should never be allowed to drop below 55% clean water, and 45% antifreeze.

If there is any doubt about the strength of the coolant solution, the system should be drained and refilled as described in the *'24 000 miles (40 000 km)'* service Section on page 100.

ELECTRICAL SYSTEM

Where applicable, check the battery electrolyte level

Refer to *'Regular checks'* on page 75.

Check and if necessary clean the battery terminals

Make sure that the terminals are secure, and clean any corrosion from the metal.

To prevent corrosion, the terminals can be coated with petroleum jelly (don't use ordinary grease).

Check the condition and adjustment of the alternator drivebelt

Refer to the procedure given in the *'6000 miles (10 000 km)'* service Section on page 94.

Check the operation of all lights, electrical equipment and accessories

Refer to *'Fault finding'* on page 127 if any problems are discovered.

If any of the bulbs need to be renewed, refer to *'Bulb, fuse and relay renewal'* on page 113.

Check the washer fluid level and the wipers and washers

Refer to *'Regular checks'* on page 75.

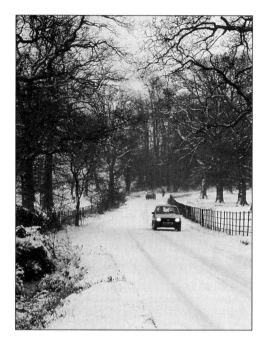

TYRES

Check tread depth and condition

Refer to *'Regular checks'* on page 73. Remember that you may be driving in slippery conditions during the winter.

BODYWORK

Thoroughly clean the car

Wash the car, and then polish it thoroughly to help protect the paint during the winter.

Spring

UNDERBODY

Thoroughly clean the underside of the car

The best time to clean the underside of the car is after the car has been driven in wet conditions, when the accumulated dirt will be softened up.

To clean the car, first of all the car must be jacked up as high as possible (making sure that it is safely supported – refer to *'Safety first!'* on page 84).

Gather together a quantity of paraffin, or water-soluble solvent, a stiff-bristle brush, a scraper, and a garden hose.

With the car jacked up and safely supported, get underneath the car, and cover the brake components at each wheel with polythene bags to stop dirt and water getting into them.

Loosen any encrusted dirt, scraping or brushing it away – the paraffin or solvent can be used where there's oil contamination. Pay particular attention to the wheel arches. Take care not to remove the underseal (a waxy substance applied to the car underbody to protect against corrosion).

When all the dirt is loosened, a wash down with the hose will remove the remaining dirt and mud.

You can now check for signs of damage to the underseal. If there's any sign of the underseal breaking away, patch it up by spraying or brushing on a suitable underseal wax (available from motor accessory shops and motor factors). Make sure the area is clean and dry before applying the wax.

Take the opportunity to check for signs of rusting. Likely places are the body sills and floor panels.

If rust is found, seek advice and have the affected area repaired before the problem gets too bad.

On completion, lower the car to the ground.

BODYWORK

Thoroughly check and clean the surfaces of the bodywork

Give the car a thorough wash and check for stone chips and rust spots. For details of how to treat these minor paint problems, refer to *'Bodywork and interior care'* on page 111.

After any repairs to the paint have been carried out (not before, otherwise the paint will not stick), give the car a polish.

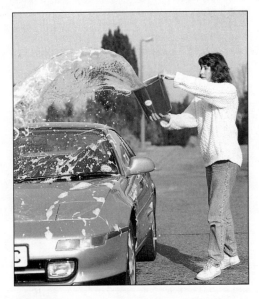

WHAT TO BUY

If you're intending to carry out your own servicing, you'll need to obtain a few basic tools. Although at first sight you may think that tools seem expensive, once you've bought them they should last a lifetime if you look after them properly.

The tools supplied with the car will enable you to change a wheel, and not much more. The absolute minimum tool kit you'll need to carry out any maintenance or servicing will be a range of metric spanners, two screwdrivers (one for crosshead or 'Phillips' type screws), and a pair of pliers. With a bit of ingenuity, these items should enable you to complete the more basic routine servicing jobs, but they won't allow you to do much else.

When buying tools, it's important to bear in mind the quality. You don't need to buy the most expensive tools available, but generally you get what you pay for. Cheap tools may prove to be a false economy, as they're unlikely to last as long as better quality alternatives.

It's very difficult to lay down hard and fast rules on exactly what you're going to need, but the following list should be helpful in building up a good tool kit. Combination spanners (ring one end, open-ended the other) are recommended because, although more expensive than double open-ended ones, they give the advantages of both types.

- *Combination spanners to cover a reasonable range of sizes (say 7 mm to 17 mm at least)*
- *Adjustable spanner*
- *Spark plug spanner (with rubber insert)*
- *Spark plug gap adjustment tool*
- *Set of feeler gauges*
- *Screwdriver (Plain) – 100 mm long blade x 6 mm diameter (approx)*
- *Screwdriver (Crosshead) – 100 mm long blade x 6 mm diameter (approx)*
- *Oil filter wrench*
- *Pliers*
- *Tyre pump*
- *Tyre pressure gauge*
- *A suitable key (Torx or Allen type, depending on model) to fit the gear-box oil filler plug (later models only)*
- *Oil can*
- *Funnel (medium size)*
- *Stiff brush (for general cleaning jobs)*
- *Tool box*
- *Hydraulic jack (ideally a trolley jack)*
- *Pair of axle stands*
- *Suitable containers for draining engine oil and coolant*
- *Inspection lamp*

This is by no means a comprehensive list of tools, and you'll probably want to gradually add to your tool box as you discover the need for other tools, especially if you decide to tackle some of the more advanced servicing jobs described in the **Owners Workshop Manual** for your particular car.

CARE OF YOUR TOOLS

Having bought a reasonable set of tools, it's worth taking the trouble to look after them. After use, always wipe off any dirt or grease using a clean, dry cloth before putting them away. Never leave tools lying around after they've been used – a tool rack, or better still a proper toolbox will prove the best way of keeping everything up together. Rags can be wrapped around loose tools to prevent them from rattling if you're going to keep them in the boot of the car.

Feeler gauges should be wiped with an oily cloth from time to time, to leave a thin coating of oil on the metal which will prevent corrosion. Screwdriver blades inevitably lose their keen edges, and a little occasional attention with a file or an oilstone will keep them in good condition.

SHF

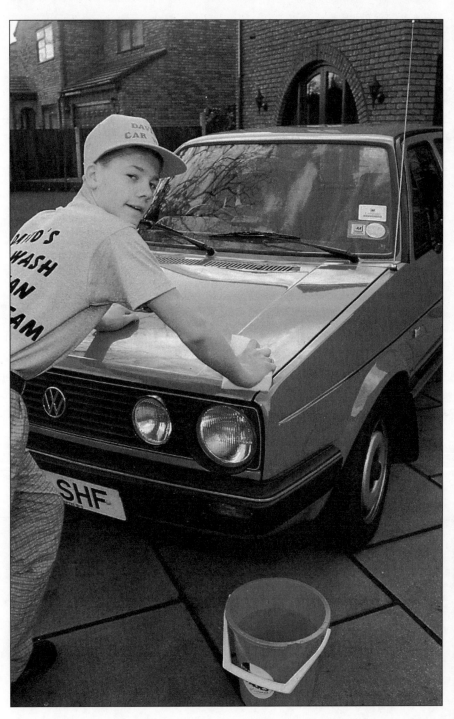

It's well worth spending the time and effort necessary to look after your car's bodywork and interior. Cleaning your car regularly will not only improve its appearance, it will also protect the bodywork against the elements and the grime encountered in everyday driving. It's worth bearing in mind that if your car looks clean and tidy, it will also be worth more money when you come to sell it or trade it in for a newer model.

This Section will help you to keep your car in 'showroom' condition. If you wish to tackle repairs to more serious bodywork damage or corrosion, comprehensive details can be found in our **'Car Bodywork Repair Manual'**.

CLEANING THE INTERIOR

It's a good idea to clean the interior of the car first, before cleaning the exterior, as this will avoid spreading the dirt from inside over the bodywork.

Start by removing all the loose odds and ends from inside the car, not forgetting the ashtrays, glovebox and any interior pockets. Take out any loose mats or carpets, which should be shaken and brushed, and if possible vacuum-cleaned.

The inside of the car can be cleaned with a brush and dustpan, or preferably a vacuum-cleaner. If you can't use your household vacuum-cleaner, it may be worth investing in one of the small 12-volt hand vacuum-cleaners which can be powered from the car battery. If the carpets are very dirty, use a suitable proprietary cleaner with a brush to remove the ingrained dirt. Ideally, it's best to remove the carpets for cleaning, but this is an involved task in most modern cars, and it will probably be easier to leave them in place.

The facia, door trim, seats, and any other items which require attention can now be wiped over with a cloth soaked in warm water containing a little washing up liquid. If the trim is particularly dirty, use one of the proprietary cleaners available from motor accessory shops – a number of different types are available, suitable for vinyl, cloth or leather upholstery, etc, as required. An old nail brush or tooth brush will help to remove any ingrained dirt. On completion, wipe the surfaces dry using a lint-free cloth, and leave the windows open to speed up drying.

The inside of the windscreen and windows should be cleaned using a proprietary glass cleaner, or methylated spirits. Be careful about using certain household products such as washing-up liquid which may leave a smeary film. Finish off by wiping with a clean, dry paper tissue.

Don't forget to clean the boot.

Check for any nicks or tears in the interior trim, seats, headlining, etc. Various repair kits are available from motor accessory shops to suit most types of trim, but if the damage is very serious, the relevant trim panel will probably have to be renewed.

CLEANING THE BODYWORK

Ideally, the car should be washed every week, either by hand (preferably using a hosepipe), or by using a local car-wash. If you're washing the car by hand, use plenty of water to loosen the dirt and dust, and if possible use a suitable car shampoo or wax additive in the water. Any stubborn dirt such as road tar or bird droppings can be removed using methylated spirit or preferably one of the special proprietary cleaning solutions (in which case make sure that the product is suitable for use on car paint) – in either case, wash the affected area down with plenty of water after removing the dirt. **Never** just wipe over a dirty car, as this will scratch the paint very effectively.

Two or three times a year, a good silicone or wax polish can be used on the paintwork. It's important to wash the car and remove all stubborn dirt, tar, etc, before using polish, as the polish will effectively seal over the top of any dirt, making it extremely difficult to remove in the future. Good polishes actually form a protective coating over the paint finish, which should help to make future accumulated dirt easier to remove. Always follow the manufacturer's recommendations closely when using polish. Try to avoid getting polish on any unpainted plastic or rubber body parts such as bumpers and spoilers, as it tends to leave a stain when dry. Chrome parts are best cleaned with a special chrome cleaner, as ordinary metal polish will wear away the finish.

Plastic or rubber body parts such as bumpers and spoilers should be cleaned using a suitable proprietary cleaner. A number of different types are available, including colour restorers, and special solvents to remove any stray polish which may have crept onto the plastic when polishing the paintwork. Make absolutely sure that any solvents or cleaners used are suitable, as certain products may attack plastic and/or rubber.

If the paint is beginning to lose its gloss or colour, and ordinary polishing doesn't seem to solve the problem, it's worth considering the use of a polish with a mild 'cutting' action to remove what is in effect a surface layer of 'dead' paint. In this case, follow the manufacturer's instructions, and don't polish too vigorously, or you might remove more paint than you intended!

DEALING WITH SCRATCHES

With superficial scratches which don't penetrate down to the metal, repair can be very simple.

Very light scratches can be polished out by carefully using a suitable 'cutting' polish. Follow the manufacturer's instructions, and take care not to remove too much of the surrounding paint.

If the scratch cannot be polished out, touch-up paint will be required. Touch-up paint is usually available in the form of a touch-up stick from the car manufacturer's dealers, or in various forms from motor accessory shops. You will probably have to quote the year and model of the car in order to make sure that you obtain the correct matching colour, and in some cases you may have to quote a paint reference number which will usually appear on the car's Vehicle Identification Number (VIN) plate under the bonnet (refer to *'Servicing'* on page 86).

Lightly rub the area of the scratch with a very fine cutting paste to remove loose paint from the scratch and to clear the surrounding bodywork of polish.

Rinse the area with clean water.

Apply suitable touch-up paint to the scratch using a fine paint brush, and continue to apply fine layers of paint until the surface of the paint in the scratch is level with the surrounding paintwork.

Allow the new paint at least two weeks to harden, then blend it into the surrounding paintwork by rubbing the scratch area with a paintwork renovator or a very fine cutting paste.

If the paint finish requires a lacquer coat (in which case the lacquer will be supplied with the touch-up paint), it should now be applied to the newly painted area and allowed to dry in accordance with the manufacturer's instructions.

Finally, apply a suitable wax polish to the affected area for added protection.

BULBS

A defective exterior light can be not only dangerous, but also illegal. Carrying spare bulbs will enable you to renew blown ones as they occur. A failed interior light bulb may be just a nuisance, but a faulty exterior light could be a life or death matter.

Before assuming that a bulb has failed, check for corrosion on the bulb holder and wiring connections, particularly around the rear light assemblies.

- **Note that as a safety precaution, the battery earth (black) lead should always be disconnected before renewing a bulb.**
- **Remember to reconnect the lead on completion.**

Bulb ratings

Always make sure that when a bulb is renewed, a new bulb of the correct rating is used.

All the bulbs are of the 12-volt type, and their ratings are as follows:

Bulb	Rating [watts]
Headlight (tungsten)	50/45
Headlight (halogen)	60/55
Front sidelight (models up to 1986)	4
Front sidelight (models from 1986)	5
Front and rear direction indicator lights	21
Front driving light	55
Front direction indicator repeater light	5
Rear brake/tail light	21/5
Reversing light	21
Rear foglight	21
Rear number plate light	5
Courtesy light	10
Luggage compartment light	10
Glovebox light	2

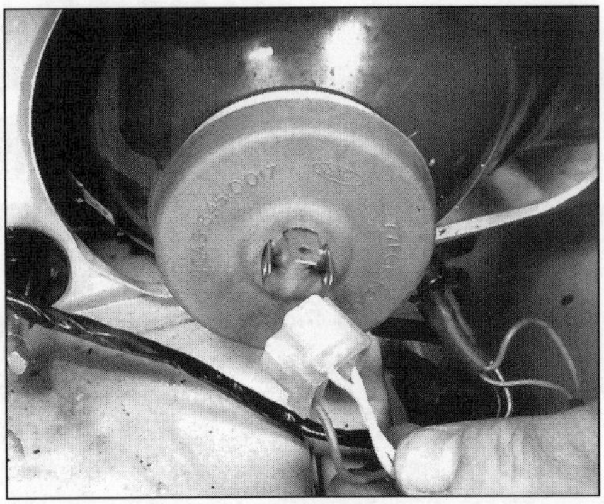

▲ *Pulling the wiring plug from the back of a headlight*

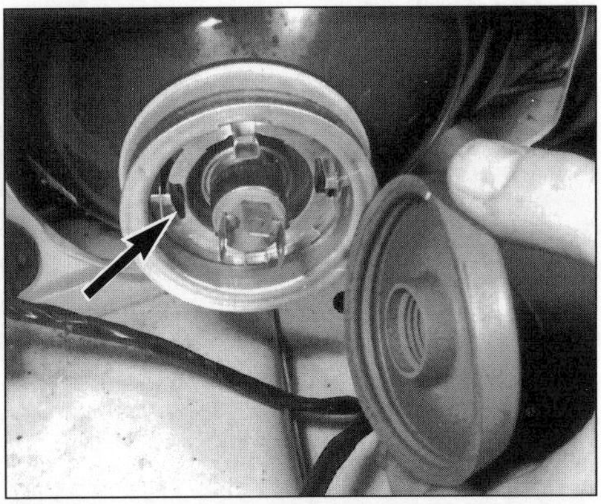

▲ *Removing the rubber cover from the back of a headlight to expose the bulb securing clip (arrowed)*

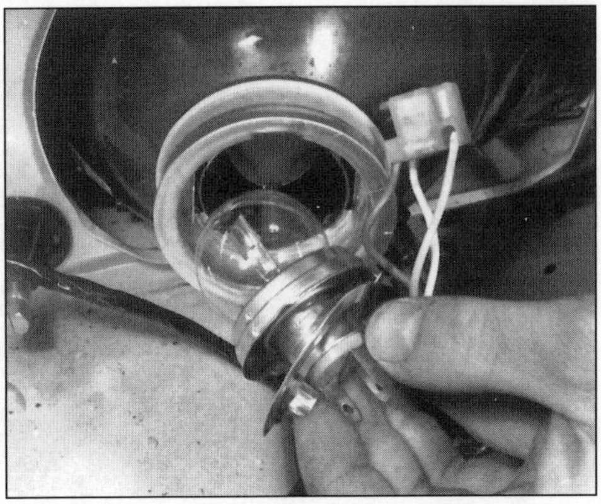

▲ *Removing a headlight bulb with securing clip*

Exterior light bulbs

HEADLIGHT

Open the bonnet. On RS Turbo models, if the left-hand (when viewed from the driver's seat) headlight bulb is to be renewed, the air cleaner must be removed for access – refer to the procedure for air cleaner element renewal in the *'24 000 miles (40 000 km)'* service Section on page 102.

Working in the engine compartment, pull the wiring plug from the back of the headlight.

Pull the rubber cover from the back of the headlight, then rotate the bulb securing clip, or release the spring clip arms from bulb housing, according to type, and withdraw the bulb. Note that the bulb may be either a tungsten or halogen type – tungsten bulbs have a conventional spherical type glass bubble, whereas halogen types have a cylindrical glass section with a tapered point at the end.

Fit the new bulb, taking care not to touch it with your fingers (hold the bulb using a clean cloth or paper tissue), using a reversal of the removal procedure. If the glass on the new bulb is inadvertently touched, wipe it with a cloth moistened with methylated spirit.

Make sure that the rubber cover is securely fitted to the back of the headlight.

FRONT SIDELIGHT

Open the bonnet, then remove the sidelight bulbholder from the side of the headlight by twisting it anti-clockwise.

Withdraw the push-fit bulb from the holder.

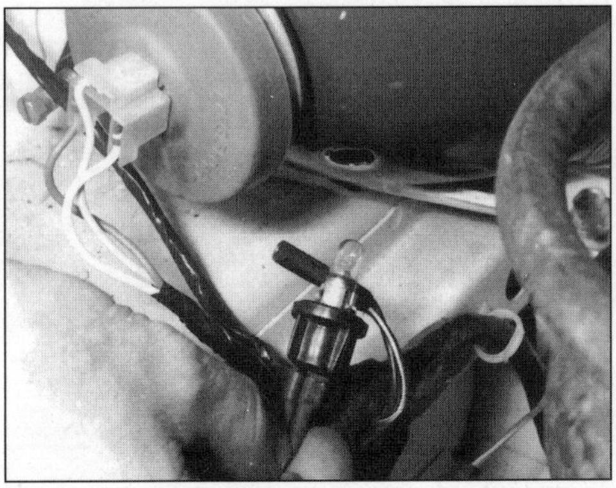

▲ *Removing a sidelight bulbholder from the side of the headlight*

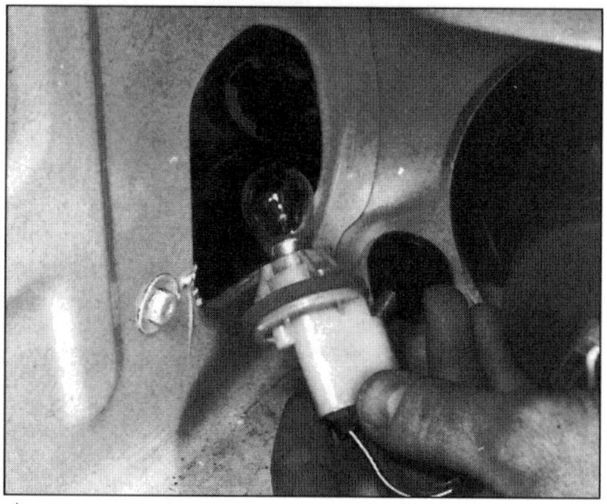

▲ Removing a front direction indicator light bulbholder

Fit the new bulb using a reversal of the removal procedure.

FRONT DIRECTION INDICATOR LIGHT

Open the bonnet, then working through the cut-out in the wing panel at the side of the engine compartment, twist the bulbholder anti-clockwise and withdraw it from the lens unit.

Press the bulb and turn it anti-clockwise to remove it from the holder.

Fit the new bulb using a reversal of the removal procedure.

FRONT DRIVING LIGHT

Remove the retaining screw at the bottom of the lens, and withdraw the lens assembly from the light.

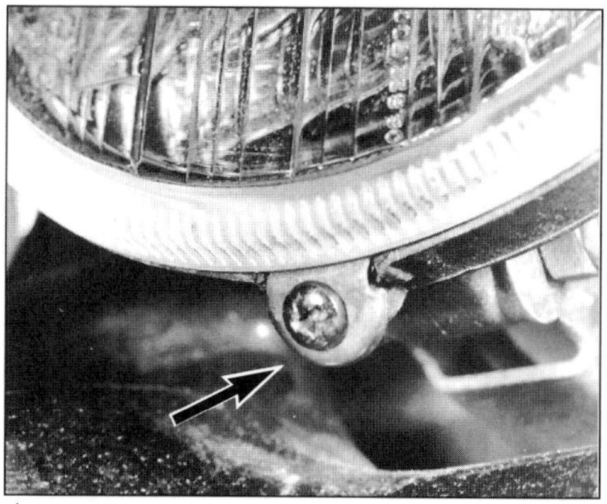

▲ Front driving light lens retaining screw (arrowed)

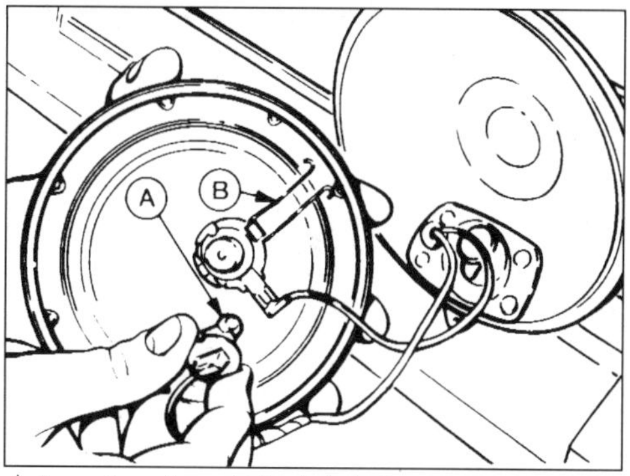

▲ Removing a front driving light bulb
A Bulb
B Spring clip

Disconnect the wires from the connectors inside the light housing, and remove the lens assembly from the car.

Release the spring clip arms from the back of the lens assembly, and withdraw the bulb (which is an H3 type with integral bulbholder and wire).

Fit the new bulb, taking care not to touch it with your fingers (hold the bulb using a clean cloth or paper tissue), using a reversal of the removal procedure. If the glass on the new bulb is inadvertently touched, wipe it with a cloth moistened with methylated spirit.

Refit the lens assembly, making sure that the wires are securely connected.

FRONT DIRECTION INDICATOR REPEATER LIGHT

Reach up behind the back of the front wheelarch and locate the back of the repeater light holder.

Squeeze the two clips on the back of the holder body, and push the assembly out through the wing panel.

Twist the bulbholder anti-clockwise to remove it from the lens, then pull the bulb from its socket.

Push a new bulb into the socket, and refit the assembly in the reverse order to removal.

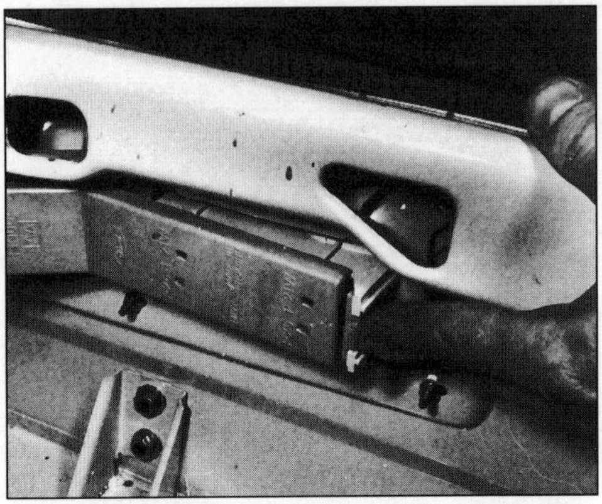

▲ *Releasing a rear light bulbholder retaining tab (Escort Hatchback model)*

REAR LIGHTS

Escort Hatchback models

Open the tailgate, and press the retaining tab on the edge of the bulbholder, then swing the bulbholder outwards to release the locating tag at the other end.

Remove the relevant bulb by pushing it down and turning it anti-clockwise.

Fit the new bulb and refit the bulbholder using a reversal of the removal procedure.

Escort Cabriolet models

Open the boot, and pull open the access flap to expose the bulbholder.

Push the upper and lower retaining tabs apart, and withdraw the bulbholder.

Remove the relevant bulb by pushing it down and turning it anti-clockwise.

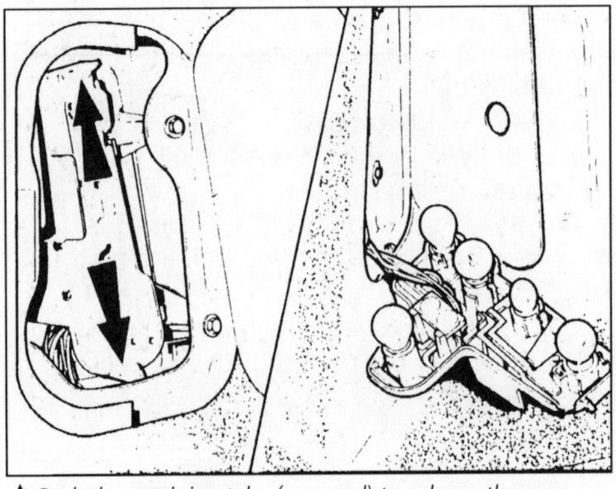

▲ *Push the retaining tabs (arrowed) to release the rear light bulbholder (Escort Cabriolet model)*

Fit the new bulb and refit the bulbholder using a reversal of the removal procedure.

Escort Estate models

Open the tailgate, then release the luggage compartment side trim panel, which covers the light assembly, by turning the four fasteners a quarter of a turn using a coin.

Pull the trim panel away to expose the bulbholder, then push the upper and lower retaining tabs apart, and withdraw the bulbholder.

Remove the relevant bulb by pushing it down and turning it anti-clockwise.

Fit the new bulb and refit the bulbholder using a reversal of the removal procedure.

Orion models

Open the boot, and press the retaining tabs on the edges of the bulbholder, then withdraw the bulbholder.

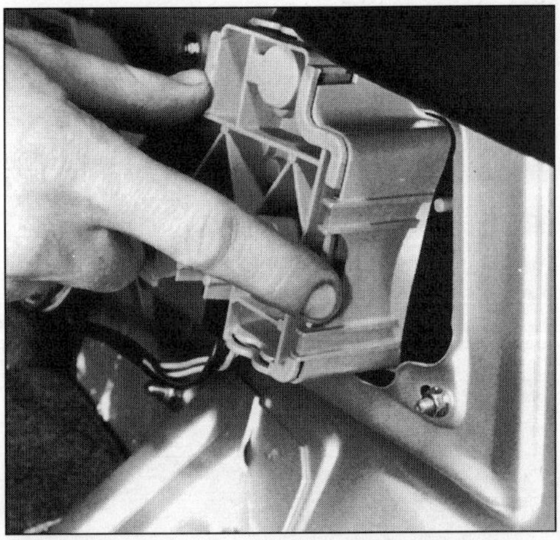

▲ *Releasing a rear light bulbholder retaining tab (Orion model)*

Remove the relevant bulb by pushing it down and turning it anti-clockwise.

Fit the new bulb and refit the bulbholder using a reversal of the removal procedure.

REAR NUMBER PLATE LIGHT

Using a small screwdriver, carefully prise the light assembly out through the top of the bumper. Take care to avoid scratching the bumper.

Models up to 1986

Turn the bulbholder anti-clockwise and remove it from the lens, then withdraw the push-fit bulb.

Fit the new bulb, then reassemble and refit the light assembly by reversing the removal operations.

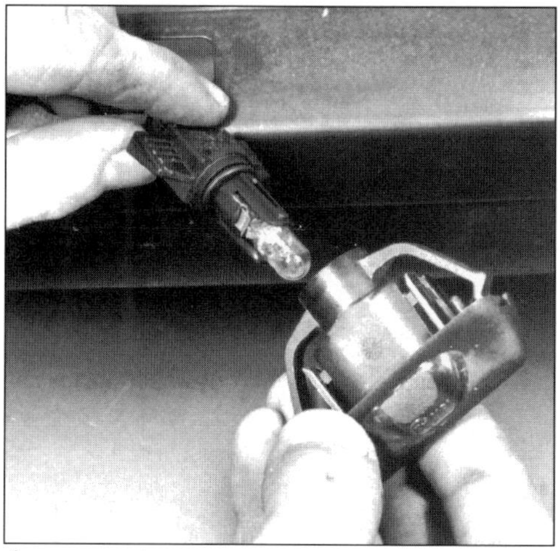

▲ *Removing the number plate light bulbholder (models up to 1986)*

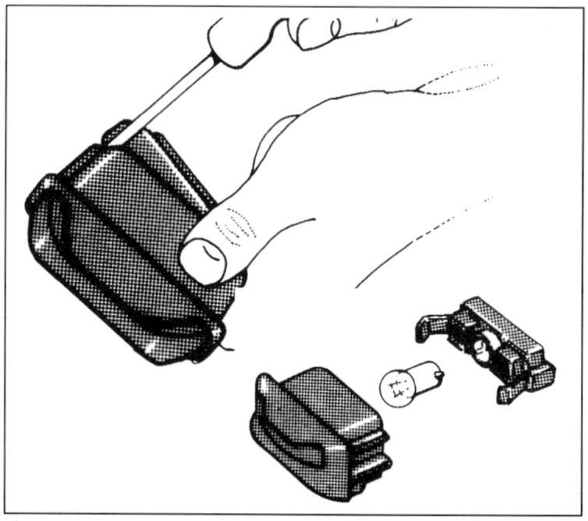

▲ *Removing the number plate light bulb (models from 1986)*

Models from 1986

Release the retaining clips by carefully inserting a screwdriver between the clips and the light housing, and withdraw the bulbholder. Remove the bulb by pushing it down and turning it anti-clockwise.

Fit the new bulb, then reassemble and refit the light assembly by reversing the removal operations.

Interior light bulbs

Note: *Renewal of the various instrument panel and facia-mounted control illumination light bulbs requires detailed explanation and in some cases extensive dismantling. Details can be found in the relevant* ***Owners Workshop Manual*** *for your particular car (OWM 686 for Escort models, or OWM 1009 for Orion models).*

COURTESY LIGHT

Carefully prise the light assembly from its location in the roof, taking care not to damage the roof trim, then pull the bulb from the spring contacts in the light body.

Fit the new bulb, making sure that it locates securely in the spring contacts, then refit the light assembly.

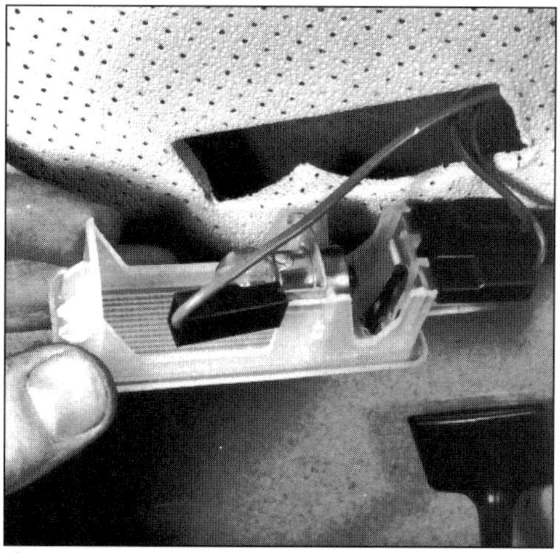

▲ *Removing the courtesy light*

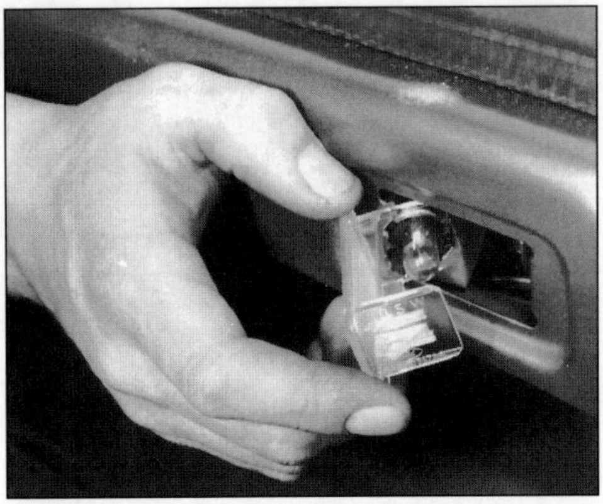

▲ *Removing the luggage compartment light*

LUGGAGE COMPARTMENT LIGHT

Using a small screwdriver, carefully prise the light assembly from its location, then (on all except Escort Cabriolet models) pull the bulb from the spring contact clip. On Escort Cabriolet models, remove the bulb by pushing it down and twisting.

Fit the new bulb, making sure that it locates securely in the spring contact clip, where applicable, then refit the light assembly.

GLOVEBOX LIGHT

Models up to 1986

Simply pull the old bulb from its socket in the glovebox, and push the new one into place.

Models from 1986

From inside the glovebox, remove the two screws securing the light switch, and withdraw the assembly.

Using a small screwdriver, carefully prise the switch from the light assembly, then remove the bulb by pushing it down and turning it anti-clockwise.

Fit the new bulb, then reassemble and refit the assembly using a reversal of the removal procedure.

FUSES

Most of the car's electrical circuits are protected by fuses which will blow when the relevant circuit becomes overloaded. This is to prevent possible damage to electrical components, or the possible risk of fire.

- **Before renewing a fuse, always make sure that the ignition and the relevant circuit are switched off.**

The fuses are housed in a plastic box located under the bonnet at the rear right-hand side of the engine compartment (when viewed from the driver's seat).

The fuses are numbered to identify the circuit which they protect, and the circuits are represented by symbols on the plastic fusebox cover.

To check a fuse, release the tab at the front of the fusebox cover, and open the cover. All fuses are a push fit in their sockets, and a blown fuse can be recognised by a break in the wire between the two terminals.

If a fuse has blown, renew it with one of identical rating. The fuses are colour-coded to show their rating as follows:

Colour	Rating [amps]
Red	10
Blue	15
Yellow	20
Clear	25
Green	30

Spare fuses are located in the fusebox cover. Always use proper fuses of the correct type and rating, and **never** use wire or any other material to bridge the gap where a fuse should be.

Note that the same fuse should never be renewed more than once without investigating the source of the trouble. Seek advice from someone suitably qualified if necessary.

The radio, and where applicable the electric aerial, have their own in-line circuit fuses (usually located in the wiring loom behind the radio), or are protected by fuses in the rear of the radio casing.

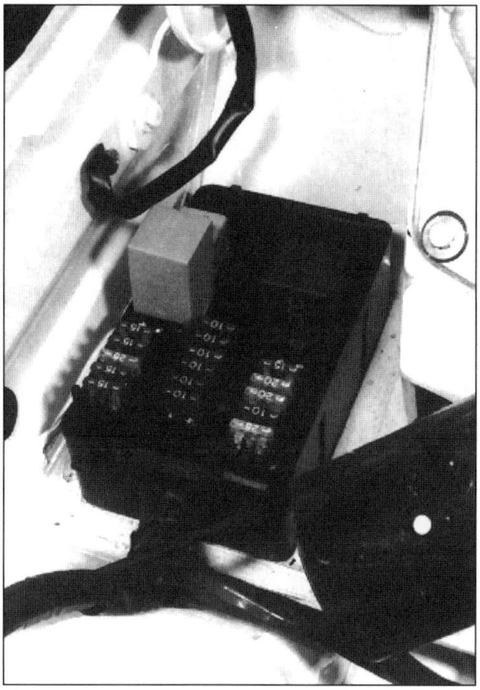

▲ *Fusebox location in engine compartment (cover removed to show fuses and relays)*

RELAYS

Various types of relays are used in some circuits, and a faulty relay may prevent one or more components from working.

- **Before renewing a relay, always make sure that the ignition and the relevant circuit are switched off.**

Relays are of the plug-in type, and most of the major relays are located in the fusebox (refer to *'Fuses'* on page 118), with symbols on the fusebox cover representing the circuit covered by each relay.

Various additional relays may be used depending on the equipment fitted, and these may be located in various positions depending on model. If a problem is suspected which may be due to a relay not located in the fusebox, it's best to seek advice from a Ford dealer who will know where on the car to find the relevant components.

To remove a relay, simply pull it from its socket.

It's difficult to tell visually whether a relay is faulty, and the best test is to substitute a known good relay to see if the relevant circuit then operates – if it does, then it's probably the relay which was causing the problem.

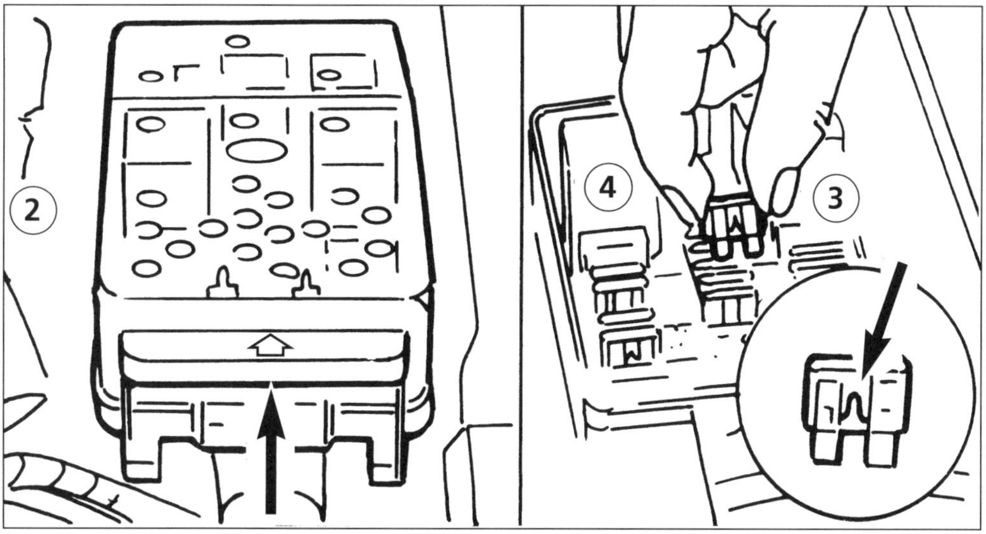

▲ *Fusebox showing cover removal* **(2)**, *fuse removal* **(3)**, *and relays* **(4)**
Check if fuse has blown by checking for a broken wire at the point indicated in inset

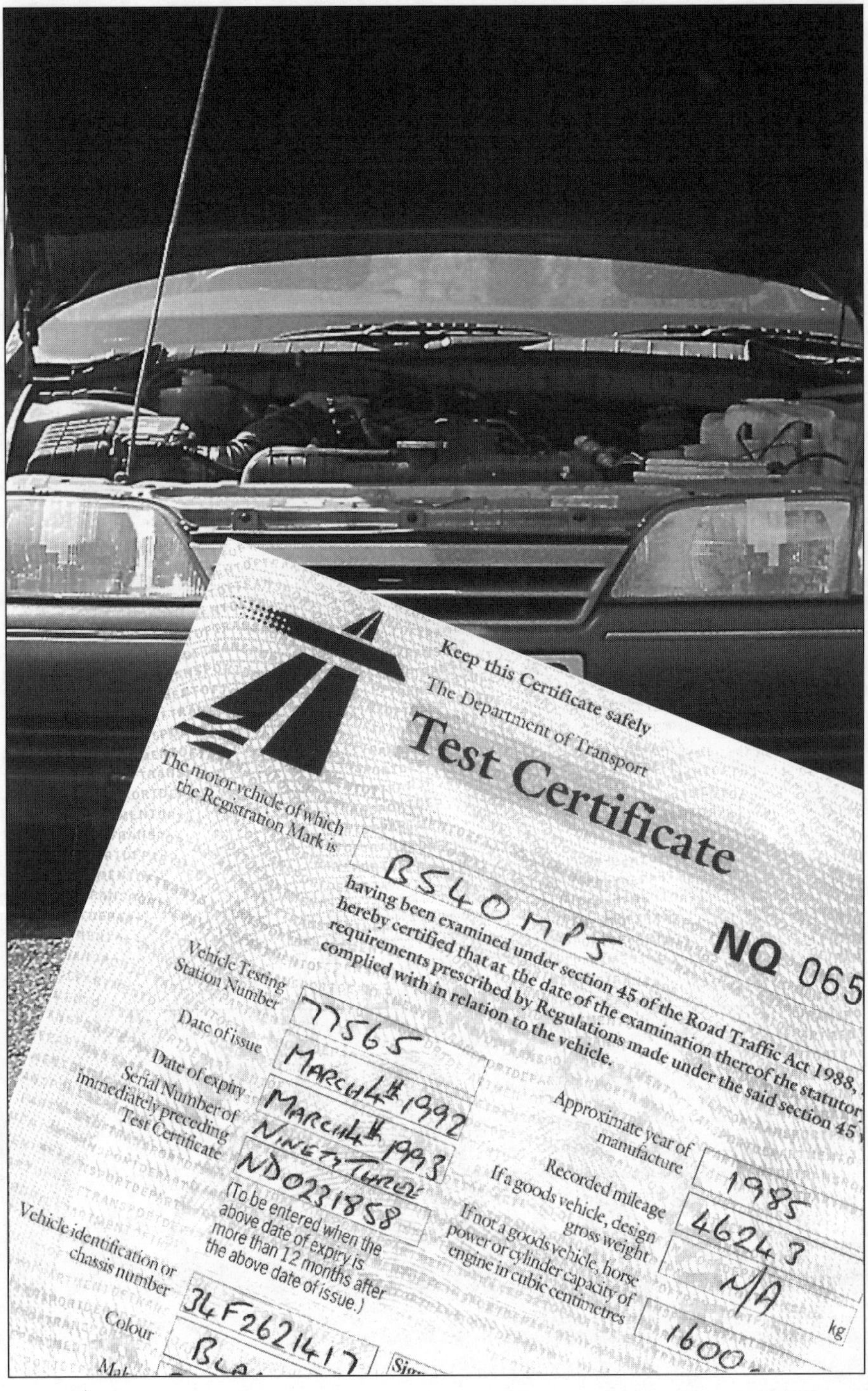
Keep this Certificate safely
The Department of Transport
Test Certificate
The motor vehicle of which the Registration Mark is
B540MPJ
NQ 065
having been examined under section 45 of the Road Traffic Act 1988,
hereby certified that at the date of the examination thereof the statutor
requirements prescribed by Regulations made under the said section 45
complied with in relation to the vehicle.
Vehicle Testing Station Number
77565
Date of issue
MARCH 4th 1992
Date of expiry
MARCH 4th 1993
Serial Number of immediately preceding Test Certificate
NINETY THREE
ND0231858
(To be entered when the above date of expiry is more than 12 months after the above date of issue.)
Approximate year of manufacture
1985
Recorded mileage
46243
If a goods vehicle, design gross weight
N/A
kg
If not a goods vehicle, horse power or cylinder capacity of engine in cubic centimetres
1600
Vehicle identification or chassis number
34F2621417
Colour

The following information is intended as a guide to enable you to spot some of the more obvious faults which may cause your car to fail the MOT test.

Obviously it isn't possible to check the car to the same standard as a professional MOT tester, who will be highly experienced and will have all the necessary tools and equipment.

Although we can't cover all the points of the test, the following should provide you with a good indication as to the general condition of the car, and will enable you to identify any obvious problem areas before submitting your car for the test.

Further explanation of most of the checks, and details of how to cure any problems discovered can be found in the relevant *Owners Workshop Manual* for your particular car (OWM 686 for Escort models, and OWM 1009 for Orion models).

Lights

- All lights must work reliably, and the lenses and reflectors must not be damaged.
- Pairs of similar lights must be of the same brightness (eg both rear lights).
- Both headlights must show the same colour, and must be correctly aimed so that they light up the road adequately, but don't dazzle other drivers.
- The brake lights must work when the brake pedal is pressed.
- The direction indicator lights must flash between one and two times per second.
- All switches and driver's tell-tale lights must be fitted, secure and in good working order.
- No lamp should be adversely affected by the operation of any other lamp.

Steering and suspension

- All the components and their mounting points must be secure, and there must be no damage or excessive corrosion.
- There must be no excessive free play in the joints and bushes, and all rubber gaiters must be secure and undamaged.
- The steering mechanism must operate smoothly without excessive free play or roughness.
- There should be no excessive free play or roughness in the wheel bearings, but there should be sufficient free play to prevent tightness or binding.
- There should be no major fluid leaks from the shock absorbers and, when each corner of the car is depressed, it should rise and then settle in its normal position.
- The driveshafts and propeller shaft (on rear wheel drive cars) must not be damaged or distorted.

Brakes

- It should be possible to operate the handbrake without excessive force or excessive movement of the lever, and it must not be possible for the lever to release unintentionally. The handbrake must be able to lock the relevant wheels on which it operates.
- The brake pedal must not be damaged, and when the pedal is pressed, resistance should be felt near the top of its travel – hard resistance should be felt, and the pedal should not move down towards the floor. The resistance should be firm and not spongy.
- There should be no signs of any fluid leaks anywhere in the braking system.
- The wheels should turn freely when the brakes are not applied.
- When the brakes are applied, the brakes on all four wheels must work, and the car must stop evenly in a straight line without pulling to one side.

- All the braking system components must be secure, and there must be no signs of excessive wear or corrosion.

Tyres and wheels

- The tyres must be in good condition, and there must be no signs of excessive wear or damage (refer to *'Regular checks'* on page 73).
- Tyres at the same end of the car must be of the same size and type. Always fit radial tyres; crossply tyres are not suitable for modern cars.

Seatbelts

- The mountings must be secure, and must not be loose or excessively corroded.
- The seatbelt webbing should not be frayed or damaged (this must be checked along the full length of the belts).
- When a seatbelt is fastened, the locking mechanism should hold securely and should release when intended.
- In the case of inertia reel seatbelts, the retractors should work properly when the belts are released.

General

- The windscreen wipers and washers must work properly, and the wiper blades must clear the windscreen without smearing.
- The swept area of the windscreen must have a zone 290mm wide, centred on the steering wheel, free of impact damage greater than 10mm across; this zone must be not encroached by any stickers by more than 10mm. Similar restrictions apply to the remainder of the swept area. Here, the damage or obstruction must not exceed 40mm across.
- The horn must work properly, be loud enough to be heard by other road users and emit a constant tone. Two-tone horns, which alternate between the two frequencies (i.e. they warble), are illegal.
- The exhaust mountings must be secure, and the system itself must be free from leaks and serious corrosion.
- There must be no serious corrosion or damage to the vehicle structure. Corrosion of body panels will not necessarily cause a car to fail the test, but there should be no serious corrosion of any of the 'load bearing' structural components.
- Door handles and locks should work properly from both inside and outside; boot lids and tailgates must close securely; seats and spare tyres must be securely mounted; petrol caps must seal and fasten properly.
- Registration plates must be securely fitted, front and rear, clearly legible, not obscured by items such as a tow bar, with the letters and figures correctly formed and spaced. (Letters or figures formed or positioned so that they are likely to be mis-read, i.e. to personalise a number plate, are now illegal – the vehicle will be failed.)
- Vehicles must display a legible Vehicle Identification Number (VIN). This is either a plate secured to the body or chassis in the engine compartment or a number stamped or etched on the vehicle.
- The exhaust gas emissions level must be within certain limits depending on the age of the car (special equipment is required to measure exhaust gas emissions), and the MOT test also includes a visual check for excessive exhaust smoke when the engine is running. Generally, the car should meet the emission regulations if regular servicing has been carried out.

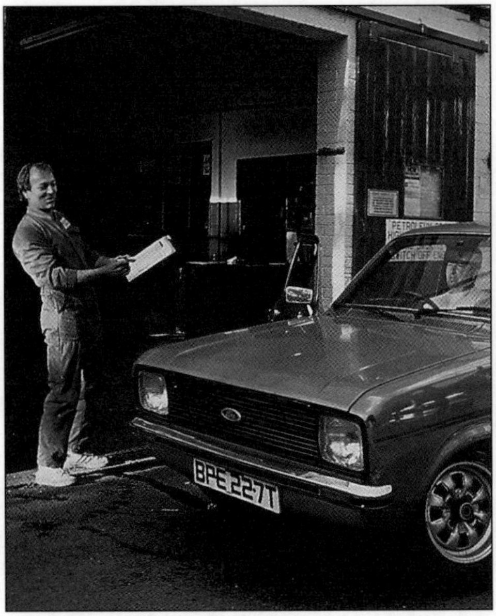

The following table isn't intended as an exhaustive guide to fault finding, but it summarises some of the more common faults which may crop up during a car's life.

Hopefully, the table should help you to find the cause of a problem, even if you can't cure it yourself.

When confronted with a fault, try to think calmly and logically about the symptom(s), and you should be able to work out what the fault *can't* be! Check one item at a time, otherwise if you do clear the fault, you may not know what was causing it.

The commonest cause of difficulty is starting, especially in the winter. Make sure that your battery is kept fully charged, and that the ignition components are in good condition, clean and dry (refer to *'Servicing'* on page 92).

Further details of fault diagnosis, along with comprehensive renewal procedures for most components can be found in our **Owners Workshop Manual** for your particular model (OWM 686 for Escort models, or OWM 1009 for Orion models).

SYMPTOM	POSSIBLE CAUSES
ENGINE	
Starter motor doesn't turn, and headlights don't come on	● Flat battery ● Loose, dirty or corroded battery connections ● Other electrical or wiring fault
Starter motor doesn't turn, and headlights dim	● Battery charge low ● Loose, dirty or corroded battery connections ● Faulty starter motor ● Other electrical or wiring fault ● Seized engine
Starter motor doesn't turn, and headlights are bright	● Loose or dirty starter motor connections ● Faulty starter motor or ignition switch ● Gear selector lever not in position **N** or **P** (automatic transmission only) ● Other electrical or wiring fault
Starter motor spins but doesn't turn engine	● Faulty starter motor ● Engine fault
Engine turns slowly but won't start	● Battery charge low ● Electrical or wiring fault ● Wrong grade of engine oil (refer to *'Service specifications'* on page 67)

SYMPTOM	POSSIBLE CAUSES
ENGINE (continued)	
Engine turns but won't fire or engine starts but won't keep running	● Fuel tank empty ● Damp or dirty ignition system components ● Dirty or loose ignition system connections ● Incorrectly adjusted or faulty spark plugs (refer to *'Servicing'* on page 96) ● Fuel system fault ● Other electrical or wiring fault
Engine idles but stalls when accelerator pedal is depressed	● Blocked or dirty air cleaner filter element (refer to *'Servicing'* on page 102) ● Fuel system fault ● Ignition system fault ● Electrical fault
Poor acceleration, misfiring or lack of power	● Incorrectly adjusted or faulty spark plugs (refer to *'Servicing'* on page 96) ● Incorrect engine valve clearances (OHV engines only) ● Fuel system fault ● Ignition system fault ● Electrical fault
Engine continues to run when ignition switched off	● Engine overheating (possibly due to low coolant level – refer to *'Regular checks'* on page 71) ● Incorrectly adjusted spark plugs or wrong type of spark plugs fitted (refer to *'Servicing'* on page 96) ● Wrong grade of petrol ● Fuel system fault ● Excessive build-up of carbon inside engine ('decoke' required) ● Faulty ignition switch ● Other electrical or wiring fault
Engine doesn't reach normal operating temperature	● Faulty cooling system thermostat ● Faulty temperature gauge or sensor

SYMPTOM	POSSIBLE CAUSES
ENGINE (continued)	
Engine overheats or temperature gauge reads too high	● Airflow to radiator obstructed ● Blocked radiator, hose or engine coolant passage ● Coolant or engine oil level low (refer to '*Regular checks*' on page 69) ● Coolant hose(s) leaking, worn or damaged ● Faulty cooling system thermostat ● Faulty water pump ● Faulty water pump drive ● Faulty temperature gauge or sensor ● Faulty electric cooling fan or switch
Ignition warning light comes on when engine is running	● Alternator drivebelt loose or broken (refer to *'Servicing'* on page 94) ● Faulty alternator ● Other electrical or wiring fault
Oil pressure warning light comes on when engine is running	● Oil level below `MIN' mark on dipstick – refer to *'Regular checks'* on page 70, (if oil level is correct, and light is still on, seek advice, but don't start the engine) ● Oil leak ● Faulty oil pressure switch ● Badly worn engine components
GEARBOX,TRANSMISSION AND CLUTCH	
Difficulty in engaging gear (manual gearbox)	● Worn or faulty gearbox components ● Worn or faulty clutch mechanism ● Engine idle speed too high
Clutch slips (car does not accelerate when engine revs increase – manual gearbox)	● Faulty clutch mechanism ● Contaminated or worn clutch
Car gearchange is harsh (automatic transmission)	● Fault in transmission
Car pull away/gear change sluggish (automatic transmission)	● Low transmission fluid level (refer to *'Servicing'* on page 98) ● Fault in transmission

SYMPTOM	POSSIBLE CAUSES
BRAKES	
Brakes feel 'spongy'	● Air in brake hydraulic system ● Fluid leak in brake system
Excessive brake pedal travel	● Faulty rear brake mechanism ● Air in hydraulic system ● Fluid leak in brake system
Brakes require excessive pedal pressure	● Damp, dirty or contaminated brake components ● Fluid leak in brake system ● Faulty or seized brake components ● Faulty brake servo
Car pulls to one side	● Incorrect tyre pressure(s) or uneven tyre wear (refer to *'Regular checks'* on page 73) ● Faulty or seized brake components ● Worn or contaminated brake friction material ● Incorrect wheel alignment ● Worn or faulty steering components ● Worn or faulty suspension components
Brakes squeal and/or judder	● Badly worn or corroded brake components ● Incorrectly assembled brake components ● Contaminated brake friction material ● Worn or faulty suspension components ● Worn or faulty steering components
Brake fluid level warning light comes on	● Low brake fluid level (refer to *'Regular checks'* on page 72) ● Faulty fluid level sensor or wiring
SUSPENSION AND STEERING	
Car becomes heavy to steer	● Low tyre pressure(s) (refer to *'Regular checks'* on page 73) ● Incorrect wheel alignment ● Worn or faulty steering components ● Worn or faulty suspension components

SYMPTOM	POSSIBLE CAUSES
SUSPENSION & STEERING (continued)	
Car pulls to one side	● *Refer to 'BRAKES' section of table*
Car wanders	● Incorrect tyre pressure(s) or uneven tyre wear (refer to *'Regular checks'* on page 72) ● Car unevenly loaded ● Incorrect wheel alignment ● Worn or faulty suspension components ● Worn or faulty steering components
Car vibrates when driving	● Loose wheel bolt(s) ● Wheel(s) out of balance ● Worn or damaged driveshaft ● Worn or faulty suspension components ● Worn or faulty steering components ● Worn or faulty brake components
Hard or 'choppy' ride	● Incorrect tyre pressure(s) (refer to *'Regular checks'* on page 72) ● Worn or faulty suspension components
Car leans excessively when cornering	● Roof rack overloaded ● Car unevenly loaded ● Worn or faulty suspension components
Uneven tyre wear	● Incorrect tyre pressure(s) (refer to *'Regular checks'* on page 72) ● Incorrect wheel alignment ● Wheel(s) out of balance ● Worn or faulty suspension components ● Worn or faulty steering components ● Brakes 'grabbing'
ELECTRICS	
Electrical systems don't work	● Loose, dirty or corroded battery connections ● Faulty earth connection ● Battery charge low ● Blown fuse (refer to *'Bulb, fuse and relay renewal'* on page 118) ● Faulty relay ● Fuse link, connecting main wiring loom to battery blown (seek advice)

SYMPTOM	POSSIBLE CAUSES
ELECTRICS (continued)	
Direction indicators don't work	● Blown fuse (refer to *'Bulb, fuse and relay renewal'* on page 118) ● Faulty earth connection ● Faulty direction indicator relay ● Faulty direction indicator switch
Bulbs burn out repeatedly	● Faulty connections at light socket ● Faulty alternator regulator
All lights dim when engine speed drops to idle	● Loose alternator drivebelt (refer to *'Servicing'* on page 94) ● Battery charge low ● Faulty alternator

This Section should help you to understand some of the odd words of phrases used at garages and by 'car enthusiasts' which you may not be familiar with.

A

ABS – Abbreviation for Anti-lock Braking System. Uses sensors at each wheel to sense when the wheels are about to lock, and releases the brakes to prevent locking. This process occurs many times per second, and allows the driver to maintain steering control when braking hard.
Accelerator pump – A device attached to many *carburettors* which provides a spurt of extra fuel to the carburettor fuel/air mixture when the accelerator pedal is suddenly pressed down.
Additives – Compounds which are added to petrol and oil to improve their quality and performance.
Advance and retard – A system for altering the *ignition timing*.
AF – An abbreviation of 'Across Flats', the way in which many nuts, bolts and spanners are identified. AF is usually preceded by an Imperial unit of measurement – eg ½ in AF. Unless otherwise stated, all metric measurements are assumed to be AF, so the abbreviation is not normally used for metric nuts, bolts and spanners.
Air cooling – Alternative method of engine cooling in which no water is used. An engine-driven fan forces air at high speed over the surfaces of the engine.
ALB – Abbreviation for Anti-Lock Braking System. See *'ABS'*.
Alternator – A device for converting rotating mechanical energy into electrical energy. In modern cars, it has superseded the dynamo for charging the battery because of its much greater efficiency.
Ammeter – A device for measuring electrical current – the current supplied to the battery by the alternator, or drawn from the battery by the car's electrical systems.
Antifreeze – A chemical mixed with the water in the cooling system to lower the temperature at which the coolant freezes, and in modern cars to prevent corrosion of the metal in the cooling system.
Anti-roll bar – A metal bar mounted transversely across the car, connecting the two sides of the suspension, which counteracts the natural tendency for the car to lean when cornering.
Aquaplaning – A word used to describe the action of a tyre skating across the surface of water.
Automatic transmission – A type of *gearbox* which selects the correct gear ratio automatically according to engine speed and load.
Axle – Spindle on which a wheel revolves.

B

Balljoint – A ball-and-socket type joint used in steering and *suspension* systems, which allows relative movement in more than one plane.
Battery condition indicator – A device for measuring electrical voltage (a voltmeter) connected via the ignition switch to the car battery. Unlike an *ammeter*, it gives an indication that a battery is close to failing. **Also**, most 'maintenance-free' batteries have a battery condition indicator fitted to their casing, which consists of a small disc which changes its colour when the battery is close to failure and requires renewal.
Bearing – Metal or other hard wearing surface against which another part moves, and which is designed to reduce friction and wear (bearings are usually lubricated).

Bendix drive – A device on some types of starter motor which allows the motor to drive the engine for starting, then disengages when the engine starts to run.
BHP – see *Horsepower*.
Big end – The end of a *connecting rod* which is attached to the *crankshaft*. It incorporates a *bearing* and transmits the linear movement of the connecting rod to the crankshaft.
Bleed nipple (or valve) – A hollow screw which allows air or fluid to be bled out of a system when it is loosened.
Brake caliper – The part of a *disc brake* system which houses the *brake pads* and the hydraulically-operated pistons.
Brake disc – A rotating disc, coupled to a roadwheel, which is clamped between hydraulically operated friction pads in a *disc brake* system.
Brake fade – A temporary loss of braking efficiency due to overheating of the brake friction material.
Brake pad – The part of a *disc brake* system which consists of the friction material and a metal backing plate.
Brake shoe – The part of a *drum brake* system which consists of the friction material and a curved metal former.
Breather – A device which allows fresh air into a system or allows contaminated air out.
Bucket tappet – A bucket shaped component used in some engines to transfer the rotary movement of the *camshaft* to the up-and-down movement required for *valve* operation.
Bump stop – A hard piece of rubber used in many *suspension* systems to prevent the moving parts from contacting the body during violent suspension movements.

C

Camber angle – The angle at which the front wheels are set from the vertical, when viewed from the front of the car. Positive camber is the amount in degrees which the wheels are tilted out at the top.
Cam follower – A piece of metal used to transfer the rotary movement of the *camshaft* to the up-and-down movement required for *valve* operation.
Camshaft – A rotating shaft driven from the *crankshaft* with lobes or cams used to operate the engine *valves* via the *valve gear*.
Carbon leads – Ignition HT leads incorporating carbon (black fibres) which eliminates the need for separate radio and TV *suppressors*.
Carburettor – A device which is used to mix air and fuel in the proportions required for burning by the engine under all conditions of engine running.
Castor angle – The angle between the front wheels pivot points and a vertical line when viewed from the side of the car. Positive castor is when the axis is inclined rearwards.
Catalytic converter – A device incorporated in the exhaust system which speeds up the natural decomposition of the exhaust gases, and reduces the amount of harmful gases released into the atmosphere. Cars fitted with catalytic converters must be operated on *unleaded petrol*, as *leaded petrol* will destroy the catalyst.
Centrifugal advance – System of ignition *advance and retard* incorporated in many *distributors* in which weights rotating on a shaft alter the ignition timing according to engine speed.
Choke – This has two common meanings. It is used to describe the device which shuts off some of the air in a *carburettor* during cold starting (in order to provide extra fuel), and it may be manually or automatically operated. It's also used as a general term to describe a carburettor throttle bore.
Clutch – A friction device which allows two rotating components to be coupled together smoothly, without the need for either rotating component to stop moving.
Coil spring – A spiral coil of spring steel used in many *suspension* systems.
Combustion chamber – Shaped area in the *cylinder head* into which the fuel/air mixture is compressed by the *piston* and where the spark from the *spark plug* ignites the mixture.
Compression ratio (CR) – A term used to describe the amount by which the fuel/air mixture is compressed as a *piston* moves from the bottom to the top of its travel, and expressed as a number. For example an 8.5:1 compression ratio means that the volume of fuel/air mixture above the piston when the piston is at the bottom of its stroke is 8.5 times

that when the piston is at the top of its stroke.
Compression tester – A special type of pressure gauge which can be screwed into a *spark plug* hole, which measures the pressure in the cylinder when the engine is turning but not firing. This gives an indication of engine wear or possible leaks.
Condenser (capacitor) – A device in a *contact breaker point distributor* which stores electrical energy and prevents excessive sparking at the contact breaker points.
Connecting rod ('con-rod') – Metal rod in the engine connecting a *piston* to the *crankshaft*.
Constant velocity (CV) joint – A joint used in *driveshafts*, where the instantaneous speed of the input shaft is exactly the same as the instantaneous speed of the output shaft at any angle of rotation. This does not occur in ordinary *universal joints*.
Contact breaker points – A device in the *distributor* which consists of two electrical points (or contacts) and a cam which opens and closes them to operate the *HT* electrical circuit which provides the spark at the *spark plugs*.
Crankcase – The area of the *cylinder block* below the *pistons* which houses the *crankshaft*.
Crankshaft – A cranked shaft which is driven by the *pistons* and provides the engine output to the *transmission*.
Crossflow cylinder head – A *cylinder head* in which the inlet and exhaust *valves* and *manifolds* are on opposite sides.
Crossply tyre – A tyre whose construction is such that the weave of the fabric material layers is running diagonally in alternately opposite directions to a line around the circumference of the tyre.
Cubic capacity – The total volume within the *cylinders* of an engine which is swept by the movement of the *pistons*.
CVH – A term applied by the Ford Motor Company to their overhead camshaft engines which incorporate a hemispherical *combustion chamber*. CVH means Compound Valve angle, Hemispherical combustion chamber.
Cylinder – Close fitting metal tube in which a *piston* slides. In the case of an engine, the cylinders may be bored directly into the *cylinder block*, or on some engines, cylinder liners are used which rest in the cylinder block and can be replaced when worn with matching pistons to avoid the requirement for *reboring* the cylinder block.
Cylinder block – The main engine casting which contains the *cylinders*, *crankshaft* and *pistons*.
Cylinder head – The casting at the top of the engine which contains the *valves* and associated operating components.

D

Damper – See *shock absorber*.
Dashpot – An oil-filled *cylinder* and *piston* used as a damping device in SU and Zenith/Stromberg CD type carburettors.
Dead axle (beam axle) – The simplest form of axle, consisting of a horizontal member attached to the car underbody by springs. This arrangement is used for the rear axle on some front-wheel-drive cars.
Decarbonising ('decoking') – Removal of all carbon deposits from the *combustion chambers* and the tops of the *pistons* and *cylinders* in an engine.
De Dion axle – A rear axle consisting of a cranked tube attached to the wheel hubs, with a separately mounted *differential* gear and *driveshafts*. *Suspension* is normally through *coil springs* between the wheel hubs and car underbody.
Derv – Abbreviation for Diesel-Engined Road Vehicle. A term often used to refer to Diesel fuel.
Diaphragm – A flexible membrane used in some components such as fuel pumps. The diaphragm spring used on *clutches* is similar, but is made from spring steel.
Diesel engine – An engine which relies on the heat generated when compressing air to ignite the fuel, and which therefore doesn't need an *ignition system*. Diesel engines have much higher *compression ratios* than petrol engines, normally around 20:1.
Differential – A system of gears (generally known as a crownwheel and pinion) which allows the *torque* provided by the engine to be applied to both driving wheels. The differential divides the torque proportionally between the driving wheels to allow one wheel to turn faster than the other, for example during cornering.

DIN – This stands for Deutsche Industrie Norm (German Industry Standard), which provides international standards for measuring engine power, torque, etc.
Disc brake – A brake assembly where a rotating disc is clamped between hydraulically operated friction pads.
Distributor – A device used to distribute the *HT* current to the individual *spark plugs*. The distributor may also contain the *advance and retard* mechanism. On some older cars, the distributor also contains the *contact breaker points* assembly.
Distributor cap – Plastic cap which fits on top of the *distributor* and contains electrodes, in which the *rotor arm* rotates to distribute the *HT* spark voltage to the correct *spark plug*.
DOHC – Abbreviation for Double Overhead Camshaft (see *'Twin-cam'*).
Doughnut – A term used to describe the flexible rubber coupling used in some *driveshafts*.
Driveshaft – Term usually used to describe the shaft (normally incorporating *universal* or *constant velocity joints*), which transmits drive from a *differential* to one wheel. More commonly found in front-wheel-drive cars.
Drive train – A collective term used to describe the *clutch/gearbox/transmission* and the other components used to transmit drive to the wheels.
Drum brake – A brake assembly with friction linings on 'shoes' running inside a cylindrical drum attached to the wheel.
Dual circuit brakes – A *hydraulic* braking system consisting of two separate fluid circuits, so that if one circuit becomes inoperative, braking power is still available from the other circuit.
Dwell angle – A measurement which corresponds to the number of degrees of *distributor* shaft rotation during which the *contact breaker points* are closed during the ignition cycle of one *cylinder*. The angle is altered by adjusting the contact breaker points gap.

E

Earth strap – A flexible electrical connection between the battery and a car earth point, or between the engine/*gearbox* and the car body to provide a return current path flow to the battery.
EFI – Abbreviation for Electronic *Fuel Injection*.
Electrode – An electrical terminal, eg in a *spark plug* or *distributor cap*.
Electrolyte – A current-conducting solution inside the battery (consisting of water and sulphuric acid in the case of a car battery).
Electronic ignition – An *ignition system* incorporating electronic components in place of *contact breaker points*, which can produce a much higher spark voltage than a contact breaker system, and is less affected by worn components.
Emission control – The reduction or prevention of the release into the atmosphere of poisonous fumes and gases from the engine and fuel system of a car. Required to different degrees by the laws of some countries, and achieved by engine design and the use of special devices and systems.
Epicyclic gears (planetary gears) – A gear system used in many *automatic transmissions* where there is a central 'sun' gear around which smaller 'planet' gears rotate.
Exhaust gas analyser – An instrument used to measure the amount of pollutants (mainly carbon monoxide) in a car's exhaust gases.
Expansion tank – A container used in many cooling systems to collect the overflow from the car's cooling system as the coolant heats up and expands.

F

Filter – A device for removing foreign particles from air, fuel or oil.
Final drive – A collective term (often expressed as a gear ratio) for the crownwheel and pinion (see *Differential*).
Flat engine – Form of engine design in which the *cylinders* are opposed horizontally, usually with an equal number on each side of the central *crankshaft*.
Float chamber – The part of a *carburettor* which contains a float and *needle valve* for

controlling the fuel level in the reservoir.
Flywheel – A heavy rotating metal disc attached to the *crankshaft* and used to smooth out the pulsing from the *pistons*.
Four stroke (cycle) – A term used to describe the four operating strokes of a *piston* in a conventional car engine. These are (1) Induction – drawing the air/fuel mixture into the engine as the piston moves down; (2) Compression – of the fuel/air mixture as the piston rises; (3) Power stroke – where the piston is forced down after the fuel/air mixture has been ignited by the *spark plug*, and (4) Exhaust stroke – where the piston rises and pushes the burnt gases out of the *cylinder*. During these operations, the inlet and exhaust *valves* are opened and closed at the correct moment to allow the fuel/air mixture in, the exhaust gases out, or to provide a gas-tight compression chamber.
Fuel injection – A method of injecting fuel into an engine. Used in *Diesel engines* and also on some petrol engines in place of a *carburettor*.
Fuel injector – Device used on *fuel injection* engines to inject fuel directly or indirectly into the *combustion chamber*. Some fuel injection systems use a single fuel injector, while some systems use one fuel injector for each *cylinder* of the engine.

G

Gasket – Compressible material used between two surfaces to provide a leakproof joint.
Gearbox – A group of gears and shafts installed in a housing, positioned between the *clutch* and the *differential*, and used to keep the engine within its safe operating speed range as the speed of the car changes.

H

Half-shaft – A *driveshaft* used to transmit the drive from the *differential* to one of the rear wheels.
Hardy-Spicer joint (Hooke's or Cardan joint) – See *Universal joint*.
Helical gears – Gears in which the teeth are cut at an angle across the circumference of the gear to give a smoother mesh between gears and quieter running.
Horsepower – A measurement of power. Brake Horsepower (BHP) is a measure of the power required to stop a moving body.
HT – Abbreviation of High Tension (meaning high voltage) used to describe the *spark plug* voltage in an *ignition system*.
Hub carrier – A component usually found at each front corner of a car which carries the wheel and brake assembly, and to which the *suspension* and steering components are attached.
Hydraulic – A term used to describe the operation of a system by means of fluid pressure.
Hypoid gear – A gear with curved teeth which transmits drive through a right-angle, where the centreline of the drive gear is offset from the centreline of the driven gear. The meshing action of hypoid gears allows a larger and therefore stronger drive gear, and the meshing noise is reduced in comparison with conventional gears.

I

Independent suspension – A *suspension* system where movement of one wheel has no effect on the movement of the other, eg independent front suspension.
Ignition coil – An electrical coil which forms part of the *ignition system* and which generates the *HT* voltage.
Ignition system – The electrical system which provides the spark to ignite the air/fuel mixture in the engine. Normally the system consists of the battery, *ignition coil*, *distributor*, ignition switch, *spark plugs* and wiring.
Ignition timing – The time in the *cylinder* firing cycle at which the ignition spark (provided by the *spark plug*) occurs. The spark timing is normally a few degrees of *crankshaft* rotation before the *piston* reaches the top of its stroke, and is expressed as a number of degrees before top-dead-centre (BTDC).
Inertia reel – Automatic type of seat belt mechanism which allows the wearer to move freely in normal use, but which locks on sensing either sudden deceleration or a sudden movement of the wearer.

In-line engine – An engine in which the *cylinders* are positioned in one row as opposed to being in a *flat* or *vee* configuration.

J

Jet – A calibrated nozzle or orifice in a *carburettor* through which fuel is drawn for mixing with air.
Jump leads – Heavy electric cables fitted with clips to enable a car's battery to be connected to another battery for emergency starting.

K

Kerb weight – The weight of a car, unladen but ready to be driven, ie with enough fuel, oil, etc, to travel an arbitrary distance.
Kickdown – A device used on *automatic transmissions* which allows a lower gear to be selected for improved acceleration by fully depressing the accelerator.
Kingpin – A device which allows the front wheel of a car to swivel about a near vertical axis.
Knocking – See *'Pinking'*.

L

Laminated windscreen – A windscreen which has a thin plastic layer sandwiched between two layers of toughened glass. It will not shatter or craze when hit.
Lead-free petrol – Contains no lead. It has no lead added during manufacture, and the natural lead content is refined out. This type of petrol is not currently available for general use in the UK, and should not be confused with *unleaded* petrol.
Leaded petrol – Normal 4-star petrol. Has a low amount of lead added during manufacture, in addition to the natural lead found in crude oil.
Leading shoe – A *drum brake* shoe of which the leading end (the one moved by the operating *pistons*) is reached first by a given point on the drum during normal forward rotation. A simple drum brake will have one leading and one trailing (the opposite) shoe.
Leaf spring – A spring commonly used on cars with a *live axle*, consisting of several long curved steel plates clamped together.
Limited slip differential – A type of *differential* which prevents one wheel from standing still while the other wheel spins excessively. Often used on high-performance cars.
Live axle – An axle through which power is transmitted to the rear wheels.
Loom – A complete car wiring system or section of a wiring system consisting of all the wires of correct length, etc, to wire up the various circuits.
LT – Abbreviation of Low Tension (meaning low voltage), used to describe battery voltage in the *ignition system*.

M

MacPherson strut – An independent front *suspension* system where the swivelling, springing and shock absorbing action of the wheels is dealt with by a single assembly.
Manifold – A device used for ducting the air/fuel mixture to the engine (inlet manifold), or the exhaust gases from the engine (exhaust manifold).
Master cylinder – A *cylinder* containing a *piston* and *hydraulic* fluid, directly coupled to a foot pedal (eg brake or *clutch* master cylinder). Used for transmitting pressure to the brake or clutch operating mechanism.
Metallic paint – Paint finish incorporating minute particles of metal to give added lustre to the colour.
Multigrade – Lubricating oil whose *viscosity* covers that of several single grade oils, making it suitable for use over a wider range of operating conditions.

N

Needle bearing – Type of *bearing* in which needle or cone-shaped rollers are used around the circumference to reduce friction.
Needle valve – A component of the *carburettor* which restricts the flow of fuel or fuel/air mixture according to the position of the valve in an orifice or *jet*.

Negative earth – Electrical system (almost universally adopted) in which the negative terminal of the car battery is connected to the car body. The polarity of all the electrical equipment is determined by this.

O

Octane rating – A scale rating for grading petrol.
ohc (overhead cam) – Describes an engine in which the *camshaft* is situated above the *cylinder head*, and operates the *valve gear* directly.
ohv (overhead valve) – Describes an engine which has its *valves* in the *cylinder head*, but with the *valve gear* operated by *pushrods* from a *camshaft* situated lower in the engine.
Oil cooler – Small *radiator* fitted in the oil circuit and positioned in a cooling airflow to cool the oil. Used mainly on high-performance engines.
Overdrive – A device coupled to a car's *gearbox* which raises the output gear ratio above the normal 1:1 of top gear.
Oversteer – A tendency for a car to turn more tightly into a corner than intended.

P

PCV (Positive Crankcase Ventilation) – A system which allows fumes and vapours which build up in the *crankcase* to be drawn into the engine for burning.
Pinion – A gear with a small number of teeth which meshes with one having a larger number of teeth.
Pinking – A metallic noise from the engine often caused by the *ignition timing* being too far *advanced*. The noise is the result of pressure waves which cause the *cylinder* walls to vibrate when the ignited fuel/air mixture is compressed.
Piston – Cylindrical component which slides in a closely-fitting metal tube or *cylinder* and transmits pressure. The pistons in an engine, for example, compress the fuel/air mixture, transmit the power to the *crankshaft*, and push the burnt gases out through the exhaust *valves*.
Piston ring – Hardened metal ring which is a spring fit in a groove running round the *piston* to ensure a gas-tight seal between the piston and *cylinder* wall.
Positive earth – The opposite of *negative earth*.
Power steering – A steering system which uses *hydraulic* fluid pressure (provided by an engine-driven pump) to reduce the effort required to steer the car.
Pre-ignition – See *'Pinking'*.
Propeller shaft – The shaft which transmits the drive from the *gearbox* to the rear axle in a front-engined rear-wheel-drive car.
Pushrod – A rod which is moved up and down by the rotary motion of the *camshaft* and operates the *rocker arms* in an *ohv* engine.

Q

Quarter light – A triangular window mounted in front or behind the main front or rear windows, usually in the front door, or behind the rear door.
Quartz-halogen bulb – A bulb with a quartz envelope (instead of glass), filled with a halogen gas. Gives a brighter, more even spread of light than an ordinary bulb.

R

Rack and pinion – Simplest form of steering mechanism which uses a *pinion* gear to move a toothed rack.
Radial ply tyre – A tyre in which the fabric material plies are arranged laterally, at right angles to the circumference.
Radiator – Cooling device through which the engine coolant is passed, situated in an air flow and consisting of a system of fine tubes and fins for rapid heat dissipation.
Radius arms (rods) – Locating arms sometimes used with a *live axle* to positively locate it in the fore-and-aft direction.
Rebore – The process of enlarging the *cylinder* bores to a very accurately specified measurement in order to fit new *pistons* to overcome wear in the engine. Not normally necessary unless the engine has covered a very high mileage.

Recirculating ball steering – A derivative of *worm and nut* steering, where the steering shaft motion is transmitted to the steering linkage by balls running in the groove of a worm gear.
Rev counter – See *Tachometer*.
Rocker arm – A lever which rocks on a central pivot, with one end moved up and down by the *camshaft*, and the other end operating an inlet or exhaust *valve*.
Rotary engine – See *'Wankel engine'*.
Rotor arm – A rotating arm in the *distributor* which distributes the *HT* spark voltage to the correct *spark plug*.
Running on – A tendency for an engine to keep on running after the ignition has been switched off. Often caused by a badly maintained engine or the use of an incorrect grade of fuel.

S

SAE – Society of Automotive Engineers (of America). Lays down international standards for the classification of engine performance and many other specifications, but is most commonly used to classify oils.
Safety rim – A special wheel rim shape which prevents a deflated tyre from rolling off the wheel.
Sealed beam – A sealed headlamp unit where the filament is an integral part and cannot be renewed separately.
Semi-trailing arm – A common form of independent rear *suspension*.
Servo – A device for increasing the normal effort applied to a control.
Shock absorber – A device for damping out the up-and-down movement of the *suspension* when the car hits a bump in the road.
Spark plug – A device with two *electrodes* insulated from each other by a ceramic material, which screws into an engine *combustion chamber*. When the *HT* voltage is applied to the plug terminal, a spark jumps across the electrodes and ignites the fuel/air mixture.
Squab – Another name for a seat cushion.
Steel-braced tyre – Tyre in which extra plies containing steel cords are incorporated with the fabric plies to give added strength.
Steering arm (knuckle) – A short arm on the front *hub carrier* to which the steering linkage connects.
Steering gear – A general term used to describe the steering components, usually refers to a steering rack-and-pinion assembly.
Steering rack – See *Rack and pinion*.
Stroboscopic light – A light switched on and off by the engine *ignition system* which is used for checking the *ignition timing* when the engine is running.
Stroke – The total distance travelled by a single *piston* in its *cylinder*.
Stub axle – A short axle which carries one wheel.
Subframe – A small frame which is mounted on the car's body, and carries the *suspension* and/or the *drivetrain* assemblies.
Sump – The main reservoir for the engine oil.
Supercharger – A device which uses an engine-driven turbine (usually driven by a belt or gears from the *crankshaft*) to drive a compressor which forces air into the engine, providing increased fuel/air mixture flow, and therefore increased engine efficiency. Sometimes used on high-performance engines.
Suppressor – A device which is used to reduce or eliminate electrical interference caused by the *ignition system* or other electrical components.
Suspension – A general term used to describe the components which suspend the car body on its wheels.
Swing axle – A *suspension* arm which is pivoted near the front-to-rear centreline of the car, and which allows the wheel to swing vertically about that pivot point.
Synchromesh – A device in a *gearbox* which synchronises the speed of one gear shaft with another to produce smooth, noiseless engagement of the gears.

T

Tachometer – Also known as a rev counter, indicates engine speed in revolutions per minute (rpm).
Tappet – A term often used to refer to the component which transmits the rotary *camshaft* movement to the up-and-down movement required for *valve* operation.

Thermostat – A device which is sensitive to changes in engine coolant temperature, and opens up an additional path for coolant to flow through the *radiator* (to increase the cooling) when the engine has warmed up.
Tie-rod – A rod which connects the *steering arms* to the *steering gear*.
Timing belt – Fabric or rubber belt engaging on sprocket wheels and driving the *camshaft* from the *crankshaft*.
Timing chain – Metal flexible link chain engaging on sprocket wheels and driving the *camshaft* from the *crankshaft*.
Timing marks – Marks normally found on the *crankshaft* pulley or the *flywheel* and used for setting the ignition firing point with respect to a particular *piston*.
Toe-in/toe-out – The amount by which the front wheels point inwards or outwards from the straight-ahead position when steering straight ahead.
Top Dead Centre (TDC) – The point at which a *piston* is at the top of its *stroke*.
Torque – The turning force generated by a rotating component.
Torque converter – A coupling where the driving *torque* is transmitted through oil. At low speeds there is very little transfer of torque from the input to the output. As the speed of the input shaft increases, the direction of fluid flow within a system of vanes changes, and torque from the input impeller is transferred to the output turbine. The higher the input speed, the closer the output speed approaches it, until they are virtually the same.
Torsion bar – A metal bar which twists about its own axis, and is used in some *suspension* systems.
Toughened windscreen – A windscreen which when hit, will shatter in a particular way to produce blunt-edged fragments or will craze over but remain intact. A zone toughened windscreen has a zone in front of the driver which crazes into larger parts to reduce the loss of visibility which occurs when toughened windscreens break, but is otherwise similar.
Track rod – See *Tie-rod*.
Trailing arm – A form of independent *suspension* where the wheel is attached to a swinging arm, and is mounted to the rear of the arm pivot.
Transaxle – A combined *gearbox*/axle assembly from which two *driveshafts* transmit the drive to the wheels.
Transmission – A general term used to describe some or all of the *drivetrain* components excluding the engine, most commonly used to describe automatic gearboxes.
Turbocharger – A device which uses a turbine driven by the engine exhaust gases to drive a compressor which forces air into the engine, providing increased fuel/air mixture flow, and therefore increased engine efficiency. Commonly used on high-performance engines.
Twin-cam – Abbreviation for twin overhead *camshafts* (see *'ohc'*). Used on engines with a *crossflow cylinder head*, usually with one camshaft operating the inlet *valves* and the other operating the exhaust valves. Gives improved engine efficiency due to improved fuel/air mixture and exhaust gas flow in the *combustion chambers*.
Two stroke (cycle) – A common term used to describe the operation of an engine where each downward *piston* stroke is a power stroke. The fuel/air mixture is directed to the crankcase where it's compressed by the descending piston and pumped into the *combustion chamber*. As the piston rises, the mixture is compressed and ignited, which forces the piston down. The burnt gases flow from the exhaust port, but the piston is now compressing another fuel/air mixture charge in the crankcase which repeats the cycle.

U

Understeer – A tendency for a car to go straight on when turned into a corner.
Universal joint – A joint that can swivel in any direction whilst at the same time transmitting *torque*. This type of joint is commonly used in *propeller shafts* and some *driveshafts*, but is not suitable for some applications because the input and output shaft speeds are not the same at all positions of angular rotation. The type in common use is known as a Hardy-Spicer, Hooke's or Cardan joint.
Unleaded petrol – Has no lead added during manufacture, but still has the natural lead content of crude oil. Generally available in the

UK, most modern cars can use this type of petrol, but seek advice first, as engine adjustments may be required. Engine damage can occur if unleaded petrol is used incorrectly. Not to be confused with *lead-free* petrol which is not currently available in the UK.
Unsprung weight – The part of the car which is not supported by the springs.

V

Vacuum advance – System of ignition *advance and retard* used in some *distributors* where the vacuum in the engine inlet *manifold* is used to act on a *diaphragm* which alters the *ignition timing* as the vacuum changes due to the throttle position.
Valve – A device which opens or closes to allow or stop gas or fluid flow.
Valve gear – A general term used for the components which are acted on by the *camshaft* in order to operate the *valves*.
16-valve – Term used to describe a four *cylinder* engine with four *valves* per cylinder (usually two inlet valves and two exhaust valves). Gives improved engine efficiency due to improved fuel/air mixture and exhaust gas flow in the *combustion chambers*.
Vee engine – An engine design in which the *cylinders* are set in two banks forming a 'V' when viewed from one end. A V8 for example consists of two rows of four cylinders each.
Venturi – A streamlined restriction in the *carburettor* throttle bore which causes a low pressure to occur; this sucks fuel into the air stream to form a vapour suitable for combustion.
Viscosity – A term used to describe the resistance of a fluid to flow. When associated with lubricating oil, it's given an *SAE* number, 10 being a very light oil and 140 being a very heavy oil.
Voltage regulator – A device which regulates the *alternator* output to a predetermined level. On most alternators the voltage regulator is an integral part of the alternator, and regulates the charging current as well as the voltage.

W

Wankel engine – A rotary engine which has a triangular shaped rotor which performs the function of the *pistons* in a conventional engine, and rotates in a housing shaped approximately like a broad-waisted figure of eight. Very few cars use this type of engine.
Wheel balancing – Adding small weights to the rim of a wheel so that there are no out-of-balance forces when the wheel rotates.
Wishbone – An 'A'-shaped *suspension* component, pivoted at the base of the 'A' and carrying a wheel at the apex. Normally mounted close to the horizontal.
Worm and nut steering – A steering system where the lower end of the steering column has a coarse screw thread on which a nut runs. The nut is attached to a spindle which carries the drop arm which, in turn, moves the steering linkage.

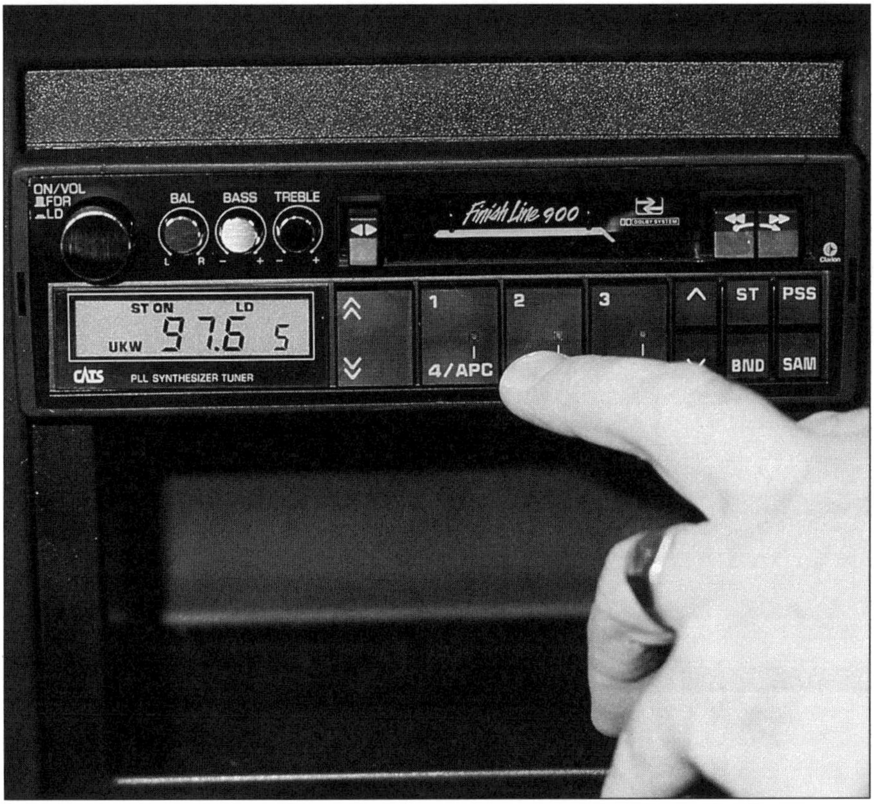

A comprehensive network of local radio stations now exists throughout the UK.

Most of these radio stations provide regularly updated reports on traffic flow and road conditions, which can be of great help to drivers. Listening to traffic reports will help you to avoid the inevitable 'jams' which occur during every day driving.

Some car radio/cassette players are now equipped with a 'Radio Data System' (RDS) which will automatically tune into special traffic information signals, interrupting normal radio or tape listening when bulletins are broadcast. An RDS-equipped radio may prove to be a worthwhile investment if you travel by car regularly, particularly when driving on business trips.

The following table provides details of all the local radio frequencies throughout the UK, region-by-region. Where stations broadcast on FM/VHF and AM/MW, it's suggested that the FM/VHF frequency is used wherever possible, as this will usually give better reception.

LOCAL RADIO FREQUENCIES

AREA	FM/VHF	AM/MW
AVON		
Bath		
BBC Bristol	104.6	1548
GWR FM	103.0	–
Bristol		
BBC Bristol	94.9	1548
Brunel Classic Gold	–	1260
Galaxy Radio	97.2	–
GWR FM	96.3	–
BEDFORDSHIRE		
Bedford		
BBC Bedfordshire	95.5	1161
Chiltern Radio	96.9	–
SuperGold	–	792
Luton		
BBC Bedfordshire	103.8	630
Chiltern Radio	97.6	–
SuperGold	–	828
BERKSHIRE		
Reading		
210 Classic Gold Radio	–	1431
210 FM	97.0	–
BBC Berkshire	104.4	–
Wokingham		
BBC Berkshire	104.1	–
BIRMINGHAM		
Birmingham		
BBC WM	95.6	1458
BRMB FM	96.4	–
Buzz FM	102.4	–
Xtra AM	–	1152
BORDERS		
Eyemouth		
Radio Borders	103.4	–
Peebles		
Radio Borders	103.1	–
Selkirk		
Radio Borders	96.8	–
BUCKINGHAMSHIRE		
Milton Keynes		
BBC Bedfordshire	104.5	630
Horizon Radio	103.3	–

AREA	FM/VHF	AM/MW
CAMBRIDGESHIRE		
Cambridge		
BBC Cambridge	96.0	1026
CN FM	103.0	–
Peterborough		
BBC Cambridge	95.7	1447
Hereward Radio	102.7	1332
CHANNEL ISLANDS		
Guernsey		
BBC Guernsey	93.2	1116
Jersey		
BBC Jersey	88.8	1026
CHESHIRE		
Echo 96	96.4	–
Chester		
BBC Merseyside	95.8	1485
Congleton		
Signal Cheshire	104.9	–
Macclesfield		
BBC Stoke	94.6	1503
Warrington		
BBC Merseyside	95.8	1485
CLEVELAND		
Middlesbrough		
BBC Cleveland	95.0	1548
TFM	96.6	–
GNR	–	1170
CLWYD		
Prestatyn		
BBC Cymru/Wales	94.2	882
Rhyl		
BBC Cymru/Wales	94.2	882
Wrexham		
BBC Cymru/Wales	93.3	657
MFM 1034	97.1/103.4	–
Marcher Gold	–	1260
CORNWALL		
Isles of Scilly		
BBC Cornwall	96.0	–
Liskeard		
BBC Cornwall	95.2	657
Redruth		
BBC Cornwall	103.9	630
CUMBRIA		
Barrow-in-Furness		
BBC Furness	96.1	837
Kendal		
BBC Cumbria	95.2	–
Windermere		
BBC Cumbria	104.2	–
Workington		
BBC Cumbria	95.6	1458

AREA	FM/VHF	AM/MW
DERBYSHIRE		
Chesterfield		
BBC Sheffield	94.7	1035
Derby		
BBC Derby	94.2	1116
Trent FM	102.8	–
Gem AM	–	945
Matlock		
BBC Derby	95.3	–
DEVON		
Barnstaple		
BBC Devon	94.8	801
Exeter		
BBC Devon	95.8	990
DevonAir	97.0	666/954
South West	103.0	–
Okehampton		
BBC Devon	96.0	801
Plymouth Area		
BBC Devon	103.4	855
Plymouth Sound	97.0	1152
Tavistock		
Radio in Tavistock	96.6	–
Torbay		
BBC Devon	103.4	1458
DevonAir	96.4	666/954
DORSET		
Poole		
BBC Solent	96.1	1359
Bournemouth		
BBC Solent	96.1	1359
2CR Classic Gold		828
2CR FM	102.3	–
Weymouth		
BBC Solent	96.1	–
DUMFRIES & GALLOWAY		
Dumfries		
BBC Scotland/Solway	94.7	585
SW Sound	97.2	–
Stranraer		
BBC Scotland	94.7	–
DURHAM		
Darlington		
BBC Newcastle	95.4	–
Durham		
BBC Newcastle	95.4	1458
DYFED		
Aberystwyth		
BBC Cymru/Wales	93.1	882

AREA	FM/VHF	AM/MW
EAST SUSSEX		
Brighton		
BBC Sussex	95.3	1485
South Coast Radio	–	1323
Southern Sound Classic Hits	103.5	–
Eastbourne		
BBC Sussex	104.5	1161
Southern Sound Classic Hits	102.4	–
Hastings		
Southern Sound Classic Hits	97.5	–
Newhaven		
Southern Sound Classic Hits	96.9	–
ESSEX		
Basildon		
BBC Essex	95.3	765
Chelmsford		
BBC Essex	103.5	765
Breeze AM		1431/1359
Essex Radio	102.6	–
Colchester		
BBC Essex	103.5	729
Mellow 1557	–	1557
Harlow		
BBC Essex	–	765
Manningtree		
BBC Suffolk	103.9	–
Southend-on-Sea		
BBC Essex	95.3	1530
Breeze AM		1431/1359
Essex Radio	96.3	–
FIFE		
Kirkcaldy		
BBC Scotland	94.3	810
GLOUCESTERSHIRE		
Gloucester		
BBC Gloucester	104.7	603
Severn Sound	102.4	
Three Counties Radio		774
Stroud		
BBC Gloucester	95.0	603
Severn Sound	103.0	–
GRAMPIAN		
Aberdeen		
BBC Scotland/Aberdeen	93.1	990
North Sound	96.9	1035
Stirling		
Central FM	96.7	–

AREA	FM/VHF	AM/MW
GWENT		
Newport		
Red Dragon Radio	97.4	–
Touch AM		1305
GWYNEDD		
Anglesey		
BBC Cymru/Wales	94.2	882
HAMPSHIRE		
Andover		
210 FM	102.9	–
Basingstoke		
210 FM	102.9	–
BBC Berkshire	104.1	–
Isle of Wight		
BBC Solent	96.1	999/1359
Isle of Wight Radio	–	1242
Portsmouth		
BBC Solent	96.1	999
Oceansound	97.5	–
South Coast Radio	–	1170
Southampton		
BBC Solent	96.1	999
Oceansound	97.5	–
Power FM	103.2	–
South Coast Radio	–	1557
Winchester		
Oceansound	96.7	–
Power FM	103.2	–
HEREFORDSHIRE		
Hereford		
BBC Here/Worc	94.7	819
Radio Wyvern	97.6	954
HERTFORDSHIRE		
Watford		
BBC GLR	94.9	1458
St Albans		
BBC Bedfordshire	103.8	630
Stevenage		
BBC Bedfordshire	103.8	630
HIGHLAND		
Inverness		
BBC Scotland	94.0	810
Moray Firth Radio	97.4	1107
Fort William		
BBC Scotland	93.7	–
Oban		
BBC Scotland	93.3	–
Thurso		
BBC Scotland	94.5	–

AREA	FM/VHF	AM/MW
HUMBERSIDE		
Kingston upon Hull Area		
BBC Humberside	95.9	1485
Classic Gold	–	1161
Viking FM	96.9	–
ISLE OF MAN		
Douglas		
Manx Radio	97.2	1368
Snaefell		
Manx Radio	89.0	–
KENT		
Ashford		
Invicta FM	96.1	–
Canterbury		
BBC Kent	104.2	774
Invicta FM	102.8	–
Dover		
BBC Kent	104.2	774
Invicta FM	97.0	–
East Kent		
Coast Classics	–	603
Folkestone		
BBC Kent	104.2	774
Maidstone & Medway		
BBC Kent	96.7	1035
Coast Classics	–	1242
Invicta FM	103.1	–
Royal Tunbridge Wells		
BBC Kent	96.7	1602
Thanet		
Invicta FM	95.9	–
LANCASHIRE		
Burnley Area		
BBC Lancashire	95.5	855
Blackpool		
BBC Lancashire	103.9	855
Red Rose Gold	–	999
Red Rose Rock FM	97.4	–
Lancaster		
BBC Lancashire	104.5	1557
Preston		
BBC Lancashire	103.9	855
Red Rose Gold	–	999
Red Rose Rock FM	97.4	–
LEICESTERSHIRE		
Leicester		
BBC Leicester	104.9	837
Gem AM	–	1260
Sound FM	103.2	–

LOCAL RADIO FREQUENCIES

AREA	FM/VHF	AM/MW
LINCOLNSHIRE		
Lincoln Area		
BBC Lincoln	94.9	1368
Lincs FM	102.2	–
LONDON		
Brixton		
Choice FM	96.9	–
Ealing		
Sunrise Radio	–	1413
Greater London		
BBC GLR	94.9	1458
Capital FM	95.8	–
Capital Gold	–	1548
Jazz FM	102.2	–
Kiss FM	100.0	–
LBC Newstalk	97.3	–
Melody Radio	104.9	–
Spectrum Int. Radio	–	558/990
Haringey		
London Greek Radio	103.3	–
WNK	103.3	–
Thamesmead		
London Talkback Radio	–	1152
RTM	103.8	–
Southall		
Sunrise Radio	–	1413
LOTHIAN		
Bathgate		
Radio Forth	97.3	–
Dunfermline		
BBC Scotland	94.3	810
Edinburgh		
BBC Scotland	94.3	810
Max AM	–	1548
Radio Forth	97.3/97.6	–
MANCHESTER		
Manchester		
BBC GMR	95.1	1458
KFM	104.9	–
Piccadilly Gold	–	1152
Piccadilly Key 103	103.0	–
Sunset Radio	102.0	–
MERSEYSIDE		
Liverpool		
BBC Mersey	95.8	1485
City Talk	–	1548
Radio City	96.7	–
MID GLAMORGAN		
Aberdare		
BBC Cymru/Wales	93.6	882
Merthyr Tydfil		
BBC Cymru/Wales	96.8	882

AREA	FM/VHF	AM/MW
MIDDLESEX		
Hounslow		
Sunrise Radio	–	1413
NORFOLK		
King's Lynn		
BBC Norfolk	104.4	873
Norwich Area		
BBC Norfolk	95.1	855
Broadland	102.4	1152
NORTHAMPTONSHIRE		
Kettering		
KCBC	–	1530
Northampton		
BBC Northampton	104.2	1107
Northants	96.6	–
SuperGold	–	1557
NORTHUMBERLAND		
Berwick-upon-Tweed		
BBC Newcastle	96.0	–
Radio Borders	97.5	–
NOTTINGHAM		
Nottingham		
BBC Nottingham	103.8	1521
Trent FM	96.2/96.5	–
Gem AM	–	999
ORKNEY		
Kirkwall		
BBC Scotland	93.7	–
OXFORDSHIRE		
Banbury		
Fox FM	97.4	–
Oxford		
BBC Oxford	95.2	1485
Fox FM	102.6	–
POWYS		
Welshpool		
BBC Cymru/Wales	94.0	882
SHETLAND		
Lerwick		
BBC Scotland	92.7	–
SIBC	96.2	–
SHROPSHIRE		
Ludlow		
BBC Shropshire	95.0	1584
RFM	97.6	–
Shrewsbury		
BBC Shropshire	96.0	–
Beacon Radio	97.2/103.1	
WABC	–	1017
Telford		
BBC Shropshire	96.0	756
Beacon Radio	97.2/103.1	
WABC	–	1017

AREA	FM/VHF	AM/MW
SOMERSET		
Mendip Area		
Orchard FM	102.6	–
Wells		
BBC Bristol	95.5	1548
SOUTH GLAMORGAN		
Cardiff		
BBC Cymru/Wales	96.8	882
Red Dragon Radio	103.2	–
Touch AM		1359
STAFFORDSHIRE		
Stafford		
Echo 96	96.9	–
Stoke on Trent		
BBC Stoke	94.6	1503
Signal Radio	102.6	1170
STRATHCLYDE		
Ayr		
West Sound	96.7	1035
Girvan		
West Sound	97.5	–
Glasgow		
BBC Scotland	94.3	810
Clyde 1	102.5	–
Clyde 2	–	1152
Radio Clyde FM	97.3	
Greenock		
BBC Scotland	94.3	810
Kilmarnock		
BBC Scotland	93.9	810
SUFFOLK		
Bury St. Edmunds		
Saxon Radio	96.4	1251
Great Barton		
BBC Suffolk	104.6	–
Ipswich		
BBC Suffolk	103.9	–
Radio Orwell	97.1	1170

AREA	FM/VHF	AM/MW
SURREY		
Guildford		
BBC Surrey	104.6	–
Delta Radio	97.1	–
First Gold Radio	–	1476
Premier Radio	96.4	–
Reigate		
Radio Mercury	102.7	1521
TAYSIDE		
Dundee		
Radio Tay	102.8	1161
BBC Scotland	92.7	810
Perth		
Radio Tay	96.4	1584
TYNE & WEAR		
Fenham		
BBC Newcastle	104.4	–
Metro FM	103.0	–
Newcastle Area		
BBC Newcastle	95.4	1458
GNR	–	1152
Metro FM	97.1	–
Sunderland		
Wear FM	103.4	–
ULSTER		
Belfast		
BBC Ulster	94.5	1341
Classic Trax BCR	96.7	–
Cool FM	97.4	–
Downtown Radio	102.6	–
Enniskillen		
BBC Ulster	93.8	873
Downtown Radio	96.6	–
Limavady		
Downtown Radio	96.4	–
Londonderry		
BBC Foyle	93.1	792
Downtown Radio	102.4	–
WARWICKSHIRE		
Leamington Spa		
Mercia FM	102.9	–

AREA	FM/VHF	AM/MW
WEST GLAMORGAN		
Swansea		
BBC Cymru/Wales	93.9	882
Swansea Sound	96.4	1170
WEST MIDLANDS		
Coventry		
BBC CWR	94.8	–
Mercia FM	97.0	–
Radio Harmony	102.6	–
Xtra AM	–	1359
Sutton Coldfield		
BBC Derby	104.5	–
Beacon Radio	97.2/103.1	–
Wolverhampton		
BBC WM	95.6	828
Beacon Radio	97.2/103.1	–
WABC	–	990
WEST SUSSEX		
Crawley		
Radio Mercury	102.7	1521
Horsham		
BBC Sussex	95.1	1368
Worthing		
BBC Sussex	95.3	1485
WESTERN ISLES		
Stornoway (Lewis)		
BBC Scotland	94.2	–
WILTSHIRE		
Chippenham		
BBC Wiltshire Sound	104.3	–
Marlborough		
GWR FM	96.5	–
Salisbury		
BBC Wiltshire Sound	103.5	–
Swindon		
BBC Wiltshire Sound	103.6	1368
Brunel Classic Gold	–	1161
GWR FM	97.2	–
West Wilts		
Brunel Classic Gold	–	936
GWR FM	102.2	–
WORCESTERSHIRE		
Worcester		
BBC Here/Worc	104.0	738
Radio Wyvern	102.8	1530

AREA	FM/VHF	AM/MW
YORKSHIRE NORTH		
Northallerton		
BBC York	104.3	–
Scarborough		
BBC York	95.5	1260
Whitby		
BBC Cleveland	95.8	–
York		
BBC York	103.7	666
YORKSHIRE SOUTH		
Barnsley		
Classic Gold	–	1305
Hallam	102.9	–
Doncaster		
BBC Sheffield	104.1	1035
Classic Gold	–	990
Hallam	103.4	–
Rotherham		
BBC Sheffield	88.6	1035
Hallam	96.1	–
Sheffield		
BBC Sheffield	88.6	1035
Classic Gold	–	1548
Hallam	97.4	–
YORKSHIRE WEST		
Bradford		
Classic Gold	–	1278
Pennine	97.5	–
Sunrise FM	103.2	–
Halifax		
Classic Gold	–	1530
Pennine	102.5	–
Huddersfield		
Classic Gold	–	1530
Pennine	102.5	–
Leeds		
Aire FM	96.3	–
BBC Leeds	92.4	774
Magic 828	–	828

CONVERSION FACTORS

Length (distance)

Inches *(in)*	x 25.4	= Millimetres *(mm)*	x 0.0394	= Inches *(in)*
Feet *(ft)*	x 0.305	= Metres *(m)*	x 3.281	= Feet *(ft)*
Miles	x 1.609	= Kilometres *(km)*	x 0.621	= Miles

Volume (capacity)

Cubic inches *(cu in; in^3)*	x 16.387	= Cubic centimetres *(cc; cm^3)*	x 0.061	= Cubic inches *(cu in; in^3)*
Pints *(pt)*	x 0.568	= Litres *(l)*	x 1.76	= Pints *(pt)*
Quarts *(qt)*	x 1.137	= Litres *(l)*	x 0.88	= Quarts *(qt)*
Gallons *(gal)*	x 4.546	= Litres *(l)*	x 0.22	= Gallons *(gal)*

Mass (weight)

Ounces *(oz)*	x 28.35	= Grams *(g)*	x 0.035	= Ounces *(oz)*
Pounds *(lb)*	x 0.454	= Kilograms *(kg)*	x 2.205	= Pounds *(lb)*

Force

Pounds-force *(lbf; lb)*	x 4.448	= Newtons *(N)*	x 0.225	= Pounds-force *(lbf; lb)*
Newtons *(N)*	x 0.1	= Kilograms-force *(kgf; kg)*	x 9.81	= Newtons *(N)*

Pressure

Pounds-force per square inch *(psi; lbf/in^2; lb/in^2)*	x 0.070	= Kilograms-force per square centimetre *(kgf/cm^2; kg/cm^2)*	x 14.223	= Pounds-force per square inch *(psi; lbf/in^2; lb/in^2)*
Pounds-force per square inch *(psi; lbf/in^2; lb/in^2)*	x 0.068	= Atmospheres *(atm)*	x 14.696	= Pounds-force per square inch *(psi; lbf/in^2; lb/in^2)*
Pounds-force per square inch *(psi; lbf/in^2; lb/in^2)*	x 0.069	= Bars	x 14.5	= Pounds-force per square inch *(psi; lbf/in^2; lb/in^2)*

Torque (moment of force)

Pounds-force feet *(lbf ft; lb ft)*	x 0.138	= Kilograms-force metres *(kgf m; kg m)*	x 7.233	= Pounds-force feet *(lbf ft; lb ft)*
Pounds-force feet *(lbf ft; lb ft)*	x 1.356	= Newton metres *(Nm)*	x 0.738	= Pounds-force feet *(lbf ft; lb ft)*
Newton metres *(Nm)*	x 0.102	= Kilograms-force metres *(kgf m; kg m)*	x 9.804	= Newton metres *(Nm)*

Power

Horsepower *(hp)*	x 0.745	= Kilowatts *(kW)*	x 1.3	= Horsepower *(hp)*

Velocity (speed)

Miles per hour *(miles/hr; mph)*	x 1.609	= Kilometres per hour *(km/h; kph)*	x 0.621	= Miles per hour *(miles/hr; mph)*

Fuel consumption*

Miles per gallon *(mpg)*	x 0.354	= Kilometres per litre *(km/l)*	x 2.825	= Miles per gallon *(mpg)*

Temperature

Degrees Fahrenheit = (°C x 1.8) + 32

Degrees Celsius (Degrees Centigrade; °C) = (°F – 32) x 0.56

* *Note: It is common practice to convert from miles per gallon (mpg) to litres/100 kilometres (l/100 km), where mpg x l/100 km = 282*

MILES

	LONDON	Aberdeen	Aberystwyth	Birmingham	Bournemouth	Brighton	Bristol	Cambridge	Cardiff	Carlisle	Chester	Derby	Dover	Edinburgh	Exeter	Fishguard	Fort William	Glasgow	Harwich	Holyhead
LONDON		806	341	179	169	89	183	84	249	484	298	198	117	608	275	422	818	634	114	420
Aberdeen	501		724	658	903	895	789	742	792	349	571	634	924	198	911	795	254	241	848	692
Aberystwyth	212	450		193	328	425	206	354	177	375	153	222	459	526	325	90	708	525	460	182
Birmingham	111	409	120		237	267	132	161	163	309	117	63	296	460	259	283	642	459	267	246
Bournemouth	105	561	204	147		148	124	251	195	554	351	306	278	705	132	375	887	703	283	463
Brighton	55	556	264	166	92		217	180	288	573	386	286	130	697	275	468	906	723	203	509
Bristol	114	490	128	82	77	135		233	71	439	237	195	314	591	121	251	722	589	314	340
Cambridge	52	461	220	100	156	112	145		290	417	269	155	204	544	351	436	750	566	106	391
Cardiff	155	492	110	101	121	179	44	180		443	237	225	385	587	192	180	776	608	359	341
Carlisle	301	217	233	192	344	356	273	259	275		222	304	602	151	571	444	333	150	523	341
Chester	185	355	95	73	218	240	147	167	147	138		114	415	373	357	243	555	372	375	137
Derby	123	394	138	39	190	178	121	96	140	189	71		315	436	315	312	637	454	261	251
Dover	73	574	285	184	173	81	195	127	239	374	258	196		726	391	539	935	752	203	538
Edinburgh	378	123	327	286	438	433	367	338	365	94	232	271	451		723	616	233	72	650	489
Exeter	171	566	202	161	82	171	75	218	119	355	222	196	243	449		372	904	721	389	460
Fishguard	262	494	56	176	233	291	156	271	112	276	151	194	335	383	231		777	594	533	272
Fort William	508	158	440	399	551	563	480	466	482	207	345	396	581	145	562	483		183	856	671
Glasgow	394	150	326	285	437	449	366	352	378	93	231	282	467	45	448	369	114		673	488
Harwich	71	527	286	166	176	126	195	66	223	325	233	162	126	404	242	331	532	418		497
Holyhead	261	430	113	153	288	316	211	243	212	212	85	156	334	304	286	169	417	303	309	
Hull	168	348	229	143	255	223	226	124	244	155	132	98	251	225	301	285	362	250	181	217
Inverness	537	105	482	445	594	590	528	497	524	253	387	430	601	159	603	529	66	176	563	463
Leeds	190	322	173	111	261	251	206	148	212	115	78	74	269	199	268	229	322	210	214	163
Leicester	98	417	151	39	166	153	112	68	139	208	94	28	171	294	187	207	415	301	134	183
Lincoln	136	382	186	85	217	191	163	86	190	180	123	51	213	259	238	245	387	273	152	208
Liverpool	205	334	104	94	235	260	164	184	164	116	17	88	278	210	239	160	323	211	250	94
Manchester	192	332	133	81	228	247	167	154	172	115	38	58	265	209	242	189	322	210	220	123
Newcastle	271	230	270	209	348	326	295	231	310	58	175	164	344	107	370	326	257	143	297	260
Norwich	107	487	267	155	212	162	221	60	237	287	210	139	169	364	277	331	494	380	63	299
Nottingham	123	388	154	50	189	178	132	84	152	185	87	16	196	265	207	210	392	278	150	172
Oxford	56	464	157	62	92	99	66	79	107	256	128	98	129	341	139	207	461	340	134	202
Penzance	282	683	313	268	193	269	186	329	230	466	333	307	354	560	111	342	673	559	353	397
Plymouth	213	614	244	199	124	213	117	260	161	397	264	238	285	491	42	273	604	490	284	328
Preston	216	302	144	105	256	271	185	198	190	85	49	100	289	179	266	200	292	180	264	125
Sheffield	162	358	158	75	227	217	163	124	176	145	78	36	235	235	248	214	352	240	190	163
Southampton	79	530	202	128	32	60	75	136	119	322	194	164	149	416	111	231	520	415	150	283
Stranraer	410	235	342	301	453	465	382	368	384	109	247	298	483	133	464	385	199	85	434	321
Swansea	196	506	76	126	162	220	85	216	41	289	151	165	280	383	160	71	496	382	264	189
Worcester	114	428	98	26	131	168	60	116	75	211	88	65	187	305	135	155	418	304	182	152
York	196	309	197	134	273	251	215	157	242	116	102	89	269	186	290	253	323	211	223	187

KILOMETRES

Hull	Inverness	Leeds	Leicester	Lincoln	Liverpool	Manchester	Newcastle	Norwich	Nottingham	Oxford	Penzance	Plymouth	Preston	Sheffield	Southampton	Stranraer	Swansea	Worcester	York	
270	864	306	158	219	330	309	436	172	198	90	454	343	348	261	127	660	315	183	315	**LONDON**
560	169	518	671	615	538	534	370	784	624	747	1099	988	486	576	853	378	814	689	497	Aberdeen
369	776	278	243	304	167	214	435	430	248	253	504	393	232	254	325	550	122	158	317	Aberystwyth
230	716	179	63	137	151	130	336	249	80	100	431	320	169	121	206	484	203	42	216	Birmingham
410	956	420	267	349	378	367	560	341	304	148	311	200	412	365	51	729	261	211	439	Bournemouth
359	950	404	246	307	418	398	525	261	286	159	433	343	436	349	97	748	354	270	404	Brighton
364	850	332	180	262	264	269	475	356	212	106	299	188	298	262	121	615	137	97	346	Bristol
200	800	238	109	138	296	248	372	97	135	127	529	418	319	200	219	592	348	187	253	Cambridge
393	843	341	224	306	264	277	499	381	245	172	370	259	306	283	192	618	66	121	389	Cardiff
249	407	185	335	290	187	185	93	462	298	412	750	639	137	233	518	175	465	340	187	Carlisle
212	623	126	151	198	27	61	282	338	140	206	536	425	79	126	312	398	243	142	164	Chester
158	692	119	45	82	142	93	264	224	26	158	494	383	161	58	264	480	266	105	143	Derby
404	967	433	275	343	447	426	554	272	315	208	570	459	465	378	240	777	451	301	433	Dover
362	256	320	473	417	338	336	172	586	426	549	901	790	288	378	669	214	616	491	299	Edinburgh
484	970	431	301	383	385	389	595	446	333	224	179	68	428	399	179	747	257	217	467	Exeter
459	851	369	333	394	257	304	525	533	338	333	550	439	322	344	372	620	114	249	407	Fishguard
583	106	518	668	623	520	518	414	795	631	742	1083	972	470	566	837	320	798	673	520	Fort William
402	283	338	484	439	340	338	230	612	447	547	900	789	290	386	668	137	615	489	340	Glasgow
291	906	344	216	245	402	354	478	101	241	216	568	457	425	306	241	698	429	293	359	Harwich
349	745	262	295	335	151	198	418	481	277	325	639	528	201	262	455	517	304	245	301	Holyhead
	615	90	145	61	196	151	190	240	148	262	663	552	180	103	412	425	433	272	63	Hull
382		579	729	673	605	604	428	842	682	816	1159	1049	555	634	925	417	872	747	552	Inverness
56	358		158	108	119	64	148	277	116	272	613	502	90	58	378	360	369	220	39	Leeds
90	453	98		82	187	138	301	187	42	119	480	369	206	105	225	510	282	109	174	Leicester
38	418	67	51		192	137	245	169	56	201	562	451	185	72	307	465	340	192	124	Lincoln
122	376	74	116	119		55	253	360	167	251	563	452	50	119	357	362	270	169	158	Liverpool
94	375	40	86	85	34		212	306	119	230	568	457	48	64	325	360	295	164	103	Manchester
118	266	92	187	152	157	132		414	254	412	774	663	203	206	518	262	517	378	127	Newcastle
149	523	174	116	105	224	190	257		198	224	626	515	354	241	299	637	439	283	293	Norwich
92	424	72	26	35	104	74	158	123		156	512	401	167	64	262	473	283	122	134	Nottingham
163	507	169	74	125	156	143	256	139	97		402	291	272	217	106	587	230	95	291	Oxford
412	720	381	298	349	350	353	481	389	318	250		126	597	560	357	925	436	396	645	Penzance
343	652	312	229	280	281	284	412	320	249	181	78		486	447	246	814	325	285	534	Plymouth
112	345	56	128	115	31	30	126	220	104	169	371	302		113	375	312	322	203	126	Preston
64	394	36	65	45	74	40	128	150	40	135	348	278	70		323	490	336	163	90	Sheffield
256	575	235	140	191	222	202	322	186	163	66	222	153	233	201		679	257	193	398	Southampton
264	259	224	317	289	225	224	163	396	294	365	575	506	194	254	422		641	515	362	Stranraer
269	542	229	175	211	168	183	321	273	176	143	271	202	200	209	160	398		161	418	Swansea
169	464	137	68	119	105	102	235	176	76	59	246	177	126	101	120	320	100		257	Worcester
39	343	24	108	77	98	64	79	182	83	181	401	332	78	56	247	225	260	160		York

A

B

C

D

E

F

G

H

I

J

L

M

N

O

P

R

S

T

U

V

W

Date	Action

Date	Action

Date	Action

Date	Action

Date	Action

Date	Action

Date	Action

Date	Action

Escort & Orion Manuals

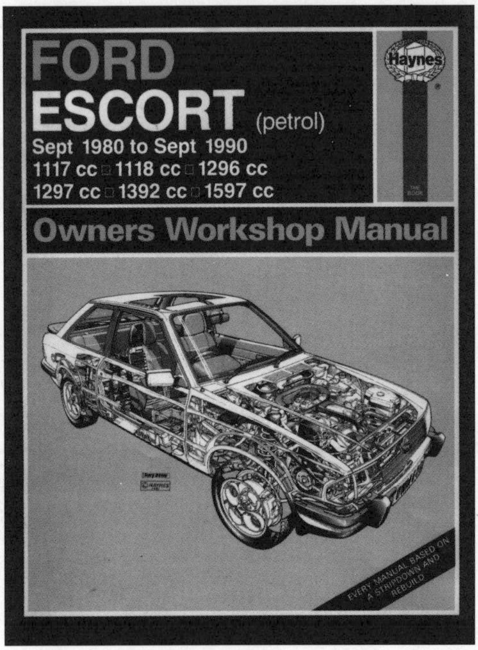

Like this Handbook, the above manuals have been written specifically for your Escort or Orion. Most models are covered from September 1980 to September 1990, the only exceptions are the diesel engines (for which a separate manual on Ford diesel engines is produced), the RS1600i model Escort and the CTX transmission.

The manuals are written in the same easy-to-follow manner as the Handbooks and enable you to tackle even major overhauls and repairs yourself. They will advise you on which jobs are suitable for the DIY mechanic and often suggest practical alternatives to the specialist tools that are so often recommended.

With the ever increasing cost of garage labour, think of the money you could save!

Haynes Manuals are available from most good motor accessory stores and bookshops or direct from the publisher.

HAYNES

Haynes Publishing, Sparkford, Nr Yeovil, Somerset BA22 7JJ Telephone 0963 440635

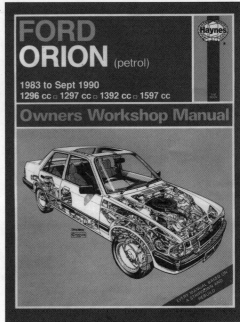